Symposium on retina
and retinal surgery

TRANSACTIONS OF THE NEW ORLEANS
ACADEMY OF OPHTHALMOLOGY

Symposium on retina and retinal surgery

TRANSACTIONS OF THE NEW ORLEANS
ACADEMY OF OPHTHALMOLOGY

WALTER D. COCKERHAM, M.D.

VICTOR T. CURTIN, M.D.

ROBERT Y. FOOS, M.D.

H. MacKENZIE FREEMAN, M.D.

ARNOLD J. KROLL, M.D.

ROBERT MACHEMER, M.D.

PROF. DR. GERD MEYER-SCHWICKERATH

EDWARD W. D. NORTON, M.D.

EDWARD OKUN, M.D.

CHARLES L. SCHEPENS, M.D.

LOUIS M. SPENCER, M.D.

BRADLEY R. STRAATSMA, M.D.

With 372 illustrations, including 12 color plates

THE C. V. MOSBY COMPANY

Saint Louis   1969

Contributors

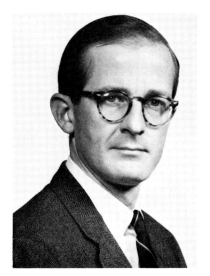

WALTER D. COCKERHAM, M.D.
Boston, Massachusetts
Retina Service Fellow, Massachusetts
Ear and Eye Infirmary

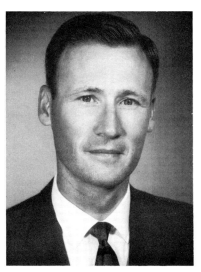

VICTOR T. CURTIN, M.D.
Miami, Florida
Associate Professor, Department of
Ophthalmology, University of Miami

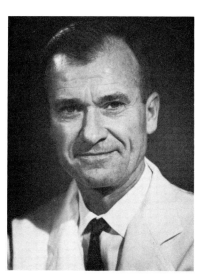

ROBERT Y. FOOS, M.D.
Los Angeles, California
Associate Professor of Pathology,
Jules Stein Eye Institute,
U.C.L.A. School of Medicine

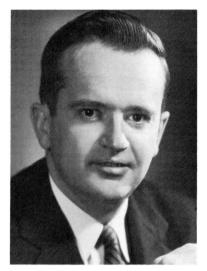

H. MacKENZIE FREEMAN, M.D.
Boston, Massachusetts
Research Associate, Assistant to the
Director, Department of Research,
Retina Foundation; Instructor in
Ophthalmology, Harvard Medical
School; Assistant in Ophthalmology,
Massachusetts Eye and Ear Infirmary

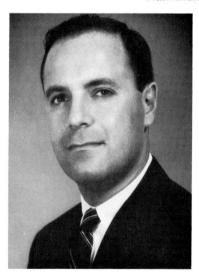

ARNOLD J. KROLL, M.D.
Miami, Florida
Assistant Professor of Ophthalmology,
Department of Ophthalmology,
University of Miami School of
Medicine

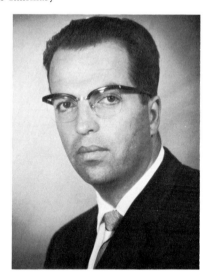

ROBERT MACHEMER, M.D.
Göttingen, Germany
Visiting Research Fellow, Department
of Ophthalmology, University of
Miami School of Medicine, Miami,
Florida; University Eye Clinic,
Göttingen

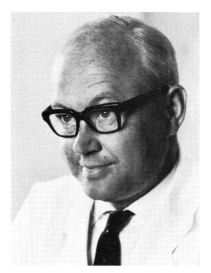

**PROF. DR. GERD MEYER-
SCHWICKERATH**
Essen, Germany
Director of the University
Eye Clinic, Essen

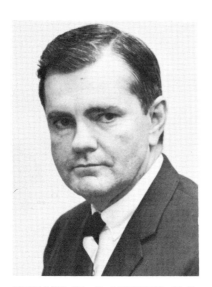

EDWARD W. D. NORTON, M.D.
Miami, Florida
Professor and Chairman, Department
of Ophthalmology, University of
Miami School of Medicine,
Bascom Palmer Eye Institute

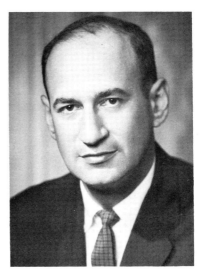

EDWARD OKUN, M.D.
St. Louis, Missouri
Clinical Assistant Professor of
Ophthalmology, Washington
University School of Medicine

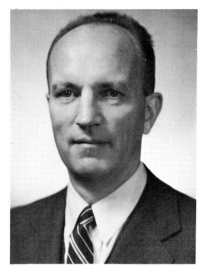

CHARLES L. SCHEPENS, M.D.
Boston, Massachusetts
Director of the Department of
Retinal Research, The Retina
Foundation

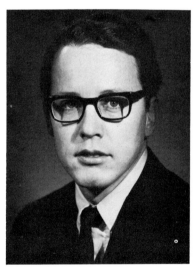

LOUIS M. SPENCER, M.D.
Los Angeles, California
Postdoctoral Research Fellow,
The Jules Stein Eye Institute,
U.C.L.A. School of Medicine

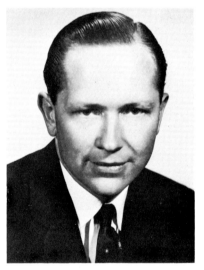

BRADLEY R. STRAATSMA, M.D.
Los Angeles, California
Professor and Chairman, Division
of Ophthalmology; Director of
The Jules Stein Eye Institute,
U.C.L.A. School of Medicine

Preface

As an extension of the annual postgraduate course in various ophthalmic oriented subjects, the New Orleans Academy of Ophthalmology presents for 1968 its course in ophthalmic retinal surgery. Both theoretical and practical considerations are covered in the lectures, and the theories of retinal disease along with research and their practical and experimental demonstration are presented. Well-recognized experts in the field have been most gracious in giving their time and knowledge toward the completion of the course and this volume, despite their already overcrowded schedules. The New Orleans Academy of Ophthalmology appreciates this time and energy and wishes not only officially but also warmly and personally to thank each of the contributors for his part in the success of this project. Since ophthalmic medicine and surgery is an advancing science of almost daily discoveries, it is necessary that ophthalmologists keep themselves knowledgeable in all fields. The New Orleans Academy of Ophthalmology hopes that this volume will help to bring together the scattered literature on modern-day retinal science.

Publications committee

J. William Rosenthal, M.D., Chairman
James H. Allen, M.D.
C. L. M. Samson, M.D.
Robert A. Schimek, M.D.
Robert E. Schoel, M.D.
N. Leon Hart, M.D.,
 Chairman, Ex officio

Contents

1 The retina—topography and clinical correlations (Bradley R. Straatsma, Robert Y. Foos, and Louis M. Spencer), 1

2 Evolution of concepts related to retinal detachment (Charles L. Schepens), 27

3 Techniques of examination of the fundus periphery (Charles L. Schepens), 39

4 Differential diagnosis of retinal detachment (Edward W. D. Norton), 52

5 Technique of vitreous cavity examination (Walter D. Cockerham and Charles L. Schepens), 66

6 Trophic degenerations of the peripheral retina (Robert Y. Foos, Louis M. Spencer, and Bradley R. Straatsma), 90

7 Tractional degenerations of the peripheral retina (Louis M. Spencer, Bradley R. Straatsma, and Robert Y. Foos), 103

8 Photocoagulation with different light sources (Gerd R. E. Meyer-Schwickerath and K. J. Pesch), 128

9 Cryotherapy in retinal detachment surgery (Edward W. D. Norton), 136

10 Pathologic changes following retinal detachment surgery (Victor T. Curtin), 147

11 Current management of giant retinal breaks (H. MacKenzie Freeman), 171

12 Lamellar undermining, diathermy, and tissue transplantation versus cryotherapy and full-thickness scleral buckling (Edward Okun), 184

13 Management of complex cases (Charles L. Schepens), 197

14 Complications of retinal detachment surgery (Edward W. D. Norton), 222

15 Six years' experience with silicone injections into the vitreous cavity (Gerd R. E. Meyer-Schwickerath, O. E. Lund, and W. Höpping), 235

16 Experimental retinal detachment and reattachment I. Methods, clinical picture, and histology (Robert Machemer), 239

17 Experimental retinal detachment and reattachment II. Electron microscopy (Arnold J. Kroll and Robert Machemer), 258

18 Therapy of retinal detachment complicated by massive preretinal fibroplasia (Long-term follow-up of patients treated with intravitreal liquid silicone) (Edward Okun and Neva P. Arribas), 278

19 Prevention of detachment and proliferation in diabetic retinopathy (Gerd R. E. Meyer-Schwickerath), 294

20 Traumatic retinal detachment: clinical and experimental study (Charles L. Schepens), 302

21 Therapy of diabetic retinal detachment (Edward Okun and Wayne E. Fung), 319

22 General summary of the symposium (Bradley R. Straatsma), 328

Round table discussion, 334

Members of the New Orleans Academy of Ophthalmology, 1968, 380

Color plates

1 Real fundus and inverted image, 81

2 Undetached vitreous showing pseudohyaloid face, 81

3 Syneresis or liquefaction, 82

4 Lattice degeneration showing syneresis or cavitation, 82

5 Posterior vitreous detachment, 83

6 Minimal detachment of vitreous in a young person, 83

7 Lattice degeneration with strands, 84

8 Vitreous attachment to the macula with a hemorrhagic lesion, 84

9 Posterior hyaloid face attached to horseshoe retinal break, 85

10 Giant retinal break with hyaloid face, 85

11 Free operculum attached to hyaloid face, 86

12 Prolapsing giant retinal break, 86

Symposium on retina and retinal surgery

TRANSACTIONS OF THE NEW ORLEANS ACADEMY OF OPHTHALMOLOGY

1

The retina—topography and clinical correlations

Bradley R. Straatsma
Robert Y. Foos
Louis M. Spencer

RETINAL TOPOGRAPHY

The retina is unique among the complex elements of the central nervous system and the special senses: It may be readily viewed during life, and it is sufficiently transparent so that alterations within and adjacent to it may be observed in vivo. For these and other reasons related to its structure, organization, and function, the retina has been of ever-increasing importance in science as a whole and in the field of ophthalmology.

Consistent with this growing importance, methods for viewing the retina have steadily improved during the more than a century since the principles of ophthalmoscopy were presented by von Helmholz. As a result, current techniques of ophthalmoscopy and biomicroscopy facilitate clinical examination of the entire human retina. Interpretations of the findings, however, depend on accurate and detailed knowledge of retinal surface characteristics, appreciation of retinal structure, and understanding of the variations and degenerations that commonly affect the appearance of the peripheral retina.

Recognizing the significance of this fundamental knowledge, we will consider in this presentation retinal topography, regional variations in retinal structure, relationships of the vitreous base, and pertinent clinical correlations. In two subsequent presentations,* variations and degenerations of the peripheral retina (i.e., retina anterior to the equator of the eye) will be classified, defined, and described.

Much of the currently available information concerning topography of the human retina stems from the fine general description of Salzmann[1] in 1912, and from the monumental work of Polyak[2] published in 1941. This information has been

---

*See Chapters 6 and 7.

supplemented by more recent careful observations by Ishii,[3] Thiel,[4, 5] Schepens,[6] Rutnin,[7-10] and others. In toto, these studies provide data regarding the expanse of the retina, size of the optic disc, position of the foveola, features of the ora serrata, and position of the vitreous base. This information is of distinct value, but the diversity of material examined, the variation in methods employed, and the absence of certain significant details prevent formation of an overall concept of retinal topography.

Interestingly, knowledge regarding retinal structure is much more extensive. This knowledge takes origin from the work of a number of scientists who utilized light microscopy,[2, 11] electron microscopy,[12-17] and special tissue preparations[18-20] to establish the general retinal architecture, the types of neuronal and glial cells in the retina, the principal synaptic patterns, and many details of vascular supply and ultrastructure. Moreover, in these studies, the human retina is topographically divided into a central area, characterized by the presence of more than a single row of cells in the ganglion-cell layer, and a peripheral area, in which the ganglion cells form only a single continuous or broken row. The central area was further divided into three zones and the peripheral retina into four regions so that the human retina was separated into seven roughly concentric zones that range from the central fovea, zone I, to the extreme periphery, zone VII.[2, 21] Defined by cell distribution and by other histologic criteria, these zones are of significance to the anatomist and, potentially, to the physiologist. They do not, however, generally correspond to gross or clinical landmarks and, consequently, do not facilitate the correlation of retinal microanatomy with clinical observations.

Also of significance in the interpretation of clinical observations is an intimate attachment of the vitreous to the retina and ciliary body in an area known as the vitreous base. This band extends anterior and posterior to the ora serrata throughout the circumference of the eye. It is described as a ring that is 2 to 3 mm. in width,[21] but, despite its obvious importance, it has not been precisely measured or located in a sizable series of human eyes.

To supply data regarding retinal topography, retinal regional microanatomy, and the vitreous base, several studies were carried out on eyes removed at autopsy.

For topographic evaluation, the general size and shape of the retina and the characteristics of the disc, foveola, and ora serrata were determined in a study of 200 postmortem eyes obtained from patients 20 years of age or more at the time of death. Average anteroposterior diameter and standard deviation in these eyes was 24.75 ± 0.74 mm., the vertical equatorial diameter was 24.1 ± 0.86 mm., and the horizontal equatorial diameter was 24.26 ± 0.82 mm.[22, 23]

The average dimension of the retina, measured as a chord, from the correspond-

Table 1-1. The retina: chord measurements in 200 eyes

	Optic disc to equator	*Equator to ora serrata*
Superior meridian	14.71 ± 1.08 mm.	5.07 ± 1.11 mm.
Inferior meridian	14.51 ± 1.01 mm.	4.79 ± 1.22 mm.
Nasal meridian	13.27 ± 1.11 mm.	5.81 ± 1.12 mm.
Temporal meridian	17.29 ± 1.60 mm.	6.00 ± 1.22 mm.

ing margin of the optic disc to the equator, was 14.71 ± 1.08 mm. in the superior meridian, 14.51 ± 1.01 mm. inferiorly, 13.27 ± 1.11 mm. nasally, and 17.29 ± 1.60 mm. temporally (Table 1-1). From the equator to the ora serrata, the average retinal dimension, measured as a chord, was 5.07 ± 1.11 mm. superiorly, 4.79 ± 1.22 mm. inferiorly, 5.81 ± 1.12 mm. nasally, and 6.00 ± 1.22 mm. temporally (Fig. 1-1).

In regard to shape, the retina expanded from the optic disc to line the posterior pole and reach the equator. At the equator, the retina had an average diameter of 24.08 ± 0.94 mm. in the vertical meridian and 24.06 ± 0.80 mm. in the horizontal meridian. At the ora serrata, the average diameter of the retina was 20.41 ± 1.09 mm. in the vertical direction and 20.03 ± 1.04 mm. in the horizontal direction. As depicted in Fig. 1-2, the retina had the shape of a cup that was expanded to its greatest diameter at the equator and was considerably reduced in diameter at its serrated anterior margin.

In the retina and the closely related optic nervehead, three areas—the optic disc, the foveola, and the ora serrata—were specially evaluated. The optic disc had an average vertical diameter of 1.86 ± 0.21 mm. and an average horizontal diameter of 1.75 ± 0.19 mm. The center of the fovea (i.e., the foveola) was located temporal to the optic disc and slightly inferior to the horizontal diameter of the disc. From the

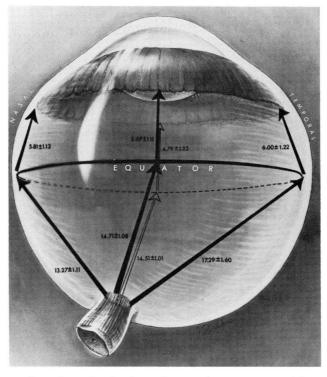

Fig. 1-1. Average dimensions of retina from disc margin to equator and from equator to ora serrata in four principal meridians. Based on 200 adult human eyes, measurements and standard deviations are recorded in millimeters.

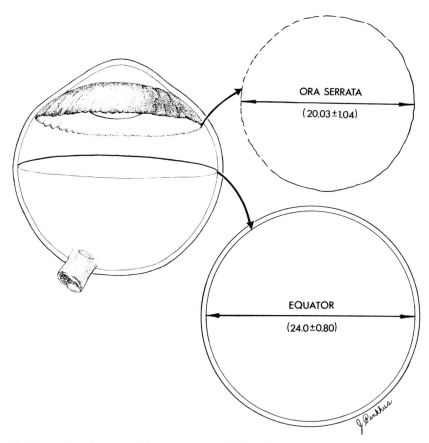

Fig. 1-2. Shape of retina resembling a cup expanded to its greatest diameter at equator and considerably reduced in diameter at its serrated anterior margin. Measurements and standard deviations are in millimeters.

horizontal meridian of the temporal disc margin to the foveola, the average dimension was 3.42 ± 0.34 mm. (Fig. 1-3).

In this study, the ora serrata, located anterior to the equator, received particular attention. The distance from the anterior limit of the retina to Schwalbe's line, which constitutes the posterior border of the limbus, was 6.14 ± 0.85 mm. superiorly, 6.20 ± 0.76 mm. inferiorly, 5.73 ± 0.81 mm. nasally, and 6.52 ± 0.75 mm. temporally (Fig. 1-4).

The relationship of the ora serrata to structures in the anterior segment of the eye was further appreciated by viewing the peripheral retina, ora serrata, and anterior ocular tissues as they appear from the posterior aspect (Fig. 1-5). Illustrated in a photograph of the right eye, the lens is shown within the circle formed by the ciliary processes. Approximately 70 ciliary processes blend with the relatively smooth and striated pars plana. The overall anteroposterior extent of the ciliary body is least on the nasal aspect of the eye, greater superiorly and inferiorly, and greatest temporally. The ciliary body merges abruptly with the ora serrata.

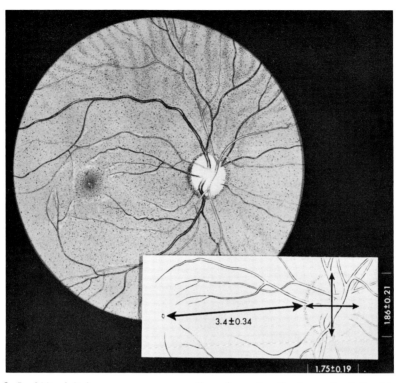

Fig. 1-3. In 200 adult human eyes, average dimensions of optic disc and relationship of disc and foveola. Measurements and standard deviations are in millimeters.

In general configuration, the ora serrata was irregularly scalloped (Fig. 1-5). The irregularities were more pronounced nasally than temporally, and the overall contour presented marked fluctuations and extreme variations. Dentate or toothlike processes extended anterior to the main contour of this border, and bays or indentations extended posterior to the main contour of the ora serrata. At the ora serrata, projections of the retina toward the vitreous body were termed *meridional folds* or *retinal tags*.

For topographic evaluation, classification of the morphologic features of the ora serrata was necessary. Therefore, the following definitions and criteria for classification were adopted:

Dentate process—an anterior extension of the retina that projects from 0.5 to 2.5 mm. anterior to the adjacent retina on both sides. To be distinguished from a fluctuation in the contour of the ora, this projection must occur in a circumferential (parallel to the ora serrata) distance of 1.0 mm. or less (Fig. 1-6, *A*).

Large dentate process—an anterior extension of the retina that projects onto the pars plana of the ciliary body more than 2.5 mm. anterior to the adjacent retina on both sides (Fig. 1-6, *B*).

Giant dentate process—a pronounced extension of the retina that projects to or onto the pars plicata of the ciliary body (Fig. 1-6, *C*).

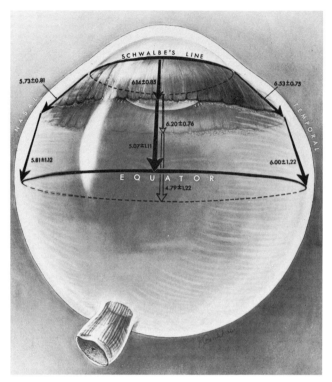

Fig. 1-4. Relationship of ora serrata to Schwalbe's line and to equator. For the four principal meridians, average measurements and standard deviations are in millimeters.

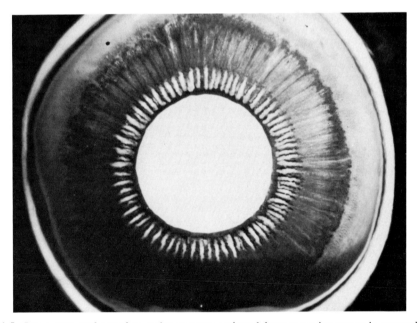

Fig. 1-5. Ora serrata and anterior ocular structures viewed from posterior aspect in gross photograph of right eye.

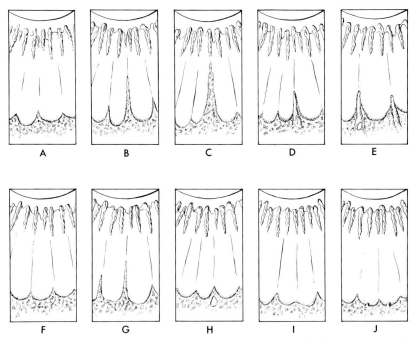

Fig. 1-6. Scale drawings of morphologic features of ora serrata: **A,** dentate process; **B,** large dentate process; **C,** giant dentate process; **D,** meridional fold; **E,** meridional fold with localized posterior retinal defect; **F,** ora bay; **G,** large ora bay; **H,** enclosed ora bay; **I,** doubled ora bay; **J,** retinal tag in ora bay.

Meridional fold—a ridgelike projection of the retina toward the vitreous body located at and perpendicular to the ora serrata (Fig. 1-6, *D*). Immediately posterior to some meridional folds is a localized retinal abnormality, usually an area of retinal thinning (Fig. 1-6, *E*).

Ora bay—a posterior indentation in the retina extending from 0.5 to 2.5 mm. posterior to the adjacent retina on both sides. To be distinguished from a fluctuation in the contour of the ora, this indentation must occur in a circumferential distance of 2.0 mm. or less (Fig. 1-6, *F*).

Large ora bay—a posterior indentation in the retina that extends more than 2.5 mm. posterior to the adjacent retina on both sides (Fig. 1-6, *G*).

Partially enclosed ora bay—a posterior indentation in the retina that extends more than 0.5 mm. posterior to the adjacent retina on both sides and, anteriorly, has a width less than one half its maximum width posteriorly.

Enclosed ora bay—a posterior indentation in the retina completely separated from the pars plana anteriorly by retinal tissue (Fig. 1-6, *H*).

Doubled ora bay—a posterior indentation in the retina that extends from 0.5 to 2.5 mm. posterior to the adjacent retina on both sides; it is divided by an abbreviated anterior extension of the retina that projects less than 0.5 mm. The entire doubled bay must occur within a circumferential distance of 4.0 mm. or less (Fig. 1-6, *I*).

Table 1-2. Morphologic features of the ora serrata (total in 200 eyes)

Dentate processes	2573
Ora bays	2037
Doubled ora bays	185
Retinal tags in ora bays	174
Giant dentate processes	109
Meridional folds	80
Large dentate processes	64
Large ora bays	63
Meridional folds with posterior abnormalities	25
Enclosed ora bays	16
Partly enclosed ora bays	10

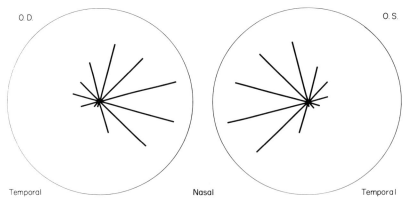

Fig. 1-7. In 200 adult human eyes, meridional distribution of dentate processes (0.5 mm. to 2.5 mm.).

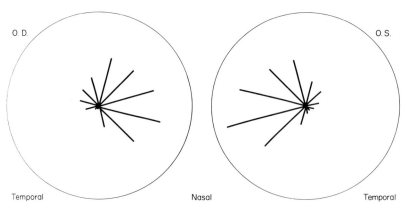

Fig. 1-8. Meridional distribution of ora bays (0.5 mm. to 2.5 mm.) in 200 adult human eyes.

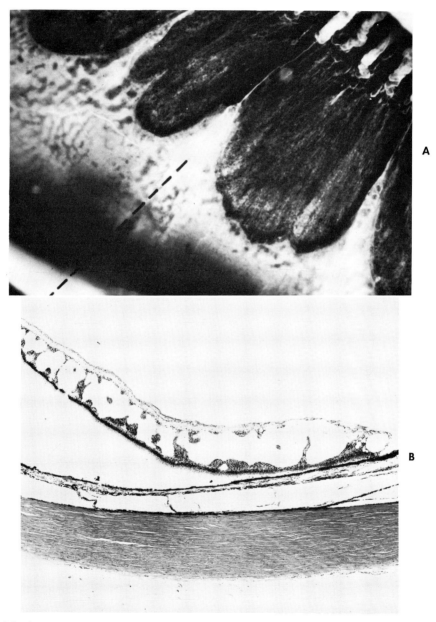

Fig. 1-9. A, Grossly, dentate process shown as triangular or awl shaped. Dotted line indicates site illustrated in *B*. **B,** In microscopic section, retina in dentate process appearing slightly thinned, markedly degenerated, and firmly joined to pigment epithelium (×35).

Retinal tag in an ora bay—a projection of the retina that originates at the posterior margin of an ora bay and extends anterior and internal to the immediately adjacent retina (Fig. 1-6, *J*).

In overall incidence, the most common morphologic features of the ora serrata were the dentate processes and the ora bays (Table 1-2). Generally less common were doubled ora bays, retinal tags in ora bays, giant dentate processes, meridional folds, large dentate processes, and large ora bays. Least common were the meridional

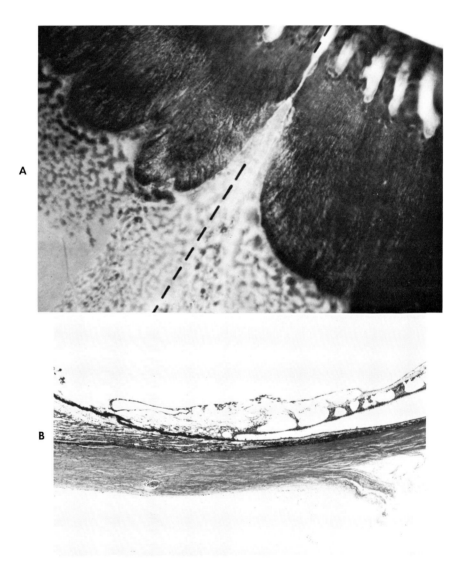

Fig. 1-10. A, Giant dentate process extending to pars plicata of ciliary body. **B,** Corresponding to dotted line in *A,* microscopic section illustrates mild retinal thinning, advanced cystoid degeneration, and broad attachment between pigment epithelium and retina (×25).

folds with posterior abnormalities, enclosed ora bays, and partly enclosed ora bays.

An analysis of distribution demonstrated that, statistically, dentate processes (Fig. 1-7) and ora bays (Fig. 1-8) were significantly most frequent in the superior nasal quadrant, less frequent in the inferior nasal quadrant, even less frequent in the superior temporal quadrant, and least frequent in the inferior temporal quadrant. Moreover, a statistical regression pattern established the peak incidence of dentate processes and ora bays in the superior nasal quadrant within 1 clock hour of the

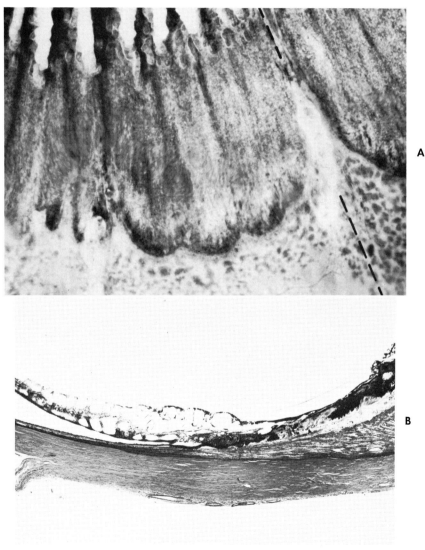

Fig. 1-11. A, Meridional fold associated with large dentate process. Dotted line corresponds to site portrayed in *B.* **B,** Microscopically, projection of internal surface of retina toward vitreous due to increase in thickness of degenerated and cystoid retina (×25).

horizontal meridian (i.e., between 2:00 and 3:00 in the right eye and between 9:00 and 10:00 in the left eye). From this point, progression clockwise or counterclockwise was associated with a decreasing incidence of processes and bays.

Other topographic features of the ora serrata were encountered, as previously noted, far less frequently than the dentate processes and ora bays (Table 1-2). Considering the distribution of these less frequent features, however, we find they were

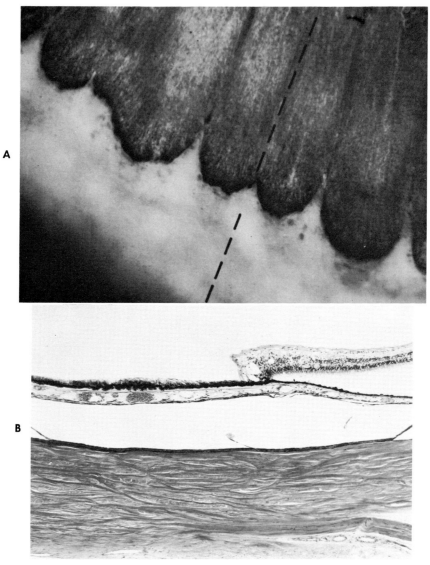

Fig. 1-12. **A,** Retina in doubled ora bay terminating abruptly. **B,** Retina in microsection, corresponding to dotted line in *A* and characterized by mild cystoid degeneration and firm localized attachment of retina to pigment epithelium (×25).

most common in the superior nasal quadrant and present in decreasing frequency in the inferior nasal, superior temporal, and inferior temporal quadrants.

Thus, the overall topography of the ora serrata is characterized by the highest incidence of processes and bays in the superior nasal quadrant and by a progressively smaller incidence of these features in the inferior nasal, superior temporal, and inferior temporal quadrants. Although this pattern is remarkably consistent, it should be emphasized that marked variations in the contour of the ora were encountered. In some eyes, the ora serrata was extremely irregular; in others, it was remarkably smooth. When both eyes of a patient were examined, these cases demonstrated a general symmetry in the configuration of the ora.

In the correlation of gross topographic features of the ora serrata with microscopic findings, dentate processes generally presented a slight thinning of the retina,

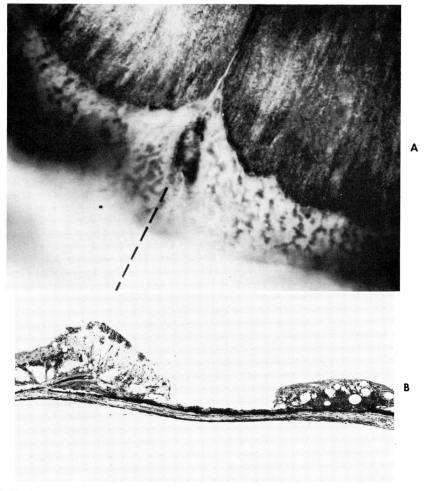

Fig. 1-13. **A,** Enclosed ora bay surrounded by extensions of sensory retina. **B,** Corresponding to dotted line in *A,* section of ciliary body epithelium in enclosed bay (×45).

a rather broad area of firm attachment between retina and pigment epithelium, and a pronounced degree of peripheral cystoid degeneration (Fig. 1-9). Dentate processes of large or giant size usually demonstrated microscopic indications of a rather large area of union between retina and pigment epithelium, progressive thinning of the retina as it approached its anterior termination, and an advanced degree of cystoid change and general retinal degeneration (Fig. 1-10).

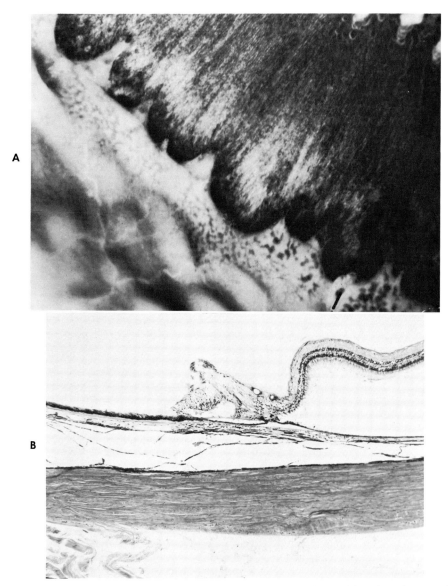

Fig. 1-14. A, Retinal tag projecting anteriorly and internally from midportion of an ora bay. **B,** Section noted by dotted line in *A* revealing degeneration and thickening of retina in this tag (×25).

Meridional folds were usually aligned with dentate processes and less often associated with ora bays. These projections of the retina toward the vitreous were related to an increase in the thickness of the degenerated and cystoid retina (Fig. 1-11). In the meridian of the fold, an enlarged ciliary process was frequently present, and posterior to the fold, an area of retinal thinning or a retinal hole was not uncommon.

In contrast to the retinal thickening and localized accentuation of retinal degeneration in the dentate processes, sectors of relatively smooth ora, ora bays, and doubled ora bays were usually characterized by an abrupt termination of the retina, a localized firm attachment of the retina to the pigment epithelium, and a variable cystoid degeneration in the adjacent retina (Fig. 1-12). Enclosed ora bays demonstrated an island of pars plana epithelium completely surrounded by extensions of the sensory retina (Fig. 1-13).

Frequently, a retinal tag projected anteriorly and internally from the midportion of an ora bay. Being suggestive of traction, this projection was histologically correlated with degeneration and thickening of the retina (Fig. 1-14).

REGIONAL RETINAL ANATOMY

In addition to retinal surface topography, regional microanatomy of the retina merits consideration. To evaluate the regional variations, retinal measurements and anatomic studies were carried out on 10 adult human eyes that were devoid of significant gross abnormality, microscopic disease, or artifact. These eyes were from four men and six women with a mean age of 57 years and an age range from 28 to 74 years at the time of death. Six specimens were right eyes and four were left eyes. Specimens were embedded in celloidin, and measurements were made with a calibrated graticule and microscope at 15 precisely located positions in the horizontal meridian. All measurements extended from the inner surface of the internal limiting membrane to the outer extremity of the rods and cones or, where these sensory cells were absent near the ora serrata, to the outer portion of the sensory retina.

Table 1-3. Thickness of the sensory retina (10 eyes)

	Mean measurement (mm.)
Temporal ora serrata	0.11
1.0 mm. posterior to temporal ora serrata	0.13
3.0 mm. posterior to temporal ora serrata	0.11
Temporal equator	0.12
Midway between temporal equator and foveola	0.14
1.0 mm. temporal to foveola	0.23
Foveola	0.10
1.0 mm. nasal to foveola	0.23
0.5 mm. temporal to temporal disc margin	0.21
0.5 mm. nasal to nasal disc margin	0.21
Midway between disc margin and nasal equator	0.14
Nasal equator	0.11
3.0 mm. posterior to nasal ora serrata	0.10
1.0 mm. posterior to nasal ora serrata	0.11
Nasal ora serrata	0.12

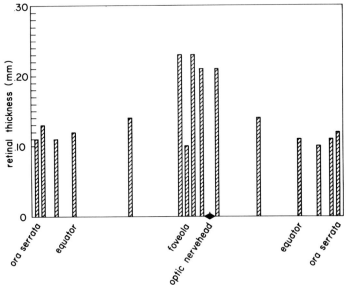

Fig. 1-15. In 10 adult human eyes, mean retinal thickness in horizontal meridian from temporal ora serrata (*left*) to nasal ora serrata (*right*).

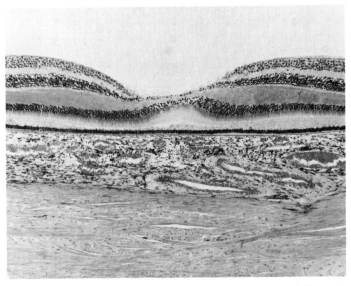

Fig. 1-16. Adjacent to foveola, relatively thick retina showing accumulation of ganglion cells arranged in more than one row (×75).

In these 10 eyes, the mean thickness of the sensory retina at the temporal ora serrata was 0.11 mm. One millimeter posteriorly, the peripheral cystoid degeneration produced a slight increase in retinal thickness, but 3 mm. posterior to the ora (approximately midway between the ora serrata and the equator) and at the temporal equator, the retina measured 0.11 and 0.12 mm., respectively (Table 1-3). Midway between the temporal equator and the foveola, the retina was 0.14 mm. thick. One millimeter temporal to the foveola, the accumulation of cells produced a retina that was 0.23 mm. from the inner limiting membrane to the external extremity of the rods and cones. This dimension decreased to 0.10 mm. at the foveola, increased to 0.23 mm. near the nasal margin of the fovea, and remained quite thick (0.21 mm.) adjacent to the optic disc. Nasally, midway between the disc and the equator, the retina reduced to 0.14 mm. and, at the equator, measured 0.11 in cross section. Three millimeters posterior to the nasal ora serrata (nearly midway between the equator and the ora), the attenuated retina extended 0.10 mm. from internal to external surface, and farther anteriorly it increased slightly in association with peripheral cystoid degeneration (Fig. 1-15).

Regionally, the thin foveola, the thick adjacent retina, and the retina near the optic disc were within the central area of the retina (Fig. 1-16). Extending somewhat asymmetrically from the foveola, this central area of the retina measured 5 to

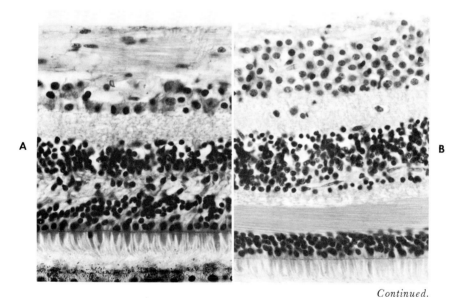

A   B

Continued.

Fig. 1-17. A, Representative portion of retina in horizontal meridian, central area, 0.5 mm. temporal to temporal margin of optic disc (×500). **B,** Representative portion of retina in horizontal meridian, central area, 1.0 mm. temporal to foveola (×500). **C,** Representative portion of retina in horizontal meridian, morphology of extracentral or peripheral retina midway between foveola and temporal equator (×500). **D,** Representative portion of retina in horizontal meridian, morphology of extracentral or peripheral retina, temporal equator (×500). **E,** Representative portion of retina in horizontal meridian, morphology of extracentral or peripheral retina, temporal ora serrata (×500).

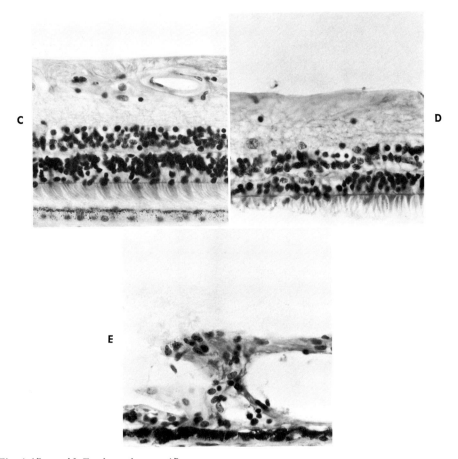

Fig. 1-17, cont'd. For legend see p. 17.

6 mm. in diameter and was distinguished morphologically by the accumulation of ganglion cells in more than one row (Fig. 1-17, *A* and *B*). Beyond this limited area (described on the basis of histologic criteria as the extracentral or peripheral retina), ganglion cells were arranged in a single continuous or interrupted row (Fig. 1-17, *C*, *D*, and *E*). This single or interrupted row of ganglion cells was noted midway between the foveola and the equator temporally, midway between the equator and disc nasally, and at all other more anterior retinal positions. Related to this attenuation in the ganglion-cell layer and in all other nuclear and plexiform layers, the retina attenuated at the equator, presented its minimum thickness 3.0 mm. posterior to the ora, and fluctuated in thickness anteriorly as a consequence of peripheral cystoid degeneration.

THE VITREOUS BASE

Internally, the retina is related to the vitreous body. This transparent gel-like tissue comprises two thirds the volume of the globe and is in contact with the optic

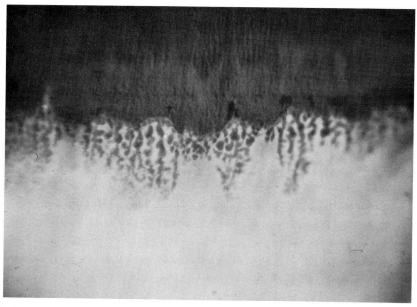

Fig. 1-18. Anterior portion of vitreous base associated with a band of increased pigmentation.

disc, retina, ciliary body, zonule, and lens. Though united to some extent with each of these tissues in the normal young adult eye,[24] the vitreous is most firmly joined with surrounding structures at the vitreous base, a circular band that extends anterior and posterior to the ora serrata.

The anterior portion of the vitreous base is the zone between the ora serrata and the origin of the anterior hyaloid membrane. Grossly, the origin of the membrane can be observed. The dimension of the anterior vitreous base was measured in 100 adult eyes removed at autopsy from patients with a mean age of 56 years and a range from 20 to 90 years at time of death. Seventy-seven of these eyes were from male patients and 23 eyes were from female patients. The series contained 43 right eyes and 57 left eyes.

The anterior vitreous base generally conformed to the contour of the ora serrata. In the temporal horizontal meridian, it had a mean value and standard deviation of 1.32 ± 0.29 mm. and a range from 0.70 to 2.50 mm. In the nasal horizontal meridian, the anterior vitreous base measured 0.26 ± 0.16 mm. with a range from 0.10 to 1.30 mm.

The posterior portion of the vitreous base is the zone of strong retinovitreal attachment that extends posterior to the ora serrata. Defined in another way, the posterior vitreous base is the area between the ora serrata and the most anterior extent to which the vitreous may be detached without causing severe disruption of the inner retinal tissue. The posterior border of the zone is somewhat variable, but it is generally parallel to the ora serrata. The location of this border cannot be measured with great precision in a statistically significant series of eyes, but a number of gross observations indicate that the posterior vitreous base extends approximately 1.5 mm.

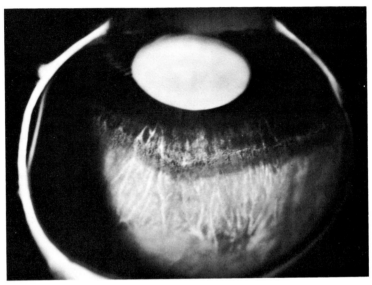

Fig. 1-19. Posterior portion of vitreous base associated with band of increased pigmentation.

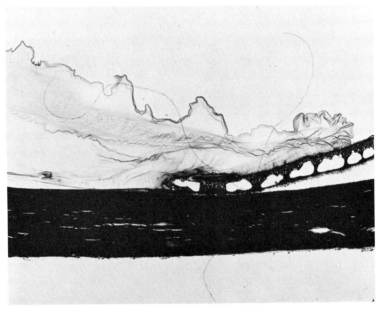

Fig. 1-20. Vitreous base in nasal horizontal meridian. Anterior portion of vitreous base extends from origin of anterior hyaloid to ora serrata. Posterior portion of vitreous base is zone of strong retinovitreal attachment immediately posterior to ora serrata (picroaniline blue, ×35).

posterior to the mean contour of the ora serrata in the temporal and nasal horizontal meridians.

Combining these observations, one may form the concept that the vitreous base straddles the ora serrata and has an overall anteroposterior dimension of approximately 2.8 mm. in the temporal horizontal meridian and 1.8 mm. in the nasal horizontal meridian.

Grossly, the vitreous base is usually associated with a band of increased pigmentation that conforms to the greater width of the vitreous base temporally and to the somewhat narrower base nasally. Anteriorly, this band rather precisely duplicates the irregularities in contour of the ora serrata (Fig. 1-18). Posteriorly, the band reflects the general contour of the ora (Fig. 1-19).

Microscopic studies, using sections stained to demonstrate vitreous structure, confirm the position and dimensions of the vitreous base (Fig. 1-20). Histologic observations also relate the grossly visible pigment band to a localized increase in the size and pigment content in corresponding portions of the pigmented retinal and ciliary body epithelium.

CLINICAL CORRELATIONS

Correlation of retinal topography, regional microanatomy, and position of the vitreous base with clinical evaluation of the retina provides concepts and guidelines of considerable practical value. With regard to topography, it should be stressed that the retina in the human eye is shaped like a cup that is considerably less in diameter and in circumference at the ora serrata than at the equator (Fig. 1-2). Conse-

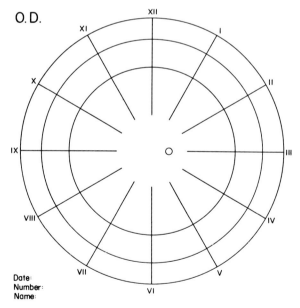

Fig. 1-21. In conventional chart of ocular fundus, peripheral circle representing anterior margin of pars plana, nearby circle representing ora serrata, and adjacent smaller circle depicting equator of the eye. Compare with Fig. 1-2.

quently, the conventional charts of the ocular fundus, which depict the ora serrata as having a diameter and circumference greater than that of the equator, are inaccurate (Fig. 1-21). In essence, these charts should be considered as diagrammatic projections in which the retina anterior to the equator is proportionately expanded.

Stated another way, features of the peripheral retina and ora serrata are actually closer together than they appear to be in the conventional fundus diagram.

For accurate dimensional relationships, quantitative measurements of the optic disc and its relationship to the fovea can be superimposed on the conventional fundus diagram along with general dimensions of the retina, converted mathematically from chord to arc measurements on the basis of a 24.0 mm. sphere. Recognizing that the disc diameter, estimated as 1.75 mm., is the standard basis of comparison in clinical examination of the retina, one may also state these general relationships in disc diameters. On this basis, the distance from the equator to the ora serrata is approximately 3.0 disc diameters and precise retinal dimensions are as noted (Fig. 1-22).

Representation of the ora serrata on the fundus diagram requires a general reproduction of the relatively smooth contour of the temporal sector and the more irregular configuration of the nasal sector as well as portrayal of specific topographic features. Illustrative of this is the correlation between a composite scale drawing depicting the ora serrata (Fig. 1-23, *A*) and its diagrammatic representation on an ocular fundus chart (Fig. 1-23, *B*).

Variation in the configuration of the ora serrata makes it difficult and somewhat misleading to describe a "typical" ora. Nonetheless, to schematically present an "average" anterior edge of the retina, one must consider the localization and inci-

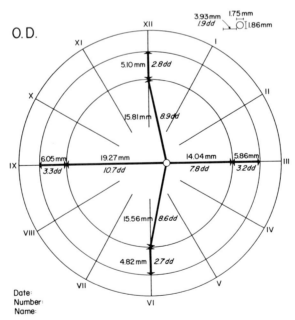

Fig. 1-22. Quantitative measurements of optic disc and retina superimposed on conventional chart of the ocular fundus. Dimensions are in millimeters (mm.) and disc diameters (dd.).

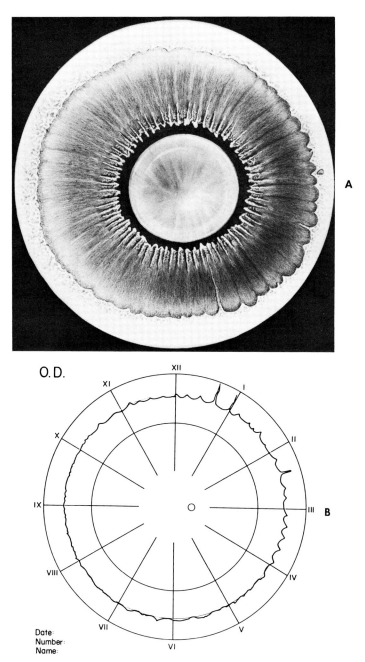

Fig. 1-23. **A,** Composite scale drawing of right eye depicting ora serrata and other anterior ocular tissues viewed from posterior aspect. **B,** Ora serrata corresponding to **A** diagrammatically portrayed on ocular fundus chart.

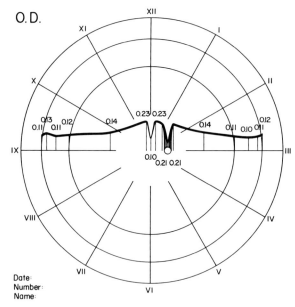

Fig. 1-24. Retinal regional microanatomy superimposed on conventional ocular fundus chart to emphasize contrast between limited area of relatively thick retina adjacent to foveola and after disc and a broad zone of relatively thin peripheral retina.

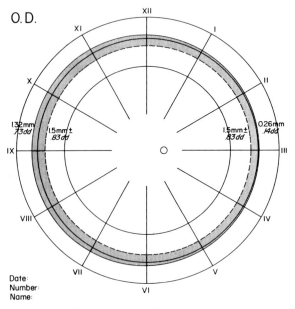

Fig. 1-25. Vitreous base extending anterior and posterior to ora serrata. On ocular fundus chart, dimensions of anterior and posterior vitreous base in temporal and nasal horizontal meridian are expressed in millimeters (mm.) and disc diameters (dd.).

dence of the topographic features. In localization there is a concentration, statistically significant at the level of $P = 0.01$, of dentate processes, ora bays, meridional folds, doubled ora bays, and retinal tags in the superior nasal quadrant. Generally, these and other features progressively decrease in incidence in the inferior nasal, superior temporal, and inferior temporal quadrants. In the full circumference of the eye, the "average" ora serrata presents approximately 16 dentate processes, 1 large or giant dentate process, 10 ora bays, 1 double ora bay, and 1 retinal tag in an ora bay. Also to be expected are such features as a meridional fold in approximately 40% of eyes, a retinal abnormality posterior to a meridional fold in 12% of eyes, and a completely enclosed ora bay, which would clinically simulate a retinal break, in 8% of eyes.

Relating regional microanatomy of the retina to the conventional fundus diagram demonstrates the limited area of relatively thick retina adjacent to the foveola and disc and the broad expanse of relatively thin retina, measuring 0.10 to 0.13 mm. in cross section, at and anterior to the equator (Fig. 1-24). This relative attenuation of the peripheral retina undoubtedly affects the course of peripheral retinal degeneration and the response of the peripheral retina to disease and injury. Finally, the variation in retinal thickness influences the response of different regions to photocoagulation, cryotherapy, and diathermy.

The position of the vitreous base is an extremely important matter. Extending anterior and posterior to the ora serrata, it incorporates approximately one third of the preequatorial retina (Fig. 1-25). This intimate retinal-vitreal union has a major effect on the localization and course of peripheral retinal degenerations.

In aggregate, retinal topography, regional microanatomy, and vitreous base anatomy described in this presentation form the basis for clinical examination of the retina, proper assessment of normal findings, and evaluation of degenerations and other retinal abnormalities.

REFERENCES

1. Salzmann, M.: The anatomy and histology of the human eyeball in the normal state: its development and senescence, Chicago, 1912, University of Chicago Press. (Translated by E. V. L. Brown.)
2. Polyak, S.: The retina, Chicago, 1941, University of Chicago Press.
3. Ishii: Acta Soc. Ophthal. Jap. 55:242, 1951.
4. Thiel, H. L.: Beiträge zur Anatomie der Ora serrata, Ber. Deutsch Ophth. Ges. 58:249, 1953.
5. Thiel, H. L.: Zur topographischen und histologischen Situation der Ora serrata, Graefe. Arch. Ophthal. 156:590, 1955.
6. Schepens, C. L., and Marden, D.: Data on the natural history of retinal detachment. Further characterization of certain unilateral nontraumatic cases, Amer. J. Ophthal. 61: 213, 1966.
7. Rutnin, U.: Fundus appearance in normal eyes. I. The choroid, Amer. J. Ophthal. 64:821, 1967.
8. Rutnin, U., and Schepens, C. L.: Fundus appearance in normal eyes. III. Peripheral degenerations, Amer. J. Ophthal. 64:1040, 1967.
9. Rutnin, U., and Schepens, C. L.: Fundus appearance in normal eyes. II. The standard peripheral fundus and developmental variations, Amer. J. Ophthal. 64:840, 1967.
10. Rutnin, U., and Schepens, C. L.: Fundus appearance in normal eyes. IV. Retinal breaks and other findings, Amer. J. Ophthal. 64:1063, 1967.

11. Cajal, R. S.: Die Retina der Wirbelthiere, Wiesbaden, 1894, Verlag v. Bergmann.
12. Sjöstrand, F. S.: Electron microscopy of the retina. In Smelser, G. K., editor: The structure of the eye, New York, 1961, Academic Press, Inc.
13. Cohen, A. J.: Some electron microscopic observations on interreceptor contacts in the human and macaque retinae, J. Anat. **99:**595, 1965.
14. Cohen, A. J.: New details of the ultrastructure of the outer segments and ciliary connectives of human and macaque retinas, Anat. Rec. **152:**63, 1965.
15. Missotten, L.: L'ultrastructures des cones de la rétine humaine, Bull. Soc. Belg. Ophtal. **132:**472, 1963.
16. Yamada, E.: Some observations on the fine structure of the human retina, Fukuoka Acta Med. **57:**163, 1966.
17. Fine, B. S.: Retinal structure: light- and electron-microscopic observations. In McPherson, A., editor: New and controversial aspects of retinal detachment, New York, 1968, Hoeber Medical Division, Harper & Row, Publishers.
18. Kuwabara, T., and Cogan, D. G.: Retinal vascular patterns: VI. Mural cells of retinal capillaries, Arch. Ophthal. **69:**492, 1963.
19. Cogan, D. G.: Development and senescence of the human retinal vasculature, Trans. Ophthal. Soc. U.K. **83:**465, 1963.
20. Ashton, N., and Cunha-Vaz, J. G.: Effect of histamine on the permeability of the ocular vessels, Arch. Ophthal. **73:**211, 1965.
21. Duke-Elder, S., and Wybar, K. C.: System of ophthalmology. Vol. II. The anatomy of the visual system, St. Louis, 1961, The C. V. Mosby Co.
22. Straatsma, B. R., Allen, R. A., Crescitelli, F., and Hall, M. O., editors: The retina: morphology, function, and clinical characteristics, UCLA Forum in Medical Sciences, no. 8, Los Angeles, University of California Press. (In press.)
23. Straatsma, B. R., Landers, M., and Kreiger, A. E.: Topography of the adult human retina, Arch Ophthal. (To be published.)
24. Zimmerman, L. E., and Straatsma, B. R.: Anatomic relationships of the retina to the vitreous body and to the pigment epithelium. In Schepens, C. L., editor: Importance of the vitreous body in retina surgery with special emphasis on reoperations, St. Louis, 1960, The C. V. Mosby Co.

2

Evolution of concepts related to retinal detachment*

Charles L. Schepens

Two fundamental elements have controlled the direction in which therapeutic efforts were developed to repair retinal detachment: methods of examination of the human fundus and concepts of pathogenesis. Possibilities of better fundus diagnosis influenced concepts of pathogenesis and, with a lag of some years, both gave treatment a more rational direction. This presentation is divided into four parts: (1) methods of examination, (2) concepts of pathogenesis, (3) treatment (each of these three parts is divided into an early and a modern period), (4) assessment of the contemporary period (with regard to methods of examination, concepts of pathogenesis, and treatment). Quotations from the literature are very selective because the number of papers that were written on the subject during the past 2 centuries is considerable.

METHODS OF EXAMINATION
Early period (1704-1851)

The early period precedes the generalized use of ophthalmoscopy. In spite of such a handicap, there were anatomic descriptions of retinal detachment. For instance, Maître-Jan[1] made two pertinent observations: the first was that in a cow autopsied in 1691 there was a dislocated lens, a total retinal detachment, and a retraction of the vitreous body; the second was that in many eyes that suffered a contusion or perforation of the globe either retinal detachment or retinal edema was noted at autopsy.

The clinical symptoms of retinal detachment were first described by de St. Yves (1772), who reported a shadow in the visual field, corresponding to the area detached.[2] In 1766, Morgagni described a retinal detachment with shriveled retina in a case of intraocular tumor.[3]

*This work was supported by Public Health Service Grant NB-03489.

Even before ophthalmoscopy accurate clinical observations of many typical signs of retinal detachment were noted by Sichel (1841) and by Desmarres (1847).[4, 5] However, little progress could be made in this area without the ophthalmoscope. To my knowledge it is Méry (1704, p. 265 of his paper) who made the first ophthalmoscopic observation of a normal fundus in a cat whose head was kept under water.[6] As the cat drowned, its pupils dilated and the fundus became easily visible because the refractive power of the cornea was neutralized by the flat surface of the water. However, Méry failed to see the importance of the phenomenon he had observed, which was explained 5 years later (1709) by de la Hire.[7]

Modern period (1851-1942)

Methods of examination include ophthalmoscopy and slit lamp microscopy of the fundus.

It was in 1851 that Helmholtz published his famous 40-page monograph describing the principles of ophthalmoscopy.[8] According to Koenigsberger, ophthalmoscopy was not initially received with enthusiasm. One distinguished eye surgeon told Helmholtz that the instrument was dangerous since it admitted the naked light into a diseased eye; another investigator was of the opinion that the mirror might be of service to ophthalmologists with defective eyesight—he himself had good eyes and wanted none of it.[9]

The first indirect ophthalmoscope[10] was designed by Ruete (1852). Inspired by the description of the first binocular microscope (1852), Giraud-Teulon designed the first direct and indirect binocular ophthalmoscope in 1861.[11] In 29 years, from 1851 to 1880, no less than 78 different ophthalmoscopes were described. In 1900, Trantas devised a method of examination of the ciliary region with a direct ophthalmoscope,[12] by depressing this region with his thumbnail. Unfortunately, this type of technique was not extensively used until almost 50 years later, when Schepens modernized and popularized it.[70]

The next important step was made by Gullstrand (1911), who studied carefully the parameters affecting ophthalmoscopy.[13] He developed reflex-free ophthalmoscopy[14] and based his work on an extremely simplified mathematical model of the optics of the human eye. No other fundamental progress was made in ophthalmoscopy until the contemporary period.

Focal illumination of the retina and deep vitreous was recommended as early as 1901[15] by Wolff who used the method with a direct electric ophthalmoscope. This optically simple method was improved in later years, but it lacked versatility: the beam of light had insufficient sharpness to form an optical section of the transparent media, and it was difficult to vary the angle formed by incident and emergent rays.

Another type of attempt to examine optical sections of the fundus consisted in using a low-power microscope. This method required that the refractive power of the eye be markedly modified. One approach derived from Méry's principle of the hydrophthalmoscope, which was later developed into a more practical instrument by Czermak (1851 and 1853).[16, 17] A further improvement was the use of a flat contact lens, originally discovered by Coccius (1853)[18] (pp. 150-156) and developed by Koeppe (1918) into the type of lens still used nowadays.[19]

A different approach was to use a strong concave lens in front of the eye rather than a contact lens. The method was originally described by Stilling (1879),[20] later developed by Lemoine and Valois (1923),[21] and further improved and popularized by Hruby (1942).[22]

Accurate observation of vitreoretinal relationships was actually impossible so long as a good slit image of the light source[23] was not available. This fact was another of Gullstrand's contributions (1912). Koeppe (1918)[19] first adapted the Gullstrand slit lamp to the examination of the fundus, thus culminating previous attempts into the slit lamp biomicroscopy of the fundus as we now know it.

Highlights of the development of methods of examination during the modern period may be summarized as follows:

Ophthalmoscopy
    1851: Monocular ophthalmoscopy (Helmholtz)
    1861: Binocular ophthalmoscopy (Giraud-Teulon)
    1900: Scleral depression (Trantas)
    1911: Reflex-free ophthalmoscopy (Gullstrand)
Slit lamp microscopy of the fundus
    1901: Ophthalmoscopy in focal illumination (Wolff)
    1912: Development of the slit lamp (Gullstrand)
    1918: Slit lamp microscopy of the fundus with a flat contact lens (Koeppe)
    1942: Slit lamp microscopy of the fundus with a concave precorneal lens (Hruby)

CONCEPTS OF PATHOGENESIS
Early period (1853-1923)

It was ophthalmoscopic observation that stimulated the development of concepts in the pathogenesis of retinal detachment. Retinal breaks were described by Coccius[18] (pp. 130-131) very soon after the discovery of the ophthalmoscope, but their importance was unrecognized. Retinal detachment was therefore attributed to a variety of causes: Arlt (1858) thought that the main cause was choroidal exudation.[24] At first (1854) von Graefe felt that retinal detachment was due to choroidal effusion or hemorrhage.[25] Later (1857) he was of the opinion that, in myopes, it was distension of the globe that stretched the retina to the point where it separated from the choroid, following the chord of the ocular sphere rather than the arc.[26] Von Graefe also regarded retinal breaks as part of the healing process. It was Iwanoff (1869) who established that vitreous detachment preceded retinal detachment and was probably a precipitating factor,[27] but he failed to understand why this was so. Yet 11 years earlier, Muller had already observed traction bands in the vitreous cavity, and he thought that they caused retinal detachment in rare cases of traumatic origin.[28] Retinal breaks were generally thought to be the result and not the cause of retinal detachment. However, as early as 1870 de Wecker and de Jaeger thought that retinal breaks were essential in causing retinal detachment, and they conceived of two fundamental mechanisms[29]: the first was felt to be most frequent in eyes with staphyloma—hypersecretion of fluid between the vitreous gel and the retina which pushed the gel forward and distended the retina. This mechanism was thought to produce retinal tears along the line of vitreoretinal attachment, and these tears in turn caused a ballooning retinal detachment. The second mechanism was felt to be operating in cases of perforating trauma or inflammation and consisted of vitreoretinal cicatricial bands causing retinal tears and detachment by traction.

The fundamental importance of retinal breaks gradually gained recognition. Developing some of de Wecker's ideas, Leber (1882) gave prime importance not to retinal distension alleged to occur in high myopia or to traction by easily identifiable vitreous bands but to retinal breaks caused by alterations of the vitreous so tenuous as to be clinically invisible.[30] In his opinion the development of visible retinal breaks always caused an acute increase of the retinal detachment. Along the same line of thinking, de Wecker (1889) insisted on the frequency of retinal breaks in cases of retinal detachment, even when the observer failed to detect them clinically.[31]

Unfortunately Leber's original hypothesis was bitterly criticized because he assumed that ophthalmoscopically invisible changes in the vitreous were causing retinal detachment. As a consequence, he gradually changed his mind. In 1908 he held that retinal breaks were not due to delicate vitreous traction bands but that they were secondary events caused by extensive preretinal organization that was visible in microscopic sections of eyes with long-standing retinal detachment.[32] Dufour and Gonin (1906), however, revived Leber's original theory and ascribed retinal breaks to isolated vitreoretinal adhesions with a normal-appearing vitreous body. It is strange that, at the time, they were the only authors still in favor of this thesis.[33]

It was Gonin (1920) who developed the modern views on the pathogenesis of retinal detachment and clearly demonstrated the relation between changes in the vitreous body and causation of retinal detachment as we conceive of it today.[34]

Modern period (1923-1950)

No new concepts of pathogenesis were developed during this period. The theses that had been proposed earlier to explain retinal detachment—such as vitreous traction, retinal distension and thinning, and preretinal organization—were gradually seen in a more realistic perspective. To a large extent, this was accomplished because of improved techniques for examination in vivo of the vitreoretinal relationships and because of the careful pathologic study of specimens with various types of retinal detachments. The gradual rearrangement of pathogenic concepts had a profound influence on methods of treatment. Gonin's thesis of the pathogenesis of retinal detachment was accepted very slowly, particularly in Anglo-Saxon countries. This was clearly ascribable to the inadequate methods of fundus examination used in these countries between 1923 and 1946: the exclusive use of direct ophthalmoscopy did not allow a sufficiently detailed examination of the fundus periphery, and slit lamp microscopy of the fundus was not popular.

The highlights of developments in concepts of pathogenesis may be summarized as follows:

1853: Discovery of retinal breaks (Coccius)

1870: Suspicion that retinal breaks make retinal detachment worse (de Wecker)

1882: Prime importance given to retinal breaks, which are ascribed to isolated almost invisible vitreoretinal adhesions (Leber)

1908: Important role of preretinal organization emphasized (Leber)

1920: First clear description of role played by vitreous in causation of rhegmatogenous retinal detachment (Gonin)

Important lessons can be learned from this historical summary. For instance, ophthalmoscopy could have become a clinically useful method 147 years before 1851, in
1704. The cause for this delay is that Méry was totally unaware of the importance
of his discovery. During the second half of the nineteenth century, Helmholtz created
a tidal wave of interest in ophthalmoscopy, but no other breakthrough was made in
ophthalmoscopy until 60 years later when a physicist and ophthalmologist named
Gullstrand established the principles of reflex-free ophthalmoscopy and of slit lamp
microscopy. Thanks to Gullstrand's work, modern fundus photography and slit lamp
microscopy of anterior segment and fundus could be developed.

After the discovery of retinal breaks (1853), it took 67 years (until 1920) to
correctly interpret their significance. This problem could have been solved much
earlier had better methods been available at that time to demonstrate the existence
of isolated vitreoretinal adhesions.

TREATMENT

As long as correct understanding of the cause of retinal detachment was lacking,
its therapy was varied but uniformly ineffective. As in the case of the methods of
examination and pathogenesis, two periods are distinguished, early and modern.

Early period (1805-1923)

The first recorded surgical attempt to repair a retinal detachment was release of
subretinal fluid by Ware (1805).[35] Vitreous injections of various materials were
started early: subretinal fluid (Weber, 1874),[36] and later air and also aqueous, saline,
and cerebrospinal fluids. Rabbit vitreous was injected into humans by Deutschmann
(1895),[37] who felt that it tended to dissolve traction bands. The same author also
advocated surgical sectioning of vitreoretinal adhesions.

Surgical operations aimed at reducing the volume of the globe were the logical
results of theories of globe distension and vitreous traction. Excision of a full-thickness
strip of sclera was first done by Alaimo (1893)[38] and later by Müller (1903).[39] The
first lamellar resection with tucking of the scleral flap was done by von Blaskowicz
(1911).[40] These resection operations were recommended exclusively for cases with
high myopia.

Attempts to reattach the retina were made by the production of chorioretinal
adhesions not aimed at closing retinal breaks. Many methods have been proposed
such as galvanocautery (1882),[41] electrolysis (1895),[42] sutures in the retina (1895),[43]
tincture of iodine injected in the vitreous (1889),[44] and later in the subretinal space
(1895).[43]

In this period during which no special effort was made to close the retinal breaks,
the rate of reattachment was estimated around 6%.[45] Accomplishments during this
period relate to surgical techniques, but they were quite ineffective in reattaching
the retina because they were not directed against the retinal breaks. Notable developments were as follows:

1805: Release of subretinal fluid (Ware)
1874: Injection into the vitreous (Weber)

1882: Chorioretinal adhesions by actual cautery (de Wecker)
1893: Scleroplastic operation (Alaimo)
1895: Injection of animal vitreous and section of vitreous bands (Deutschmann)
1911: Lamellar scleral resection (von Blaskowicz)

Modern period (1923-1950)

The modern period was characterized by attempts to close the retinal breaks. Gonin (1923) was first[46] to cause intentionally a localized chorioretinal reaction over the area of the breaks; for this purpose he used an actual cautery. Heim[47] and then Weve (1930)[48] started separately to use diathermy, which was less violent and produced more extensive reaction than did the actual cautery. Vogt (1934) modified electrolysis,[49] a method originally described in 1895,[42] and he called it catholysis. In 1931 Guist[50] improved Galezowski's method[43] of chemical irritation by placing the irritant in the subchoroidal rather than the subretinal space and by using a different substance. The barrage method for walling off weak portions of the retina was described simultaneously and separately by Gonin[51] and Lindner[52] in 1931.

In order to combat vitreous traction, procedures aimed at reducing the ocular volume, without much regard for the location of the retinal breaks, were revived separately by Lindner[53] and Hildesheimer[54] (1933), who used a modification of Alaimo's technique.[38] Similar cases were first reported in the United States[55] by Pischel and Miller (1939). Von Blaskowicz's lamellar scleral resection[40] was revived in 1951 by three authors independently, Dellaporta,[56] Paufique,[57] and Shapland.[58] Weve (1949) originally suggested making an infolding of full-thickness sclera,[59] and he recommended placing the infolding under star-shaped retinal folds. Ocular volume was reduced by Strampelli with subchoroidal injections of blood plasma (1933)[60] and later by implantation of gelatin sponge (1954),[61] and Smith (1952) used air in the subchoroidal space[62] for the same purpose.

Injections into the vitreous continued to be performed. Lenz (1922) suggested the possibility of injecting human vitreous,[63] but it was Cutler (1946) who was first to use the procedure for the correction of retinal detachment.[64, 65]

As soon as surgery was directed against the retinal breaks, surgical results improved drastically from 6% to over 50%.[45] For instance, Gonin[51] in his first series of 221 cases had 53% success (1931). From that time on, the percentage improved slowly but steadily.

Two currents were apparent in the modern period: Gonin,[66] and later Vogt,[49] Arruga,[67] and Weve[68] were the champions of methods aimed at closing the retinal breaks; on the other hand, Lindner,[53] Strampelli,[60, 61] and Cutler[64, 65] advocated

Table 2-1. Evolution of concepts related to retinal detachment

	Methods of examination	Pathogenesis	Treatment
Early period	1704 - 1851	1853 - 1920	1805 - 1923
Modern period	1851 - 1942	1920 - 1950	1923 - 1950

methods in which less careful closure of the retinal breaks were associated either with techniques reducing the total ocular volume or increasing the vitreous volume with injections. Success with the latter techniques often depended on a barrage of chorioretinal reaction that isolated the retinal breaks from the viable portions of the fundus.

Highlights of this period are listed as follows:

1923: Closure of retinal breaks by cautery (Gonin)
1930: Cautery replaced by diathermy (Heim, Weve)
1931: Barrage technique popularized (Gonin, Lindner)
1933: Revival of full-thickness scleral resections (Lindner, Hildesheimer)
1946: First injections of human vitreous (Cutler)
1949: Infolding of full-thickness sclera (Weve)
1951: Revival of lamellar scleral resections (Dellaporta, Paufique, Shapland)

As Table 2-1 indicates, the development of methods of fundus examination had preceded by 69 years (from 1851 to 1920) the development of correct concepts of pathogenesis on which to base effective treatment methods. The great obstacle to progress has been the lack of methods for adequate visualization in vivo of translucid vitreoretinal adhesions. This has required improvements in ophthalmoscopy and the development of slit lamp microscopy of the fundus.

ASSESSMENT OF THE CONTEMPORARY PERIOD

The contemporary period started between 1942 and 1950. It has been marked by keen interest and progress in the field of retinal detachment.

Methods of examination

Methods of examination have advanced both in ophthalmoscopy and in slit lamp microscopy. The indirect stereoscopic ophthalmoscope[11] of Giraud-Teulon (1861) was modernized by Schepens (1947),[69] who also improved and popularized scleral depression.[70] Today, indirect stereoscopic ophthalmoscopy with scleral depression is the method of choice to examine a fundus with retinal detachment. Recently a further improvement of the scleral depressor was described[71] that helps in making the method more accurate and more comfortable for the patient.

The greatest contribution to ophthalmoscopy since Gullstrand (1911)[13, 14] is that of Pomerantzeff and his associates who used new methods to design a more accurate mathematical model of the human eye, with the help of a high-speed computer.[72] This model served as a tool to develop a small-pupil indirect stereoscopic ophthalmoscope,[73] which has the following advantages: better illumination; maximum stereopsis; good fundus visibility, even at the periphery, through a small pupil; and greater versatility.

Instrumentation for slit lamp microscopy of the fundus has been considerably improved also. Slit lamp ophthalmoscopy in focal illumination was revived by Rotter[74] who compared results obtained with two methods: that of Hruby, who uses a strong concave lens,[22] and that of El Bayadi, who utilizes a strong convex lens.[75] The latter method is recommended in examining a highly myopic eye.

The greatest advance in slit lamp microscopy was made by Schmidt,[76] who devised a much improved slit lamp biomicroscope (model 900 of Haag-Streit), and by Goldmann,[77] who developed a special 3-mirror contact lens to be used for slit lamp microscopy of the vitreous cavity and fundus, including the periphery.

Concepts of pathogenesis

Ideas about pathogenesis of retinal detachment have been reassessed, and the precise role played by retinal breaks, vitreous traction, and high myopia has been reevaluated. With improved slit lamp microscopy of the vitreous cavity, it has been possible to relate more directly preretinal organization with fixed retinal folds.[78] Of interest is the fact that collie dogs suffer from posterior staphyloma and giant retinal breaks without detectable vitreoretinal adhesion.[79] This may be an animal model of rhegmatogenous retinal detachment caused by stretching of poorly vascularized peripheral retina. There is now evidence that the paramount role ascribed to retinal breaks in the pathogenesis of retinal detachment has been overemphasized in some respects. For instance, in one series of normal subjects, retinal breaks were found in 7.84% of the eyes.[80] Obviously, the majority of these asymptomatic subjects with retinal breaks will never develop retinal detachment, and these observations call for a reassessment of pathogenic factors as well as of criteria for preventive treatment of retinal detachment.[81]

A substantial contribution toward a better understanding of the nature of the vitreous body has been made by Balazs[82] and a number of others. The vitreous body was shown to be a collagen gel reinforced with highly polymerized molecules of hyaluronic acid. Someday this work may help us understand the pathogenesis of retinal detachment on the molecular level.

Treatment

In the contemporary period, the treatment of retinal detachment has been characterized by three main tendencies:

1. A search for more effective, less traumatic methods of obtaining a chorioretinal reaction is illustrated, for instance, by the use of crystal-controlled diathermy machines, electrodes with a small surface of contact with the sclera, and applications made over thinned sclera.[83] The development of photocoagulation by Meyer-Schwickerath[84] and later improvements in the instrument[85, 86] contributed considerably to making certain operations less traumatic. The same is true for cryosurgery originally described by Bietti,[87] and revived by Cooper[88] who introduced the use of liquid nitrogen as coolant. Recently, Amoils[89, 90] devised a very simple and effective cryosurgical machine, using carbon dioxide.

2. Surgical techniques were devised that successfully combined in one surgical step the closure of retinal breaks and the relaxation of vitreoretinal adhesions. This was accomplished with the scleral buckling operations in which an indentation is made where the chorioretinal adhesion is induced, namely over the retinal breaks. The first effort in this direction[91] was by Jess (1937), who sutured a gauze pad on the sclera overlying the retinal breaks. Custodis (1951) used Polyviol for the same purpose.[92] In 1957, Schepens and others first described scleral buckling procedures, which were modified in subsequent years.[83, 93, 94] An important result of these procedures was to shorten or eliminate preoperative bed rest, to limit postoperative bed rest to 1 day, and to shorten the total hospital stay to about 1 week.

Scleral buckling with a circling element brought about a drastic improvement of results in cases of poor prognosis.

3. Multiple efforts were made to improve the effect obtained by vitreous injections. Saline and air injections, which had been used for many years in combination with various surgical procedures for reattaching the retina, were found useful with scleral buckling operations when dealing with unfavorable cases of retinal detachment.[94] In addition, air injections became adjuncts when combined with positioning of the patient's head to evert the inverted flap of giant retinal breaks.[95] The management of giant retinal breaks was revolutionized by new pre- and postoperative techniques and by improved surgical methods.[95]

Vitreous surgery in phakic patients, which had been started by Deutschmann[37] and later revived by Cibis,[96] was developed into a relatively harmless and effective procedure.[97, 98]

In conclusion, the contemporary period is witnessing a successful effort at synthesizing our past knowledge regarding the subject of retinal detachment. The present status of research augurs well for the future. Great strides are expected in the field of molecular biology related to retinal detachment and in the development of more efficient instrumentation to diagnose and treat this condition.

REFERENCES

1. Maître-Jan, A.: Traité des maladies de l'oeil et des remèdes propres pour leur guérison, Paris, 1722, Laurent d'Houry.
2. de St. Yves, C.: Nouveau traité des maladies des yeux, Paris, 1722. English translation, London, 1741.
3. Morgagni, J. B.: De sedibus, et causis morborum per anatomen indigatis, Louvain, Belgium, 1766, Typographia Academica, vol. 1.
4. Sichel: Mémoire sur le glaucome; deuxième partie. XIII. L'hydropisie sous-choroidienne, Ann. Oculist. 5:243, 1841.
5. Desmarres, L. A.: Traité théorique et pratique des maladies des yeux, Paris, 1847, Germer Baillière.
6. Méry: Des mouvements de l'iris, Mém. Acad. Roy. Sci., p. 261, Nov. 12, 1704.
7. de la Hire: De quelques faits d'optique, et de la manière dont se fait la vision, Mém. Acad. Roy. Sci., p. 95, March 30, 1709.
8. Helmholtz, H.: Beschreibung eines Augenspiegels, Berlin, 1851, A. Förstner.
9. Koenigsberger: Hermann von Helmholtz, London, 1906, Henry Frowde. (Translated by F. A. Welby.)
10. Ruete, C. G. T.: Der Augenspiegel und das Optometer für practische Aerzte, Göttingen, 1852, Dieterichschen Buchhandlung.
11. Giraud-Teulon: Ophtalmoscopie binoculaire ou s'exerçant par le concours des deux yeux associés, Ann. Oculist. 45:233, 1861.
12. Trantas, A.: Moyens d'explorer par l'ophtalmoscope et par translucidité la partie antérieure du fond oculaire, le cercle ciliaire y compris, Arch. Ophtal. 20:314, 1900.
13. Gullstrand, A.: Einführung in die Methoden der Dioptrik des Auges der Menschen, Leipzig, 1911, S. Hirzel.
14. Gullstrand, A.: Die reflexlose Ophthalmoskopie, Arch. Augenheilk. 68:101, 1910-11.
15. Wolff, H.: Ophthalmoskopische Beobachtungen mit dem elektrischen Augenspiegel. Supplement: Ueber die fokale Beleuchtung der Netzhaut und des Glaskörpers, Z. Augenheilk. 5:101, 1901.
16. Czermak, J.: Ueber eine neue Methode zur genaueren Untersuchung des gesunden und kranken Auges, Vjschr. f. Praktische Heilk. 31:154, 1851.
17. Czermak, J.: Beiträge zur Ophthalmoskopie, Vjschr. Praktische Heilk. 37:137, 1853.

18. Coccius, A.: Ueber die Anwendung des Augen-Spiegels nebst Angabe eines neuen Instrumentes, Leipzig, 1853, Immanuel Müller.

19. Koeppe, L.: Die Mikroskopie des lebenden Augenhintergrundes mit starken Vergrösserungen im fokalen Lichte der Gullstrandschen Nernstlampe.
I. Die Theorie, Apparatur und Anwendungstechnik der Spaltlampenuntersuchung des Augenhintergrundes im fokalen Licht, Graefe Arch. Ophthal. **95**:282, 1918.
II. Die Histologie des lebenden normalen Augenhintergrundes und einiger seiner angeborenen Anomalien im Bilde der Nernstlampe, Graefe Arch. Ophthal. **97**:347, 1918.

20. Stilling, J.: Notiz über Orthoskopie des Augengrundes, Klin. Mbl. Augenheilk. **17**:52, 1879.

21. Lemoine and Valois: Ophtalmoscopie microscopique (sans verre de contact), La Clinique Ophtalmologique **12**:423, 1923.

22. Hruby, K.: Spaltlampenmikroskopie des hinteren Augenabschnittes ohne Kontaktglas. Klin. Mbl. Augenheilk. **108**:195, 1942.

23. Gullstrand, A.: Die Nernspaltlampe in der ophthalmologischen Praxis, Klin. Mbl. Augenheilk. **50**:483, 1912.

24. Arlt, F.: Krankheiten des Auges für praktische Aerzte geschildert, Prague, 1858 (vol. 2), 1859 (vol. 3), F. A. Credner.

25. von Graefe, A.: Notiz über die Ablösungen der Netzhaut von der Chorioidea, Arch. f. Ophthal. **1**(1):362, 1854.

26. von Graefe, A.: Zur Prognose der Netzhautablösung, Arch. f. Ophthal. **3**(2):394, 1857.

27. Iwanoff: Beiträge zur normalen und pathologischen Anatomie des Auges. I. Beiträge zur Ablösung des Glaskörpers, Arch. f. Ophthal. **15**:1, 1869.

28. Muller, H.: Anatomische Beiträge zur Ophthalmologie. 7. Beschreibung einigen von Prof. v. Graefe extirpirten Augäpfel, Arch. f. Ophthal. **4**(1):363, 1858.

29. de Wecker, L., and de Jaeger, E.: Traité des maladies du fond de l'oeil et atlas d'ophtalmoscopie, Paris, 1870, Adrien Delahaye.

30. Leber, T.: Ueber die Entstehung der Netzhautablösung, Ber. 14 Versammlung Ophth. Ges., pp. 18-45, 1882.

31. de Wecker, L., and Landolt, E.: Traité complet d'ophtalmologie, Paris, 1889, Lecrosnier & Babé, vol. IV.

32. Leber, T.: Ueber die Entstehung der Netzhautablösung, Ber. 35 Versammlung Ophth. Ges., p. 120, 1908.

33. Dufour, M., and Gonin, J.: Maladies de la rétine. Décollement rétinien. In Lagrange, F., and Valude, E., editors: Encyclopédie française d'ophtalmologie, Paris, 1906, Octave Doin, vol. VI.

34. Gonin, J.: Pathogénie et anatomie pathologique des décollements rétiniens, Bull. Soc. Franc. Ophtal. **33**:2, 1920.

35. Ware, J.: Chirurgical observations relative to the eye, London, 1805, J. Mawman.

36. Weber, A.: Quoted by Arlt, F. In Engelmann, W., editor: Handbuch der gesammten Augenheilkunde, ed. 1, Leipzig, 1874, vol. 3.

37. Deutschmann, R.: Ueber ein neues Heilverfahren bei Netzhautablösung, Beitr. Augenheilk. **2**:849, 1895.

38. Alaimo: Cura chirurgica del distacco retinico, Ann. Ottal. **22**:542, 1893.

39. Müller, L.: Eine neue operative Behandlung der Netzhautabhebung, Klin. Mbl. Augenheilk. **41**:459, 1903.

40. von Blaskowics, L.: Szemészet, no. 2, 1911. (Quoted by Török, E. In The treatment of detachment of the retina, with special reference to Müller's resection of the sclera, Arch. Ophthal. **46**:466, 1917.)

41. de Wecker, L., and Masselon, J.: Emploi de la galvanocaustique (galvano-puncture) en chirurgie oculaire, Ann. Oculist. **87**:39, 1882.

42. Terson: Quelques considérations sur l'application de l'électrolyse à douze cas de décollement de la rétine, Ann. Oculist **114**:22, 1895.

43. Galezowski, X.: Du décollement de la rétine et de son traitement par ophtalmotomie postérieure, Recueil Ophtal. **17**:385, 1895.

44. Schoeler, H. L.: Zur operativen Behandlung und Heilung der Netzhautablösung, Berlin, 1889, Hermann Peters.

45. Binkhorst, P. G.: Resultaten der diathermische behandeling van netvliesloslating over de jaren 1935 tot 1939 in het nederlandsch gasthuis voor ooglijders te Utrecht, Amsterdam, 1940, J. K. Smit & Zonen.

46. Gonin, J.: Guérisons opératoires de décollements rétiniens, Rev. Génér. Opht. 37:337, 1923.

47. Heim, H.: Quoted by Gonin, J.: In Le décollement de la rétine, Lausanne, 1934, Payot.

48. Weve, H. J. M.: Over netvliesloslating en den gloeiprik van Gonin, Nederl. T. Geneesk. 74:2354, 1930.

49. Vogt, A.: Die operative Therapie und die Pathogenese der Netzhautablösung, Stuttgart, 1936, F. Enke.

50. Guist, G.: Eine neue Ablatioperation, Z. Augenheilk. 74:232, 1931.

51. Gonin, J.: Le résultat de la thermo-ponction oblitérante des déchirures rétiniennes, Ann. Oculist. 168:689, 1931.

52. Lindner, K.: Ein Beitrag zur Entstehung und Behandlung der idiopatischen und der traumatischen Netzhautabhebung, Graefe Arch. Ophthal. 127:177, 1931.

53. Lindner, K.: Heilungversuche bei prognostisch ungünstigen Fällen von Netzhautabhebung, Z. Augenheilk. 81:277, 1933.

54. Hildesheimer, S.: Ablatio-Operation mit Streifenförmiger Elektroexcision der Sklera und chemischer Aetzung, Acta 14 Concilium Ophthalmologicum (Hispania) 2(2):52, 1933.

55. Pischel, D. K., and Miller, M.: Retinal detachment cured by an eyeball shortening operation, Arch. Ophthal. 22:974, 1939.

56. Dellaporta, A.: Die Verkürzung des Bulbus mittels Sklerafaltung, Klin. Mbl. Augenheilk. 119:135, 1951.

57. Paufique, L., and Hugonnier, R.: Traitement du décollement de la rétine par la résection sclérale, Bull. Soc. Franc. Ophtal. 64:435, 1951.

58. Shapland, C. D.: Scleral resection—lamellar, Trans. Ophthal. Soc. U.K. 71:29, 1951.

59. Weve, H. J M.: Bulbusverkürzung durch Reffung der Sklera, Ophthalmologica 118:660, 1949.

60. Strampelli, B.: Trattamento del distacco di retina con iniezioni sottoretiniche di plasma sanguigno, Boll. Oculist. 12:629, 1933.

61. Strampelli, B.: Introduzione di spugna di gelatina nello spazio sopracoroideale nella operazione del distacco di retina non riducibile con il riposo, Ann. Ottal. 80:275, 1954.

62. Smith, R.: Suprachoroidal air injection for detached retina, Brit. J. Ophthal. 36:385, 1952.

63. Lenz, G.: Die Behandlung der Netzhautablösung. In Saemisch, T., editor: Graefe-Saemisch Handbuch der gesammten Augenheilkunde, Augenärztliche Operationslehre, ed. 3, Berlin, 1922, Julius Springer, vol. 2.

64. Cutler, N. L.: Transplantation of human vitreous, Arch. Ophthal. 35:615, 1946.

65. Cutler, N. L.: Vitreous transplantation, Trans. Amer. Acad. Ophthal. Otolaryng. 51:253, 1947.

66. Gonin, J.: Le décollement de la rétine, Lausanne, Switzerland, 1934, Payot.

67. Arruga, H.: Le décollement de la retine, Barcelona, 1936. (Published privately.)

68. Weve, H. J. M.: Zur Entstehung und Behandlung der Netzhautablösung, Klin. Mbl. Augenheilk. 102:609, 1939.

69. Schepens, C. L.: A new ophthalmoscope demonstration, Trans. Amer. Ophthal. Otolaryng. 51:298, 1947.

70. Schepens, C. L.: Examination of the ora serrata region: its clinical significance, Acta XVI Concilium Ophthalmologicum (Britannia) 2:1384, 1950.

71. Hovland, K. R., Tanenbaum, H. L., and Schepens, C. L.: A new scleral depressor, Amer. J. Ophthal. 66:117, 1968.

72. Pomerantzeff, O., Brasseur, J., and Shefler, G.: Study of binocular indirect ophthalmoscopy by ray tracing. (Submitted for publication.)

73. Hovland, K. R., El Zeneiny, I. H., and Schepens, C. L.: Clinical evaluation of the small-pupil binocular indirect ophthalmoscope. (In press. Arch. Ophthal.)

74. Rotter, H.: Zur Theorie der Spaltlampenmikroskopie des Augenhintergrundes, Graefe Arch. Ophthal. **152:**689, 1952; **156:**503, 1955.

75. El Bayadi, G.: New method of slit-lamp micro-ophthalmoscopy, Brit. J. Ophthal. **37:**625, 1953.

76. Schmidt, T.: Zur Theorie und Praxis der Spaltlampe, Acta XVIII Concilium Ophthalmologicum (Belgica) **2:**1818, 1958.

77. Goldmann, H.: Les techniques générales d'examen. In Busacca, A., Goldmann, H., and Schiff-Wertheimer, S., editors: Biomicroscopie du corps vitre et du fond de l'oeil, Paris, 1957, Masson et Cie.

78. Tolentino, F. I., Schepens, C. L., and Freeman, H. M.: Massive preretinal retraction, Arch. Ophthal. **78:**16, 1967.

79. Freeman, H. M., Donovan, R. H., and Schepens, C. L.: Retinal detachment, chorioretinal changes, and staphyloma in the collie, Arch. Ophthal. **76:**412, 1966.

80. Rutnin, U., and Schepens, C. L.: Fundus appearance in normal eyes. IV. Retinal breaks and other findings, Amer. J. Ophthal. **64:**1019, 1967.

81. Schepens, C. L.: The preventive treatment of idiopathic and secondary retinal detachment. Surgical indications, Acta XVIII Concilium Ophthalmologicum (Belgica) **1:**1019, 1958.

82. Balazs, E. A.: The molecular biology of the vitreous. In McPherson, A., editor: New and controversial aspects of retinal detachment, New York, 1968, Hoeber Medical Division, Harper & Row, Publishers.

83. Schepens, C. L., Okamura, I. D., and Brockhurst, R. J.: The scleral buckling procedures. I. Surgical techniques and management, Arch. Ophthal. **58:**797, 1957.

84. Meyer-Schwickerath, G.: Lichtkoagulation, Klin. Mbl. Augenheilk. **33:**Suppl.: 1, 1959.

85. Pomerantzeff, O., Schepens, C. L., and Freeman, H. M.: Studies in photocoagulation. I. The photocoagulating beam, Brit. J. Ophthal. **48:**298, 1964.

86. Pomerantzeff, O., and Schepens, C. L.: Studies in photocoagulation. II. The observation beam, Brit. J. Ophthal. **48:**306, 1964.

87. Bietti, G. B.: Criocausticazioni episclerali con mezzo di terapia nel distacco retinico, Boll. Oculist. **12:**1427, 1933.

88. Cooper, I. S.: Principles and rationale of cryogenic surgery, St. Barnabas Hosp. Med. Bull. **1:**5, 1962.

89. Amoils, S. P., and Walker, A. J.: The thermal and mechanical factors involved in ocular surgery, Proc. Roy. Soc. Med. **59:**1056, 1966.

90. Amoils, S. P.: The Joule Thomson retinal cryopencils, Arch. Ophthal. **80:**128, 1968.

91. Jess, A.: Temporäre Skleraleindellung als Hilfsmittel bei der Operation der Netzhautabhebung, Klin. Mbl. Augenheilk. **99:**318, 1937.

92. Custodis, E.: (a) Beobachtungen bei der diathermischen Behandlung der Netzhautablösung und ein Hinweis zur Therapie der Amotio Retinae, Ber. Deutsch. Ophth. Ges. **57:**227, 1951.
   (b) Bedeutet die Plombenaufnähung auf die Sklera einen Fortschritt in der operativen Behandlung der Netzhautablösung? Ber. Deutsch. Ophth. Ges. **58:**102, 1953.

93. Schepens, C. L.: Scleral buckling with circling element, Trans. Amer. Acad. Ophthal. Otolaryng. **68:**959, 1964.

94. Schepens, C. L., and Freeman, H. M.: Surgery of retinal detachment. In Sorsby, A., editor: Modern trends in ophthalmology, London, 1967, Butterworths.

95. Schepens, C. L., and Freeman, H. M.: Current management of giant retinal breaks, Trans. Amer. Acad. Ophthal. Otolaryng. **71:**474, 1967.

96. Cibis, P. A.: Vitreoretinal pathology and surgery in retinal detachments, St. Louis, 1965, The C. V. Mosby Co.

97. Freeman, H. M., Schepens, C. L., and Anastopoulou, A.: Vitreous surgery. II. Instrumentation and technique, Arch. Ophthal. **77:**681, 1967.

98. Schepens, C. L., and Freeman, H. M.: Vitreous surgery, Trans. Amer. Acad. Ophthal. Otolaryng. **72:**399, 1968.

3

Techniques of examination of the fundus periphery

Charles L. Schepens

The fundus periphery is generally defined as that area located anterior to the globe's equator. The equator corresponds roughly to a circle passing through the anterior portion of the vortex ampullae. Since these structures are not always easily identifiable, it is more practical to define the posterior limit of the fundus periphery as a circle that passes through the posterior extremities of the choroidal portion of the vortex veins (Fig. 3-1). The entrance sites of the vortex veins into the sclera are among the most constant and conspicuous landmarks in the human fundus. They are located 2 disc diameters (3 mm.) posterior to the equator.

The fundus periphery is itself divided into an equatorial and an oral zone. The limit between the two is located halfway between equator and ora serrata, or 2 disc diameters posterior to the ora serrata. The oral zone extends, one each side of the ora serrata, posteriorly to the limit of the equatorial zone and anteriorly to the posterior border of the ciliary processes.

The fundus periphery can seldom be seen clearly by direct ophthalmoscopy, particularly in phakic patients. Even the scleral entrances of the vortex veins are sometimes difficult to see by this method. Three techniques are found useful to examine the fundus periphery: indirect stereoscopic ophthalmoscopy with scleral indentation, transillumination, and slit lamp microscopy with a 3-mirror lens.

INDIRECT STEREOSCOPIC OPHTHALMOSCOPY WITH SCLERAL INDENTATION[1-5]

Maximal pupillary dilatation is advisable. It is obtained by repeated instillations of a mydriatic mixture.* If drops fail to dilate the pupil sufficiently, a subconjunc-

---

*Cyclogyl   50   mg.
Phenylephrine hydrochloride   0.5 gm.
Aq. Dest.   5   ml.

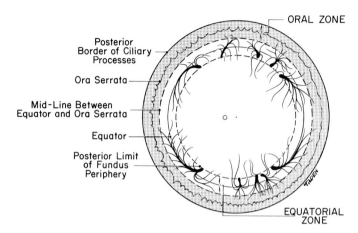

Fig. 3-1. Division of the fundus into two areas, posterior and peripheral. The limit is a circle (inner dashed line) located on the scleral entrances of the vortex veins, which is two disc diameters posterior to the equator. The fundus periphery is itself divided into an equatorial and an oral zone. The equatorial zone extends from the scleral entrances of the vortex veins (inner dashed circle) to halfway between equator and ora, or 2 disc diameters posterior to the ora serrata (outer dashed circle). The oral periphery extends from the peripheral limit of the equatorial zone to the posterior border of the ciliary processes, which is represented by the outer continuous circle. (Modified from U. Rutnin.)

tival injection of 0.1 or 0.2 ml. of mydriatic mixture* may be used. The patient must lie down comfortably in a darkened room. The posterior pole is examined first, and the main landmarks are recorded on a special fundus chart (Fig. 3-2). Recording is made with color pencils according to the following code:

Blue: Detached retina, retinal veins

Red: Attached retina, retinal arteries, hemorrhage in retina

Red lined with blue: Retinal breaks

Black: Retinal pigmentation, choroidal pigmentation when seen through attached retina

Brown: Choroidal pigmentation seen through detached retina

Green: Opacities in media—including vitreous hemorrhage

Yellow: Chorioretinal exudation, macular edema

The fundus chart is clipped on a board that rests on the patient's chest. It is oriented upside down so that 12 o'clock on the chart is toward the patient's feet and 6 o'clock toward his chin. In this way, the observer may record findings on the chart as he sees them through the ophthalmoscope.†

It is essential that what is drawn in the fundus sketch should represent without possible ambiguity what it is meant to show. Doing so is often impossible with the

---

*Phenylephrine hydrochloride   25   mg.
 Homatropine hydrobromide   20   mg.
 Procaine hydrochloride   50   mg.
 Aq. Dest.   5   ml.
†The image formed by the indirect ophthalmoscope is inverted.

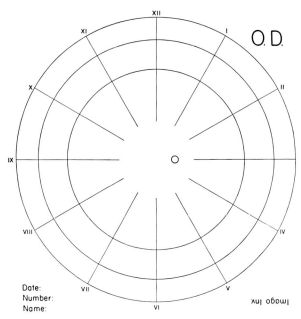

Fig. 3-2. Special chart for recording fundus details. The inner circle corresponds to the equator, the middle circle to the ora serrata, and the outer circle to the anterior limit of the pars plana ciliaris. The best charts are printed on pale gray paper which avoids glare to the ophthalmologist and from which colors are better reproduced photographically.

above color code; for instance, green may be vitreous haze, lens opacities, or corneal opacities. In order to help clear up any misunderstanding, sketches should be labeled clearly in black pencil whenever indicated. Sometimes an additional large-scale sketch or cross-section of complicated structures is helpful.

After examination of the posterior pole, examination of the periphery is started. The patient's pupil appears circular to the examiner when he studies the posterior pole, but it becomes elliptic when he looks at the fundus periphery. The best view of the periphery is always obtained if the observer is at the other end of the meridian in which the area examined is located. For example, to examine the periphery at 6 o'clock, the observer must place himself at 12 o'clock, the patient gazing toward his own feet. In order to see the periphery at 3 o'clock, the examiner must place himself at 9 o'clock, the patient gazing toward 3 o'clock, and so on. It is in this way that the observer can take best advantage of the patient's elliptic pupil, by placing the images of his own pupils on the long axis of the ellipse, thus obtaining better stereopsis (Fig. 3-3).

When the fundus periphery is observed, an increase of astigmatism and other aberrations make clear viewing progressively more difficult. As a result, better definition is obtained by using a fairly strong condensing lens (+18 D), which gives a relatively small magnification. It is for this reason that the greater magnification obtained with the direct ophthalmoscope makes it difficult to see the fundus periphery clearly.

Another problem that arises in studying the fundus periphery is to obtain sufficient illumination. In ordinary stereoscopic indirect ophthalmoscopes the light source forms a relatively large image in the patient's pupillary plane. Even when the posterior pole is examined through a pupil that is not fully dilated, the image of the light source may be so large that it cannot entirely enter the patient's pupil

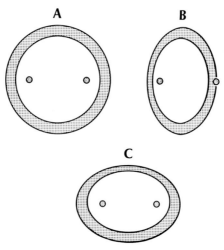

Fig. 3-3. Patient's dilated pupil as it appears to the observer. The two small circles represent the images of the observer's pupils. **A,** View during examination of the posterior pole. **B,** View during examination of the fundus periphery if, for instance, the patient is sitting and looks from either side—observer's view is monocular in this case. **C,** View during examination of the fundus periphery if observer places his eyes at other end of the meridian to be examined; view remains stereoscopic.

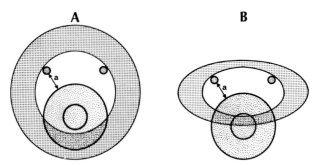

Fig. 3-4. Imaging of the light source in the patient's pupillary plane by existing types of binocular indirect headband ophthalmoscopes. The image of the light source is composed of two parts, forming two concentric circles: a bright center (image of the filament) and a halo (image of the condenser). **A,** Even when the posterior pole is examined, the total image of the light source cannot enter the patient's pupil if the latter is not fully dilated. **B,** When the fundus periphery is examined, only a small portion of the image of the light source enters the patient's elliptic pupil. The two small circles represent images of the observer's pupils. Separation (a) between images of the patient's pupils and image of the light source is necessary to avoid disturbing corneal reflections.

(Fig. 3-4). When one examines the fundus periphery, a large portion of the image of the light source necessarily falls outside the patient's elliptic pupil. It is therefore important to use as strong a light source as possible.

Small-pupil ophthalmoscope[6-8]

The small-pupil ophthalmoscope incorporates two improvements not included in any of the existing instruments: The first improvement relates to the light source that forms a small and very luminous image in the patient's pupil. The position of the image of the light source in the patient's pupil is adjustable. Regardless of the patient's pupillary size, this adjustment enables the observer to place the image of the light source in the patient's pupil near the pupillary edge (Fig. 3-5, *A*). When the fundus periphery is examined through a dilated pupil, the image of the light source can be brought closer to the center of the elliptic pupil, thereby improving considerably illumination of the fundus periphery (Fig. 3-5, *B*).

The second improvement incorporated into the small-pupil ophthalmoscope refers to positioning of the images of the observer's pupils in the patient's pupil. Most commercially available instruments are adjusted to give a binocular image through a patient's pupil that is at least 3.5 mm. in diameter. If the pupil is smaller, only a monocular view can be obtained. If the patient's pupil is larger, stereopsis of

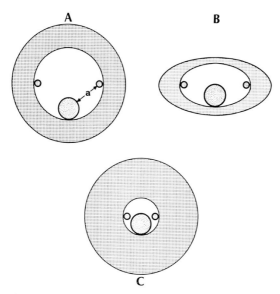

Fig. 3-5. **A,** In the small-pupil opthalmoscope, the source used for illumination forms a small and bright image in the observer's pupils; all reflections from the patient's eye are avoided when distance (a) can be made at least equal to 4 mm. **B,** When examining the fundus periphery through a patient's dilated pupil, the images of the observer's pupils are kept separated, but the image of the light source can be brought near the center of the patient's pupil, thereby improving fundus illumination. **C,** If the patient's pupil is small, the three images are brought close together. Conversely, if the patient's pupil is widely dilated, best viewing is obtained by separating the three images as much as practical.

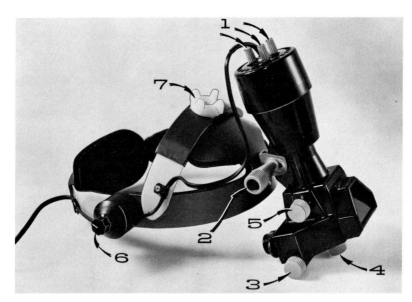

Fig. 3-6. General view of the new small-pupil indirect stereoscopic ophthalmoscope with the following adjustments: (1) three screws move the lamp's filament (as in slit lamp), (2) screw to position instrument in front of observer's eyes, (3) screw for interpupillary distance, (4) screw for positioning images of observer's pupils in patient's pupils, (5) screw to position image of light source in patient's pupil, (6) rheostat for decreasing lamp brightness, (7) one of two headband adjustments.

the fundus picture is less than it would be if the images of the observer's pupils were further apart. In the new instrument, these images can be so adjusted that they are always on the edge of the patient's pupil, regardless of its size (Fig. 3-5, *C*). With such an adjustment, it is possible in every case to obtain the maximum stereopsis permissible by the diameter of the patient's pupil; in addition, a binocular view of the patient's fundus can be obtained even through a pupil as small as 1.5 mm.

When the fundus periphery is examined, stereopsis is of particular importance because the optical quality of the images is rather poor. Adjustment of the position of the images of the observer's pupils is not only useful to improve stereopsis, but it may also help to avoid localized opacities in the media that often hinder adequate viewing of the fundus periphery. Fig. 3-6 gives a general view of the small-pupil ophthalmoscope and of its adjustments.

Use of scleral indentation

Examination of the oral region nearly always requires the use of scleral depression, which brings the peripheral fundus structures into view. The technique of scleral depression was originally suggested by Trantas,[9] who used direct ophthalmoscopy and pressed on the globe with his thumbnail. The thimble depressor of Schepens[3] permits easier and more accurate depression. It is usually worn on the middle finger of the right hand. The tip of the depressor is placed on the skin of

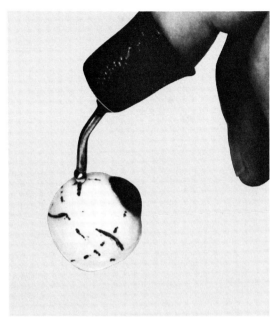

Fig. 3-7. Incorrect method of scleral depression with tip applied perpendicular to the globe. (Modified from R. J. Brockhurst.)

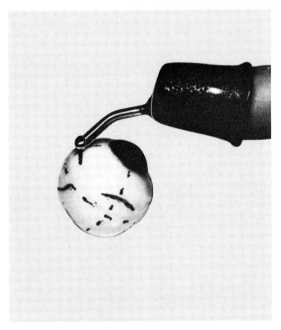

Fig. 3-8. Correct method of scleral depression with tip applied tangentially to the globe. (Modified from R. J. Brockhurst.)

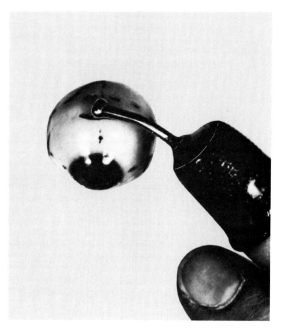

Fig. 3-9. Incorrect method of scleral depression with tip of depressor introduced from the side. (Modified from R. J. Brockhurst.)

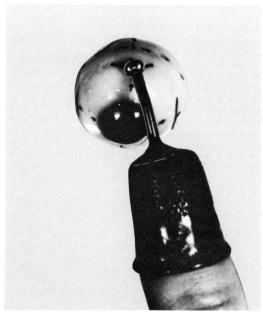

Fig. 3-10. Correct method of scleral depression with tip of depressor introduced close to the meridian of observation. (Modified from R. J. Brockhurst.)

the eyelid over the area of sclera to be indented. When the upper fundus periphery is examined, the eyelid should be closed, the depressor tip being applied to the lid at the upper edge of the tarsus. When the patient opens the lid and looks up, the tip of the depressor slides easily under the orbital margin. The whole fundus periphery can be examined usefully by indentation.

Many examiners make the mistake of pushing the depressor perpendicularly against the globe in order to bring the periphery into view (Fig. 3-7). This method invariably causes pain and induces the patient to squeeze his lids. The scleral depressor must be used tangentially to the globe, with slight flexing of the finger to cause indentation (Fig. 3-8). It should be introduced as meridionally as possible. If introduced from the side (Fig. 3-9), the tip, hidden by the lid, may not be in the meridian that is being observed and the periphery will not be seen. When inserted in a direction closely parallel to the line of observation, the tip is more likely to be in the proper meridian (Fig. 3-10).

The inferior fundus periphery is more difficult to see by scleral indentation since the lower lid is generally tighter and many patients have difficulty in looking downward. The depressor tip should be placed on the skin of the lower lid about 3 to 4 mm. from the lid margin; with a gentle movement of the depressor, the lower lid and depressor can be made to slide together back and forth as necessitated by the examination.

In order to depress the sclera at 3 or 9 o'clock, in the palpebral fissure, it is usually necessary to apply pressure directly on the bulbar conjunctiva. Some patients tolerate this procedure well without topical anesthesia, but in others it is best to anesthetize the conjunctiva with 0.5% tetracaine drops. If topical anesthesia is necessary, this portion of the examination is performed last, since tetracaine may cause edema of the corneal epithelium and hazing of the fundus view.

When scleral depression is performed, the pressure tends to push the globe back toward the primary position of gaze. The patient is then urged to hold his eyes in extreme gaze more forcefully. It is a popular misconception that considerable pressure must be applied with the scleral depressor in order to see the ora serrata. The rise of intraocular pressure caused by correctly performed scleral depression has been measured.[10] When the ora serrata is viewed with scleral indentation applied to the temporal conjunctiva, the measured increase of ocular pressure averaged 7 mm. of mercury. It was 10 mm. of mercury if indentation was exerted over the patient's eyelid.

The information obtained by scleral depression is of two kinds[11]: First, it allows one to view clearly structures in the extreme fundus periphery, as far anteriorly as the posterior border of the ciliary processes. Equally important is the fact that scleral depression permits one to see the peripheral fundus in profile, thereby giving more accurate information on the relations between retina and choroid on one side and retina and vitreous on the other.

Improved scleral depressor[12]

With the scleral depressor of Schepens,[3] it is difficult to keep the examiner's hand out of the viewing axis unless the thimble is held between thumb and index finger instead of being worn on the median finger. The short shaft of the depressor

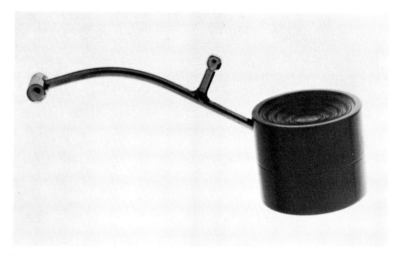

Fig. 3-11. Improved scleral depressor. The cylinder is held between thumb and index finger. The small post serves to depress the shaft with the middle finger. (From Hovland, Tanenbaum, and Schepens: New scleral depressor, Amer. J. Ophthal. **66:**117, 1968.)

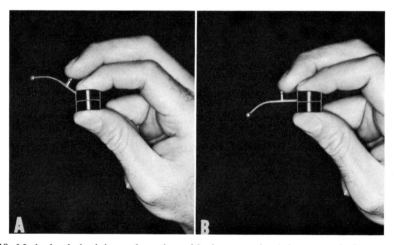

Fig. 3-12. Methods of obtaining indentation with the new scleral depressor. **A,** By a movement of the wrist. **B,** By the middle finger pressing on the small post. (From Hovland, Tanenbaum, and Schepens: New scleral depressor, Amer. J. Ophthal. **66:**117, 1968.)

makes its use difficult in deep-set eyes, and it is not easy to gauge variations of applied pressure without a great deal of practice.

An articulated scleral depressor that offers a number of improvements in design and function has been developed (Fig. 3-11). It has a movable depressor arm mounted with a spring action in a small metal cylinder. Both ends of the cylinder are serrated and slightly depressed to give the examiner a good grip. The depressor is held between the thumb and index finger (Fig. 3-12). In this fashion, the hand of the examiner and the cylinder of the depressor are completely out of the way.

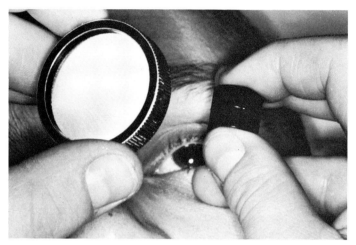

Fig. 3-13. Improved scleral depressor in use.

There are two techniques of using this instrument: Depression can be exerted with a wrist action similar to that employed with the thimble depressor (Fig. 3-12, *A*). With the other technique, the observer's middle finger presses on the small post attached to the shaft (Fig. 3-12, *B*). The amount of pressure applied to the globe can be gauged more accurately by the latter method. If excessive pressure is used with the new depressor, not only will the patient complain of pain, but the pressure of the small post onto the middle finger will cause the examiner discomfort. With either of these methods, the fourth finger can easily be used to move the eyelid out of the way, especially while one views temporal or nasal areas.

Because of the length of the depressor arm and its relationship to the holding device, a better view of the fundus periphery can be obtained while its axis is held close to that of the observer's line of view (Fig. 3-13). This affords more accurate localization of retinal breaks. The above features are particularly beneficial in examining patients with deep-set eyes or children under anesthesia.

TRANSILLUMINATION

Transillumination may give information about the fundus periphery when ophthalmoscopy is difficult or impossible. It is particularly useful when a space-taking lesion is suspected in an eye with vitreous hemorrhage.

The pupil is fully dilated and topical anesthesia with drops of 0.5% tetracaine is applied. I prefer to use a powerful transilluminator with a light that is strong, cold, and available either at the end of a probe or on its side (Fig. 3-14). The transilluminator tip is sterilizable in ethylene oxide. The patient lies down in a darkened room, and transillumination is performed via both the transcorneal and transcleral routes.

The tip that gives side illumination may safely be moved over the cornea without danger of scratching the epithelium. The patient is requested to look in the direction that will expose the portion of sclera to be examined. The transilluminator

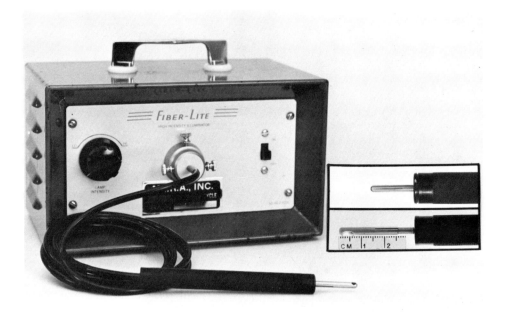

Fig. 3-14. Powerful transilluminator used for fundus examination in the presence of vitreous hemorrhage. *Inset:* the straight and right-angle transilluminator tip. (Modified from H. M. Freeman and C. L. Schepens.)

is slipped between eyelid and cornea and gently applied against the cornea. When properly positioned, it will transilluminate the scleral area under examination. In normal cases, the dark outline of the ora serrata is well visible, and pigmentary degeneration of the fundus periphery is seen as an irregular dark zone adjacent to the ora line. A lesion opaque to light and located close to the sclera will appear as a dark zone. However, it is impossible by this method to distinguish between a cellular lesion, extravasated blood, or a coagulated exudate. The fundus periphery should be examined a full 360 degrees by this procedure.

Transillumination should also be performed by applying the luminous tip over the bulbar conjunctiva, in the region of the fundus periphery. The light is then observed through the pupil, by an observer wearing a headband indirect stereo-scopic ophthalmoscope, with the ophthalmoscope light *turned off*. The red glow produced by the transilluminator is studied by ophthalmoscopy. This technique yields two types of information: First, if the red glow is interrupted, a light-absorbing lesion is present. Second, if a large vitreous hemorrhage is present, it is often im-possible to see useful fundus details by ordinary ophthalmoscopy, but the fundus periphery may become visible by scleral transillumination.

SLIT LAMP MICROSCOPY OF THE FUNDUS

Information obtained by slit lamp microscopy completes data yielded by indirect stereoscopic ophthalmoscopy. The latter is the method of choice for two purposes:

first, for scanning the fundus periphery, studying the extent and geographic distribution of changes, and establishing relationships between peripheral alterations and more centrally located landmarks; and, second, to investigate pathologic details in the retina and choroid, particularly in the fundus periphery. Once this survey is completed, further detailed study of important changes should be performed by slit lamp microscopy, which is particularly useful to establish the relation existing between retina and vitreous and to study fine structural detail in the retina. Neither method is designed to supplant the other, both being complementary, somewhat like low- and high-power magnification in light microscopy. (See Chapter 5, "Technique of Vitreous Cavity Examination.")

REFERENCES

1. Schepens, C. L.: A new ophthalmoscope demonstration, Trans. Amer. Acad. Ophthal. Otolaryng. **51**:298, 1947.
2. Schepens, C. L., and Bahn, G.: Examination of the ora serrata: its importance in retinal detachment, Arch. Ophthal. **44**:677, 1950.
3. Schepens, C. L.: Progress in detachment surgery, Trans. Amer. Acad. Ophthal. Otolaryng. **55**:607, 1951.
4. Schepens, C. L.: Examination of the ora serrata region: its clinical significance, Acta XVI Concilium Ophthalmologicum (Britannia) **II**:1384, 1950.
5. Brockhurst, R. J.: Modern indirect ophthalmoscopy, Amer. J. Ophthal. **41**:266, 1965.
6. Schepens, C. L.: Recent developments in the management of retinal detachment, Trans. Amer. Acad. Ophthal. Otolaryng. **69**:896, 1965.
7. Pomerantzeff, O., and Schepens, C. L.: Binocular indirect ophthalmoscopy. In Schepens, C. L., and Regan, C. D. J., editors: Controversial aspects of the management of retinal detachment, Boston, 1965, Little, Brown & Co.
8. Pomerantzeff, O.: A new stereoscopic indirect ophthalmoscope. In McPherson, A., editor: New and controversial aspects of retinal detachment, New York, 1968, Hoeber Medical Division, Harper & Row, Publishers.
9. Trantas, A.: Moyens d'explorer par l'ophtalmoscope et par translucidité la partie intérieure du fond oculaire, le cercle ciliaire y compris, Arch. Ophtal. **20**:314, 1900.
10. Freeman, H. M.: General discussion of preoperative examination. In Schepens, C. L., and Regan, C. D. J., editors: Controversial aspects of the management of retinal detachment, Boston, 1965, Little, Brown & Co.
11. Schepens, C. L., Tolentino, F., and McMeel, J. W.: Diagnostic and prognostic factors as found in preoperative examination. In Pischel, D. K., et al.: Retinal detachment, Trans. Amer. Acad. Ophthal. Otolaryng. **69**:51, 1965.
12. Hovland, K., Tanenbaum, H. L., and Schepens, C. L.: A new scleral depressor, Amer. J. Ophthal. **66**:117, 1968.

4

Differential diagnosis of retinal detachment

Edward W. D. Norton

In the developing eye, when the optic vesicle becomes invaginated to form the optic cup, the neuroectoderm is folded upon itself and develops into two layers, with a potential space between them. The outer layer forms the pigment epithelium, the inner layer differentiates into the retina proper, and the potential space persists throughout life unless some disease process causes an accumulation of fluid in this space. When this occurs, it is commonly called a retinal detachment or, better, an intraretinal separation. The etiologies for this event are numerous and diversified; the outline below includes some of these. In this discussion no attempt will be made to be all-inclusive; instead, the more common and often more difficult-to-recognize entities will be discussed and helpful clinical aids presented.

Differential diagnosis
I. Primary tumor
 A. Melanoma
 B. Hemangioma
 C. Retinoblastoma
II. Choroidal or combined detachments
III. Retinoschisis
 A. Adult
 B. Juvenile
IV. Vitreous hemorrhage
 A. Spontaneous
 B. Traumatic
V. Inflammatory detachment
 A. Scleritis
 B. Diffuse choroiditis
 C. Uveal effusion
 D. Toxocara
 E. Lymphoid hyperplasia uveal tract
VI. Developmental and congenital
 A. Retrolental fibroplasia

    B. Coloboma
    C. Pit optic nerve
VII. Exudative detachment associated with retinal or choroidal vascular disease
    A. Von Hippel's
    B. Coats'
        1. Juvenile
        2. Adult
    C. Central serous choroidopathy
    D. Detachment pigment epithelium
    E. Subpigment epithelial hemorrhage
    F. Eales'
    G. Postirradiation
VIII. Detachment associated with systemic disease
    A. Toxemia
    B. Uremia
    C. Diabetes
    D. Sickle cell
    E. Lupus

TECHNIQUES OF EXAMINATION

Before a discussion of specific entities is embarked upon, a few general statements about the techniques of examination and available diagnostic aids would seem appropriate.

Ophthalmoscopy

Without question, the single most important examination of any patient with a retinal separation is the viewing of the entire fundus with the binocular indirect ophthalmoscope, with and without scleral depression. I prefer the +30 aspheric lens but often supplement this with the +20 and +14 aspheric lenses. There is no way a person can learn to use this instrument except by hours of practice, but Havener[1] has set forth many useful hints for the beginner. This instrument, as developed by Schepens, gives the following advantages:
    1. A bright light source
    2. A large field of view
    3. A large depth of field
    4. A stereoscopic view of the fundus
    5. An ease of combining scleral depression with the examination
These advantages enable the examiner to view the fundus better, despite hazy media, large refractive errors, and large differences in fundus elevations. The addition of scleral depression enables the examiner to vary his perspective, particularly of peripheral lesions. Any resident finishing his training today unskilled in the use of this instrument is already a generation behind.

Biomicroscopy

Biomicroscopy of the fundus has been a much-neglected tool and should be used routinely in the study of the vitreous, retina, subretinal space, and underlying pigment epithelium and choroid. Although I believe the Goldmann 3-mirror lens is the best way to study the periphery, the Hruby lens is excellent for examination of the posterior polar area. The Hruby lens may not be quite as good as the Goldmann, but it is so easy to use with the Zeiss slit-lamp that it becomes a routine part of every examination. The binocular, magnified, variable slit-illuminated view of the disc, macula, retina, and posterior vitreous is so superior to routine ophthalmoscopy that once mastered the examination will seem incomplete without it. It is particularly useful in the study of the principal diagnostic problems of retinal separation.

Transillumination

Transillumination is a technique that has been neglected and even maligned in recent years. I believe it is a very valuable adjunct in the differential diagnosis of retinal separation. The technique I presently use (Fig. 4-1, *A* and *B*) was introduced to me by Dr. Jose A. Berrocal and consists of indirect ophthalmoscopy (with the light turned off) by retroillumination. A fiber-optic light source is useful because of its variable intensity and "cold light." With a clear lens, choroidal vessels, retinal vessels, the optic disc, chorioretinal lesions, and vitreous opacities are seen against a red-glow background. Any decrease in transmission indicates increased pigment, either blood or melanin. Even in the face of a mature cataract, some idea of the state of the vitreous and presence or absence of a mass can be determined. This technique is especially useful in differentiating serous choroidal detachments from solid lesions. Like most tests its real value exists when it is positive.

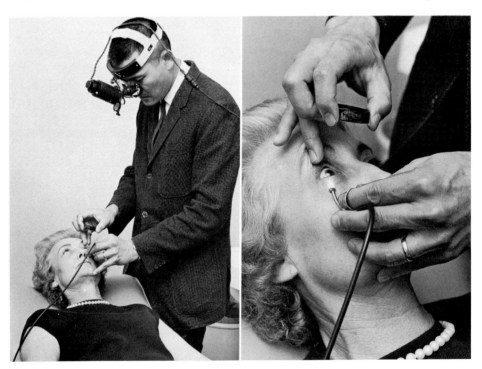

Fig. 4-1

Phosphorus-32 uptake studies

P[32] uptake studies have been in use in ophthalmology for almost 20 years and for some reason have never become popular. I can remember an occasion when this test gave the only diagnostic information. The patient's eye was filled with blood and could not be examined, but the probe located an area of high uptake, suggesting a tumor that was subsequently confirmed pathologically. The use of

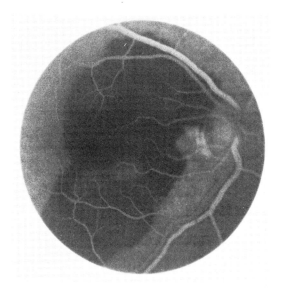

Fig. 4-2

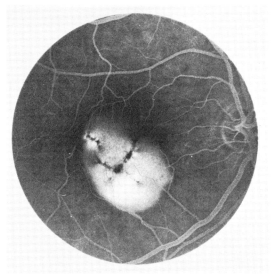

Fig. 4-3

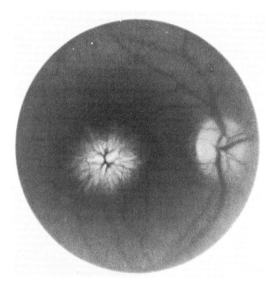

Fig. 4-4

this and subsequent tests to be mentioned requires special instrumentation, technical help, and personal interest in their diagnostic value if they are to be used to any extent. Like all clinical tests, they do not make the diagnosis but merely supplement the clinical information that must then be synthesized into the final diagnosis.

Fluorescein angiography

Fluorescein angiography has been an exciting addition to our diagnostic armamentarium. It has added to our anatomic observations since it is an indication of rate of blood flow and vascular permeability. Its greatest contribution, however, has been the stimulation to examine the fundus in greater detail with all available techniques, including stereoscopic photography. Its present value in the differential diagnosis of retinal separation will be discussed below along with the specific entities, but its greatest clinical value to date has been its aid in the recognition of posterior polar hemorrhage, i.e., subpigment epithelial hemorrhage, where it completely blocks out the choroidal background fluorescence (Fig. 4-2), in the recognition of pigment epithelial detachments (Fig. 4-3), where the pocket of fluid lights up with the accumulation of fluorescein, and in the recognition of cystoid changes in the macula in the aphakic patient (Fig. 4-4).

Ultrasound

Ultrasound is a recent addition to our diagnostic techniques but my experience is insufficient to justify comments at this time.

SPECIFIC PROBLEMS
Malignant melanoma

The most serious misdiagnosis of retinal separation is the failure to recognize an underlying malignant melanoma of the choroid as the cause of the retinal elevation.

Once the patient is subjected to retinal surgery and the integrity of the sclera disrupted, the patient's life is in jeopardy. On the other hand, removal of an eye with an idiopathic retinal detachment because of misinterpretation of the fundus changes is a similar tragedy.

The following list gives the features usually considered in any suspected melanoma case. The more important of these will be discussed below:

1. Age
2. Dark mass—pigment at base
3. Retina often attached to surface of tumor
4. Overlying retina degenerated
5. Neovascularity of mass
6. Surrounding retinal detachment: May be total with shifting fluid
7. Absence of retinal breaks
8. Iris nevi
9. Vitreous normal
10. Visual field defect
11. Defect to transillumination
12. Hemorrhage uncommon—especially when small and posterior
13. P^{32} uptake
14. Fluorescein

Age

Although one usually associates the occurrence of melanomas with the fifth decade or more of life, it is not uncommon in the late teens and early twenties. In 1 year we had six such patients proved pathologically.

Mass

Ophthalmologically, there is a mass in the choroid, elevating the overlying retina. The retina is usually attached to the dome of the tumor but detached on the slopes and around the base. It is especially adherent to the tumor if the tumor has broken through Bruch's membrane and has formed the characteristic collar-button growth. Occasionally the retina is not attached to the underlying tumor but rather highly detached, and if one does not recognize the underlying choroidal lesion—most likely located inferiorly—a disaster will ensue. This is particularly likely to occur if one does not use the binocular indirect ophthalmoscope and position the patient so as to shift fluid (Fig. 4-5, *A* and *B*).

The mass almost always has some pigment at its base. When examining with the slit lamp, one can sometimes see degenerative changes in the overlying retina, orange-brown pigment on the surface of the tumor and even migrating into the retina, and large vascular channels in the tumor itself. Indirect illumination promptly reveals a defect in transillumination that can be readily confirmed with the more conventional techniques of examination.

Hemorrhage

Hemorrhage certainly occurs with this type of tumor, but given a small posterior lesion with clear-cut evidence of bleeding, one should proceed slowly and watch the evolution of the hemorrhage.

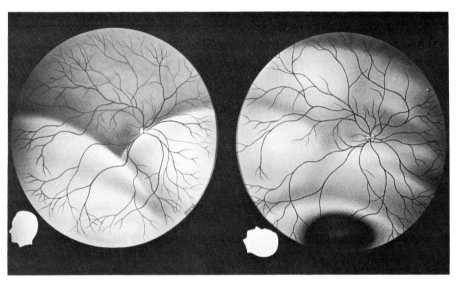

Fig. 4-5

Fluorescein

Fluorescein angiography usually shows beginning fluorescence in the arterio-venous phase and late fluorescence corresponding with shallow detachments over-lying and surrounding the tumor (Fig. 4-6, *A* and *B*). The one exception is in the classical collar-button tumor, which tends to show little or no fluorescence early and very little late, except around its base (Fig. 4-7, *A* and *B*).

Hemangioma

Hemangioma is a comparatively rare tumor of the choroid, and one must see a few of these before becoming skilled in diagnosing them. The following list gives the points to be considered, some of which will be discussed below:

1. Age
2. Located posterior polar area
3. Pink, low elevation
4. Choroidal pattern gone
5. Degeneration of overlying retina with field defect
6. Migration of pigment into clumps
7. Surrounding retinal detachment extending into macula
8. Retinal detachment may be total
9. Absence of breaks, hemorrhage
10. Transillumination
11. Fluorescein

Age

Although one usually considers the hemangioma as a congenital type of tumor, we have seen two patients with localized hemangiomas whose first symptoms began

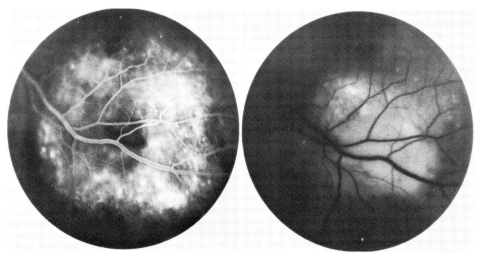

Fig. 4-6

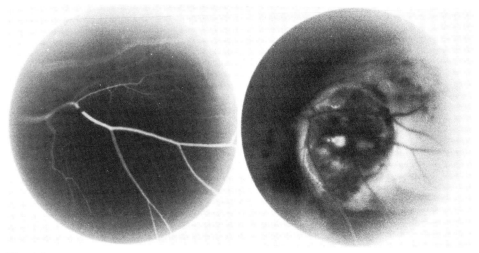

Fig. 4-7

in the latter half of the seventh decade. On the other hand, the condition may be seen in infants associated with features of the Sturge-Weber syndrome. In this situation it is usually diffuse rather than localized.

Ophthalmoscopically, the localized lesion is usually pink in color, of only moderate elevation, located within three to four disc diameters of the disc, more often temporal, with the overlying retina usually attached to its surface, and with a variable amount of surrounding subretinal fluid.

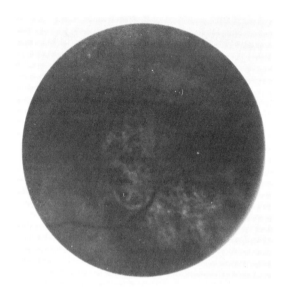

Fig. 4-8

Loss of choroidal pattern

The tumor itself is characterized by the loss of the normal choroidal pattern; there may be some disturbance of the pigment epithelium with migration into clumps, and its surface may be covered with variable areas of white fibrous proliferation. On biomicroscopic examination the overlying retina is seen to be degenerative with extensive cystoid changes, and the vascular nature of the tumor is apparent on indirect illumination.

In my experience, compression to demonstrate the vascular component has generally been unsatisfactory. Although the lesion is visible on transillumination, it does not give rise to the type of defect usually seen with melanomas and hematomas.

The diffuse choroidal hemangioma may be seen with or without an overlying retinal detachment and can best be recognized by comparing the choroidal pattern of the two eyes. In this type of lesion no recognizable normal choroidal vessels are seen, merely a diffuse pink reflex.

Fluorescein

Fluorescein angiography has been described elsewhere[2] but is characterized by the following features:

1. Early arterial fluorescence of the tumor, even before the retinal circulation (Fig. 4-8)
2. Irregular early filling that gives rise to a multilake-like pattern (Fig. 4-8)
3. Honeycomb type of staining of the retina presumably due to the secondary cystoid degeneration (Fig. 4-9)

As far as we know, none of the preceding signs are characteristic for hemangioma

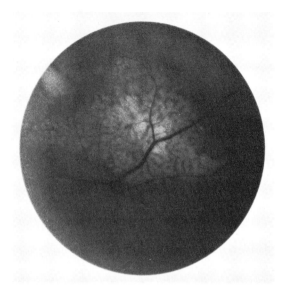

Fig. 4-9

of the choroid, but the combination of all three features with a localized nonpigmented lesion in the choroid is extremely suggestive.

Metastatic tumors

Metastatic tumors are among the most difficult lesions to recognize when the overlying retina is detached. I have often been concerned that I might miss such a lesion, particularly in an elderly aphakic patient in whom retinal breaks are difficult to find. Some of the features are listed below:

1. History
2. White, mottled, flat mass
3. Bronchogenic metastasis may be quite elevated
4. Posterior polar area
5. Multifocal, often bilateral
6. Overlying retinal detachment, often extensive with shifting fluid
7. Absence: hemorrhage, transillumination defect, breaks
8. Fluorescein

White, mottled, flat mass

Ophthalmoscopically, the lesions are relatively flat, grayish white to orange-white, usually located in the posterior polar area but often in the far periphery, multiple in location, and often bilateral. The pigment in the choroid is disturbed so that a checkerboard type of mottling may be seen. The overlying retina is not attached to the tumor and becomes detached early. In some cases the subretinal fluid is localized and opaque, giving a very white appearance to the lesion; in other cases it is clear and abundant so that when the patient is examined at the slit lamp the retina is in contact with the back surface of the lens. Shifting fluid may be a prominent feature.

There is usually no defect on transillumination and hemorrhage is a rare accompaniment.

Fluorescein

Fluorescein angiography gives very diverse patterns. In the early lesion confined to the choroid without overlying detachment, fluorescein will show little or no varia-

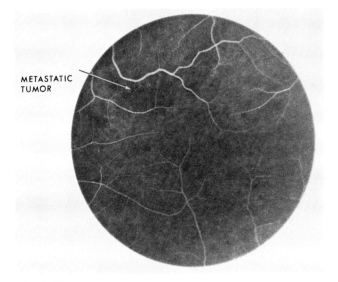

Fig. 4-10

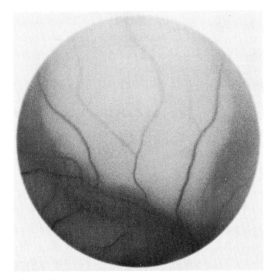

Fig. 4-11

tion from the normal (Fig. 4-10). Once the overlying retina becomes locally detached, fluorescein will pool in the subretinal fluid and there will be late staining (Fig. 4-11). In the later stages, with extensive retinal separation, there is often marked disturbance in the pigment epithelium so that one sees a prominent choroidal pattern, often mottled, during the arteriovenous phase (Fig. 4-12).

A small nonpigmented tumor of the choroid that fails to light up with fluorescein in the early phases and fails to stain in the late phases is strong evidence for a metastatic lesion.

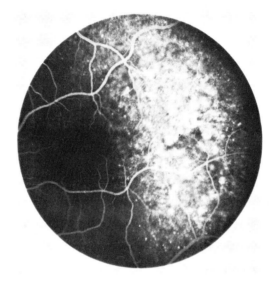

Fig. 4-12

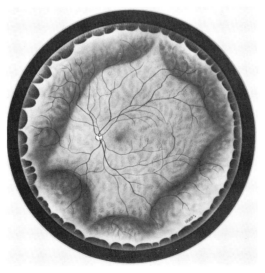

Fig. 4-13

Choroidal detachments

Choroidal detachments (Fig. 4-13) rarely should confuse the examiner if he considers the following features:
1. Usually postoperative or associated with inflammation or trauma
2. Eye usually soft
3. Typical pattern
4. Color varies with pigmentation and elevation
5. Demarcation lines
6. Transillumination

Retinal schisis
Senile retinal schisis

Retinal schisis of the senile type often presents a problem in differential diagnosis of idiopathic retinal separation. This fact is not surprising since it, too, represents a form of intraretinal separation and may be accompanied by a classical retinal separation. Its features are listed below and do not need elaboration:
1. Age, sex
2. Asymptomatic
3. Vitreous normal
4. Peripheral, 360°, more inferior temporally
5. Bilateral
6. Smooth transparent dome without folds
7. Flecks of white on or within inner surface of dome
8. White lines on vessels
9. Absence of demarcation lines
10. Breaks in inner and outer layers
11. Absolute field defect
12. Demonstration of outer layer with scleral depression, or photocoagulation
13. Slow progression unless detachment develops

Juvenile retinal schisis

The juvenile form is rare unless one is fortunate or unfortunate enough to encounter a large family reservoir. Its features are listed below:
1. Age at onset less than 20 years
2. Hereditary in male
3. Extensive Swiss cheese appearance to retina
4. Inferior retina most involved
5. Secondary macular changes
6. Diagnosis as in senile type

• • •

To discuss further the differential diagnosis of the lesions listed on pages 52 and 53 would require a textbook. The opththalmologist must approach each retinal problem with the full utilization of available diagnostic tools and, in fact, must strive to develop new ones if we are to understand the great variety of conditions manifested by the accumulation of fluid between the layers of the neuroepithelium of the ocular fundus.

REFERENCES

1. Havener, W. H.: Atlas of diagnostic techniques and treatment of retinal detachment, St. Louis, 1967, The C. V. Mosby Co.
2. Norton, E. W. D., and Gutman, F.: Fluorescein angiography and hemangiomas of the choroid, Arch. Ophthal. **78:**121, Aug. 1967.

5

Technique of vitreous cavity examination*

Walter D. Cockerham
Charles L. Schepens

GENERAL CONSIDERATIONS

Clinical examination of the vitreous cavity to establish vitreoretinal relationships is often neglected even by specialists of retinal detachment and retinal diseases. Many rely almost wholly on indirect ophthalmoscopy and few use slit lamp microscopy of the vitreous cavity to best advantage. The indirect ophthalmoscope with scleral depression has been thoroughly described by Schepens[1, 2] and is in wide use. Biomicroscopy performed routinely with the best instruments available, such as the Haag-Streit model-900 slit lamp (Fig. 5-1)[3] and the Goldmann 3-mirror contact lens (Fig. 5-2),[4] adds invaluable information to the data obtained by indirect ophthalmoscopy. Many changes in the retina can be explained by alterations in the vitreous that cannot be detected without biomicroscopic examination. Also, many alterations of the retina and vitreous that appear localized with ophthalmoscopy are actually quite extensive when studied by biomicroscopy. Subtle vitreoretinal relationships are best seen in optical sections produced by a slit lamp under conditions that give maximum contrast. The most comprehensive evaluation of a case is obtained only by correlating the findings of indirect ophthalmoscopy with those of biomicroscopy.

The Haag-Streit model-900 slit lamp allows great versatility by virtue of a rotating slit (Fig. 5-1, *K*) that can be oriented in any desired meridian, and an inclinable illumination column effecting upward inclination of the slit beam from 0 to 20 degrees in relation to the observation plane (Fig. 5-3). These two features allow otherwise impossible inspection of horizontal and oblique optical sections. In the model 900, the angle between the observation axes of the microscope objectives is 13 degrees. This angle was changed from 15 degrees in older models to improve binocular viewing through small pupils.

The Goldmann 3-mirror contact lens with mirrors inclined at 73, 67, and 59

*This work was supported by grant NB-05691 of the National Institute of Neurological Diseases and Blindness, U. S. Public Health Service.

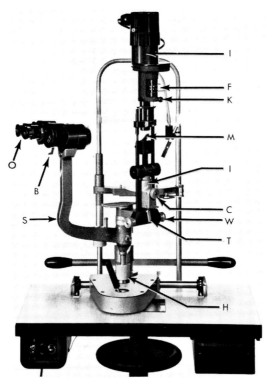

Fig. 5-1. Haag-Streit model-900 slit lamp. *K,* slit rotation knob; *I,* illumination column; *S,* microscope arm; *C,* center lock screw; *M,* slit lamp mirror; *T,* thumb latch; *H,* height adjustment screw; *W,* knob controlling slit width; *F,* controls for filters and slit length; *B,* objective selector; *O,* oculars.

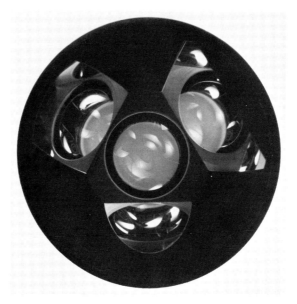

Fig. 5-2. Goldmann contact lens with a central portion and three mirrors with different inclinations.

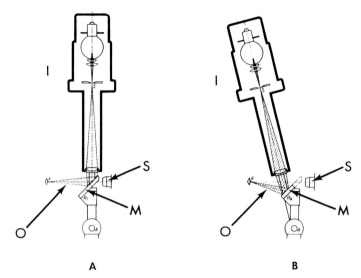

Fig. 5-3. Optics of Haag-Streit 900 slit lamp. **A,** When the illumination column *(I)* is vertical, the optical section *(O)* is horizontal after reflection by the slit lamp mirror *(M)*; **B,** when the illumination column *(I)* is inclined forward the optical section *(O)* is reflected upward by the slit lamp mirror *(M)*; *S,* microscope.

degrees allows a more extensive view of the ocular fundus than do other contact lenses or precorneal lenses. For instance, the commonly used Hruby lens is less effective because of its lower magnification, its more disturbing light reflections, difficulties encountered in keeping the lens centered at all times, and problems it causes in examining the extreme periphery.

This report describes our technique in detail. Much of these procedures can be profitably applied to equipment similar to the Haag-Streit model-900 slit lamp and the Goldmann 3-mirror contact lens.

PREPARATION OF THE OBSERVER

Biomicroscopy of the vitreous cavity is more productive if the observer first studies the case carefully with indirect ophthalmoscopy and scleral depression using a +18 or +20D condensing lens. Lesions near the posterior pole are profitably surveyed with a +14D condensing lens because of its higher magnification. A detailed fundus drawing is necessary for reference during slit lamp examination. Paper and colored pencils for sketching should be available for use during the slit lamp examination and while the contact lens is in the patient's eye. An elbow rest may be helpful for steadying the hand holding the contact lens in place at the proper height.

Darkness in the examination room should be as complete as possible, particularly for detecting barely visible structures. A small red light is useful to illuminate the fundus drawing and the sketching material on the slit lamp table. Dark adaptation with red goggles for 5 or 10 minutes seems to be helpful, especially if the observer enters the dark room from a brightly lit area.

PREPARATION OF THE PATIENT

Maximum dilation of the pupils is even more important for biomicroscopy of the vitreous cavity than for indirect ophthalmoscopy with scleral depression. Optimum height of the patient's chair and chin rest is essential for his comfort during prolonged examination. Children may be allowed to stand, and occasionally infants can be held sufficiently still by the parents or an assistant to permit this type of examination. The patient's forehead must remain in contact with the headrest to prevent difficulty in focusing. The patient should be informed of the length of the examination since some people become fatigued and restless.

Biomicroscopy of the vitreous cavity should not be performed after intravenous administration of fluorescein because the dye clouds the intraocular fluids, preventing adequate examination. This clouding effect may last several days. When edema of the corneal epithelium is present, sometimes it may be sufficiently cleared with glycerin to permit useful examination.

DESCRIPTION OF THE SLIT LAMP BIOMICROSCOPE AND CONTACT LENS
Slit lamp biomicroscope (Fig. 5-1)

The slit beam must be controlled so that it is always oriented in the position that provides the best view of the vitreous cavity and ocular fundus. The illumination-observation angle can be varied from 0 to 90 degrees by moving either the microscope arm (Fig. 5-1, *S*) or the illumination arm (Fig. 5-1, *I*). Once this angle is set, the illumination-observation angle can still be varied a little by loosening the center lock screw (Fig. 5-1, *C*) and rotating the illumination column (Fig. 5-1, *I*) and the mirror (Fig. 5-1, *M*) on its vertical axis. This second method is used for precise projection of the slit beam and for obviating bothersome light reflexes from the contact lens surfaces.

The slit beam may be inclined upward from 0 to 20 degrees by varying the angle of incidence of the light beam on the mirror (Fig. 5-3). This is done by releasing the thumb latch (Fig. 5-1, *T*) and tipping the illumination column forward. Two mirrors—short and long—are provided with the slit lamp. When the illumination column is vertical, part of its beam does not strike the short mirror and is lost. As the illumination column is inclined forward 6 to 8 degrees, all the light falls on the short mirror and hence effective illumination is increased. Since the greater portion of the examination is conducted with the illumination column inclined forward, this factor is relatively unimportant. Practically no light is lost at any time during use of the long mirror. A disadvantage of the long mirror is that it blocks the view through one of the microscope objectives when the illumination-observation angle is about 6 degrees. In practice either mirror serves quite well. The mirror should be cleaned before each examination since it becomes surprisingly dusty. Care must be exercised not to scratch its front surface silvering.

The slit rotation control (Fig. 5-1, *K*) orients the slit at any desired angle for 360 degrees. When control (*K*) is in its central position, the slit is vertical. The height adjustment screw (Fig. 5-1, *H*) serves to move the entire slit lamp either up or down. This screw can also be displaced horizontally to move the whole slit lamp as the joystick does. Using the screw in this dual fashion eliminates the need for the joystick.

The most frequently used controls of illumination-observation angle, slit beam inclination, mirror rotation, and slit beam width are easily manipulated from one convenient hand position (Fig. 5-4). The correct grip on this part of the slit lamp is important and is obtained by placing either the index finger or the middle finger on the horizontal part of the illumination arm and the thumb on the thumb latch. When the right hand is operating the slit lamp (the other hand holding the contact lens), the illumination arm must be passed at times from the right side of the microscope to the left side while the hand still maintains this grip. In this situation, the hand fits between the supporting arm of the microscope and the illumination column. Occasionally, it may be necessary to relinquish this grip and pass the right hand between the supporting arm of the microscope and the observer in order to retain control of the illumination arm when it is on the left side. When the left hand is controlling the slit lamp, the reverse positions are used.

The other two most frequently used controls are the slit rotation knob (Fig. 5-1, *K*) and the height adjustment screw (Fig. 5-1, *H*). All these controls require such frequent adjustments that the hand not holding the lens is rarely still.

The slit beam width control is generally adjusted (Fig. 5-1, *W*) to produce a fine slit giving just enough light for adequate viewing. Maximum slit length (Fig. 5-1, *F*) should be used since it is best for defining extensive, irregular surfaces. The voltage

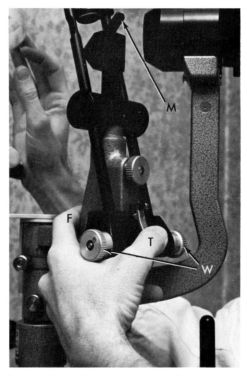

Fig. 5-4. Correct grip for control of illumination-observation angle, slit beam inclination, slit lamp mirror rotation, and slit beam width. *F,* finger on illumination arm; *T,* thumb on latch; *M,* slit lamp mirror; *W,* knob controlling slit width.

selector should be set at the maximum of 7.5 volts, even though bulbs burn out more frequently than at lower settings. The advantages are that luminosity at this setting is approximately twice that obtained with 6 volts and the view is better, especially with a narrow slit. The light filters (Fig. 5-1, *F*) are seldom used since they reduce illumination excessively.

For teaching, the observer must lean away from the microscope while holding the contact lens. This allows a second observer to obtain a binocular view and control the focus with the height adjustment screw. The method is adequate only for rapid demonstration of specific findings.

Two sets of oculars (Fig. 5-1, *O*) provide 10 and 16 magnifications. The 10× oculars are most useful and provide magnifications of 10× and 16× by selection of the proper permanently mounted objectives (1× and 1.6×) (Fig. 5-1, *B*). A magnification of 16× is best for general use. A magnification of 10× is useful for rapid scanning and orientation. The 16× oculars provide magnifications of 16× and 25× by the selection of the proper pair of permanently mounted objectives. The 25× magnification is useful only occasionally. Each eyepiece should be independently and carefully focused on the cornea or on the target provided with the instrument. The interpupillary distance should be adjusted for the observer. Slight readjustment of the interpupillary distance during examination will frequently improve the view.

Contact lens

The 3-mirror lens is a solid piece of plastic with mirror surfaces cut on three sides. Each mirror serves to view an area of the fundus that is located at the opposite

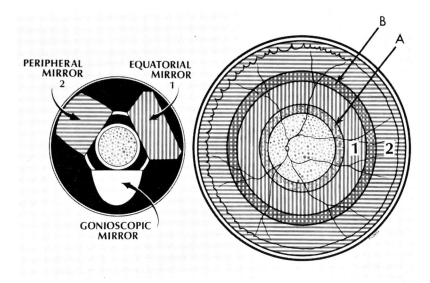

Fig. 5-5. Areas of ocular fundus viewed by 3-mirror lens. *Dots,* center of lens views from macula to 30 degrees; *1 (equatorial mirror),* views from 30 degrees to equator (vertical stripes); *2 (peripheral mirror),* views from equator to the far periphery (horizontal stripes); *A* and *B,* areas of overlapping view; remaining mirror is for gonioscopy.

end of the meridian in which the mirror is placed. There are two types of 3-mirror lenses—the old and the new. The new lens has longer mirrors than the old and is superior because it permits a wider field of view, which extends more peripherally and allows a binocular view more frequently.

The center of the lens (Fig. 5-5) provides a view of 30 degrees around the macula. The equatorial mirror (1) serves to see the area from 30 degrees to the equator. With the peripheral mirror (2) one views from the equator to the pars plana ciliaris. The areas seen with each mirror overlap considerably. The third mirror is used for gonioscopy and also serves occasionally to view the extreme fundus periphery.

The anterior surface of the contact lens is plane, and the posterior surface conforms to the patient's cornea. One percent methylcellulose is placed in the corneal portion; a higher concentration may cause epithelial clouding.

The lens must be clean before insertion. The best method is to clean it immediately after use. Methylcellulose is best removed with running water, and the lens is dried by blotting it with soft tissue paper. Finger marks require gentle washing with soap or detergent. The lens should never be wiped since it easily scratches to the extent that a clear view of the fundus cannot be obtained. When the lens is to be inserted in an eye that was recently operated on, it must be sterilized, and ethylene oxide gas is recommended for this purpose. Soaking in a sterilizing solution is more complicated since it requires rinsing in sterile water and blotting with sterile gauze or tissue paper.

EXAMINATION PROCEDURE

Slit lamp examination of the anterior segment and the anterior vitreous should be performed first without the contact lens. This method affords greater magnification, which is useful in assessing minute details in the anterior vitreous gel, such as condensation of fibers and membranes or particulate matter that may result from bleeding, inflammation, or degenerative processes.

Insertion of lens

After topical anesthesia with 0.5% proparacaine hydrochloride, the patient's chin is placed in the chin rest and the slit lamp and microscope are moved to one side. The lens is held in the right hand with its corneal portion up to prevent spilling the methylcellulose until the last moment. The left hand holds the lids apart with the thumb and index finger. Another method is to hold the upper lid with the left thumb and the lower lid with the ring finger of the right hand. Occasionally, it is useful to lift the upper lid by its cilia. After the patient has been instructed to look up, the lower edge of the lens is placed into the lower cul-de-sac. The lens is then rotated gently until its corneal portion is in contact with the globe, after which the patient is instructed to look straight ahead. In patients with deep-set globes or prominent eyebrows and in patients who tend to squeeze their lids, it may be preferable to direct their gaze straight ahead during insertion. After insertion, tissue paper is placed between the patient's cheek and the hand holding the lens to prevent dripping of methylcellulose and tears down the patient's face.

An air bubble under the lens may sometimes be expelled by slight pressure on

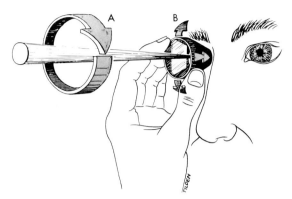

Fig. 5-6. Movements of 3-mirror lens. *A,* rotation of lens on its anteroposterior axis; *B,* displacement of lens on cornea.

the contact lens with tipping and rotation. If this is ineffectual, it may be necessary to repeat the entire insertion procedure. Patients who squeeze their eyelids, have chemotic conjunctivas, or have symblepharon tend to get bubbles under the lens. Such bubbles usually can be prevented by applying constant gentle pressure on the lens during examination.

When examining the patient's right eye, most observers hold the lens with their left hand throughout the examination (and vice versa for the left eye). Some observers switch grips on the lens from one hand to the other when the illumination arm of the slit lamp is changed from one side of the microscope to the other.

During the examination the lens is held and manipulated with the thumb, index finger, and middle finger (Fig. 5-6). For best control, the index finger should rest slightly on the front surface of the lens. A useful way to allow another observer to take hold of the lens is to place a fingernail against the front of the lens for support, a method that avoids smudging the front surface. With one hand the lens can be rotated 360 degrees around its anteroposterior axis (Fig. 5-6, *A*). It is most important to master this technique since the other hand is continuously manipulating the slit lamp. Pressing the lens too hard against the globe may cause folds in the cornea and a poor view. Surprising improvement in clarity of view often results from relaxation of one's grip on the lens, allowing it to maintain corneal contact by capillarity. A correctly performed examination causes minimal discomfort to the patient. A sterile lens usually can be inserted the first or second day after a retina operation if chemosis is not too marked.

Performing the examination

The central portion of the contact lens is used first to examine the vitreous cavity from the crystalline lens to the retina. One starts with a vertical slit, followed by horizontal and oblique slits with the optical section inclined upward. The anterior vitreous cavity is best viewed with a large observation-illumination angle, since it provides an excellent view against a dark background. As the focus is moved posteriorly, this angle must be reduced so that both axes can enter the pupil. As the focus approaches the attached retina, a view against a dark background becomes less

possible because the light scattered by the choroid produces a red glow. Clear definition of structures near the retina requires careful focusing and optimum orientation
of the slit beam. It is noteworthy that the illumination-observation angle can be
made too large to obtain the best view. Retroillumination may be helpful to detect
structures near the retina. The thickness of the retina itself can be clearly discerned
as a parallelepiped formed by the optical section. To appreciate this and to obtain
the best focus, the illumination-observation angle and the contact lens inclination
must be optimal, as determined by trial and error, and the slit must be narrow. This
also applies when using the contact lens mirrors.

A frequent error is to concentrate attention on either the vitreous or the retina
and neglect the other. Attention must be focused on both or significant details will
be missed.

The view through the center of the lens can be extended peripherally by directing
the patient's gaze in the appropriate direction. In this case, the cornea slides to a
slightly eccentric position in relation to the corneal portion of the lens. Excessive
deflection of gaze makes the view poor, both through the center of the lens and
through the mirrors.

A routine technique for detecting and tracing the extent and configuration of
surfaces, such as the posterior hyaloid face, preretinal membranes, proliferative
retinopathy of diabetes, and atrophic detached retina, is *sweeping* or *oscillation* of

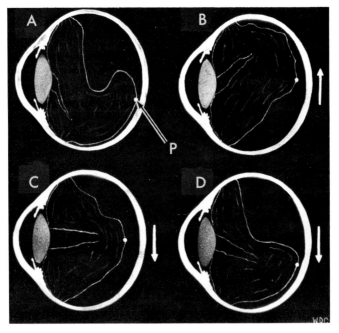

Fig. 5-7. Ascension phenomenon. **A,** Detached vitreous body in the resting state; **B,** vitreous
body displaced upward by eye movement; **C** and **D,** vitreous body settling downward. The
white dot, *P,* on posterior hyaloid face is an imaginary point to indicate how a structure in
that location would move during the ascension phenomenon. The white arrows show direction
of displacement of white dot.

the slit beam across such surfaces, which in effect shows successive cross sections. This may be accomplished as follows: (1) the illumination arm may be moved to and fro; (2) the slit lamp mirror may be rotated on its vertical axis; (3) the entire slit lamp may be raised and lowered for horizontal and oblique positions of the slit or moved laterally for vertical slits; (4) the slit rotation control can be moved; (5) the contact lens may be rotated on its anteroposterior axis, a motion which changes the angle of incidence of the slit beam on the mirrors of the contact lens; (6) the optical section may be left stationary and the structure in question may be moved by use of the *ascension phenomenon* (Fig. 5-7).[5] In this phenomenon, the vitreous body is moving while the globe is stationary. To elicit this effect, the patient is instructed to look rapidly up (right, left, or down) and back to the primary position of gaze. These saccadic movements disturb the configuration of the vitreous body. As the vitreous body settles back to its resting position, it "flows" past a horizontal or oblique optical section. This technique is frequently the only way a minimal detachment of the posterior hyaloid face can be seen. It is also useful in demonstrating discrete attachments of the vitreous body to the retina (Fig. 5-8), especially in the inferior quadrants and in the region of the macula and optic disc.

After completion of observations through the central portion of the contact lens, attention is directed to examination of the periphery through the mirrors. The equatorial mirror (1) is used first, followed by the peripheral (2) mirror. Each is employed to examine 360 degrees of peripheral fundus by rotating the contact lens on its anteroposterior axis. Upward inclination of the optical section obtained by forward inclination of the illumination column (Fig. 5-3) is employed at all times, except during examination near the 12 o'clock meridian, because the extent of the peripheral view at 12 o'clock is reduced by tilting the illumination column. In all other meridians, peripheral viewing is easier when the column is tilted. Thus, as soon as the point of observation is away from the 12 o'clock meridian, the illumination column must be inclined forward. The degree of inclination must be varied to keep it in optimum relation to the illumination-observation angle, the degree of slit rotation, and the orientation of the contact lens mirror. These optimum relationships

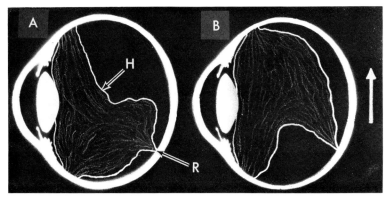

Fig. 5-8. A, Isolated vitreoretinal adhesion *(R)*; H, posterior hyaloid face; **B,** effect of adhesion on ascension phenomenon.

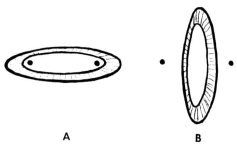

Fig. 5-9. A, Elliptic shape of patient's pupil when periphery is examined at 12 or 6 o'clock; **B,** same when periphery is examined at 9 or 3 o'clock; *dots,* images of observer's pupils.

are determined by trial and error. The slit inclination must be greatest during examination at or near the horizontal meridian. The slit beam must be kept parallel to the meridian examined, that is, parallel to the long axis of the mirror of the contact lens that is used.

To increase the peripheral range of view through one of the contact lens mirrors, the patient is instructed to look in the direction of the desired view, with the mirror of the contact lens moved in the opposite direction. For example, for a more peripheral view at 12 o'clock, the patient looks up and the contact lens is tilted down. The opposite movements provide an increase in the extent of a mirror's view toward the posterior pole. For example, for a more central view in the 12 o'clock meridian, the patient looks down and the contact lens is tilted up.

When one observes the peripheral fundus, the patient's pupil becomes elliptic. In the horizontal meridian, it is more difficult to obtain a binocular view because the observer's eyes are horizontally situated and his two lines of sight must enter the patient's pupil along the short axis of the elliptic pupil (Fig. 5-9, *B*). A binocular view at 12 or 6 o'clock is easier than at 9 or 3 o'clock because the observer's lines of sight enter the patient's pupil along the long axis of the elliptic pupil (Fig. 5-9, *A*).

The image seen in any mirror of the contact lens is inverted along the meridian being examined, but structures on either side of the meridian remain on the same side as in reality (Plate 1). During examination it is not necessary to mentally transpose mirror images as long as an accurate fundus drawing is available for orientation. The peripheral portion of the fundus is imaged in the portion of the mirror that is closest to the observer. If a structure appears in the middle of the mirror, it is located in the same meridian exactly 180 degrees away. If it is placed even slightly off center, its position corresponds to a large degree of displacement in the fundus and accurate localization is impossible.

In the majority of cases, the pars plana ciliaris cannot be seen adequately. Goldmann has devised a scleral depressor[6] that is part of the 3-mirror lens and helps to visualize the extreme periphery through the peripheral mirror (2) or sometimes through the gonioscopy mirror. It has been modified by Eisner (Fig. 5-10)[7] and is useful for studying the ora serrata, pars plana ciliaris, and vitreous base.

As the mirrors are rotated through 360 degrees, a *pattern* emerges for the optimum position of the slit lamp controls and contact lens mirrors. This pattern is the same for the right or left eye.

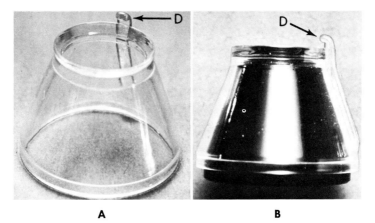

Fig. 5-10. A, Scleral depressor *(D)* supported by plastic cone; **B,** cone fitted on 3-mirror lens.

Superior and inferior views (12 and 6 o'clock). In the superior and inferior views (Figs. 5-11, *A* and *B*), the mirror must be below for 12 o'clock and above for 6 o'clock observation, and the illumination arm placed on either side of the microscope. The illumination column is inclined forward when viewing the 6 o'clock area and is vertical for 12 o'clock. The slit rotation knob is placed in its center position, creating a vertical slit.

Horizontal views (3 and 9 o'clock). In the horizontal views (Fig. 5-11, *C* and *D*), the contact lens mirror must be placed to the observer's left for 3 o'clock and to his right for 9 o'clock observation. The forwardly tilted illumination column is placed in line with the microscope (illumination-observation angle of 0 degrees). The optical section is made horizontal by turning the slit rotation knob fully either to the right or to the left.

Oblique views (1:30 and 7:30, 10:30 and 4:30). In oblique views (Fig. 5-11, *E* to *H*), the mirror of the contact lens must be at the opposite end of the meridian being examined and the slit beam must be parallel to that meridian. The illumination column must be tilted forward and located in such a position that the optimum view is obtained. This position is determined by trial and error. The slit rotation knob must be turned to the correct side. For these purposes, the slit lamp arm with the illumination column should be to the right of the microscope in viewing up and to the observer's right (Fig. 5-11, *E*) (up and nasal for OD, up and temporal for OS) or in viewing down and to the observer's left (Fig. 5-11, *F*) (down and temporal for OD, down and nasal for OS). In both cases, the slit rotation knob must be turned to the right. Conversely, the illumination column should be to the left of the microscope in viewing up and to the observer's left (Fig. 5-11, *G*) (up and temporal for OD, up and nasal for OS) or in viewing down and to the observer's right (Fig. 5-11, *H*) (down and nasal for OD, down and temporal for OS). In these cases, the slit rotation knob must be turned to the left.

At least 30 minutes should be spent in the average examination; complex cases require more time. In simple cases, experienced observers may obtain essential information in about 10 minutes. It must be emphasized that each detail of the examina-

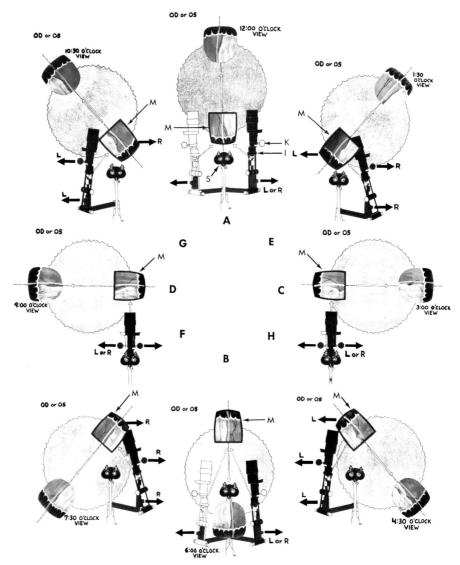

Fig. 5-11. A, 12 o'clock view. *M,* mirror; *I,* illumination column; *S,* microscope; *K,* slit rotation knob. **B,** 6 o'clock view. **C,** 3 o'clock view. **D,** 9 o'clock view. **E,** 1:30 view. **F,** 7:30 view. **G,** 10:30 view. **H,** 4:30 view.

tion procedure is important and can affect the quality of results. During the examination, almost continuous adjustment is required of the illumination-observation angle, degree of upward inclination of the optical section, slit rotation, slit lamp mirror rotation, and focus and height of the entire slit lamp. Only in this way can the slit beam and the attitude of the contact lens complement each other for optimal view of the vitreous cavity. It is difficult for the beginner to master these maneuvers, but they become second nature after months of practice.

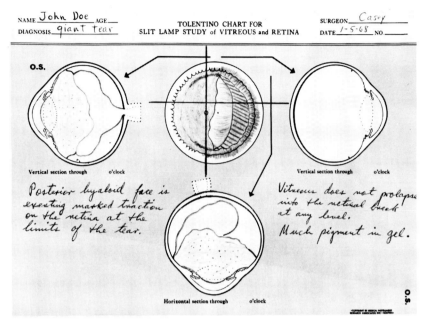

NAME *John Doe* AGE___
DIAGNOSIS *giant tear*

TOLENTINO CHART FOR
SLIT LAMP STUDY of VITREOUS and RETINA

SURGEON *Casey*
DATE *1-5-68* NO___

O.S.

Vertical section through _____ o'clock   Vertical section through _____ o'clock

Posterior hyaloid face is exerting marked traction on the retina at the limits of the tear.

Vitreous does not prolapse into the retinal break at any level. Much pigment in gel.

Horizontal section through _____ o'clock

O.S.

Fig. 5-12. Chart for recording findings.

RECORDING OF FINDINGS

Findings are usually committed to memory until the examination is finished, when they can be recorded on a Tolentino chart (Fig. 5-12). However, some sketching during examination may be helpful. A small fundus drawing and cross sections of the globe at appropriate orientation are drawn. The cross sections are indicated by straight lines across the small fundus drawing. Sketches of cross sections should show findings such as attached and detached retina; attached and detached vitreous; presence of membranes, bands, and blood in the vitreous cavity; and location of scleral implants, buckles, or tumors.

Large-scale drawings and cross sections of the macular area can be added as necessary. The color code is that used for the fundus drawing, the vitreous body and opacities of the media being drawn in green. Written comments recording information that cannot be drawn adequately are important. For instance, characteristics of the vitreous gel, vitreous membranes and bands, hemorrhages, and exudates can be better described in writing than graphically.

SOME OF THE CHANGES OBSERVED

The following is a description of vitreoretinal relationships that are best appreciated by biomicroscopy.

Normal vitreous. Vitreous gel in optical section is visible by the Tyndall effect, which renders it grayish blue and opalescent (Plate 2). In the young it is quite homogeneous and in some cases difficult to see (Plate 6). In most instances, the gel contains thin curtains or sheets that appear to be composed of bundles of fibers.

In phakic eyes, the anterior hyaloid face is generally invisible in the lenticular area, and the vitreous gel appears optically continuous with the posterior lens capsule. The anterior and posterior plicate membranes of Cloquet's canal may be seen, especially in the young, inserting onto the posterior surface of the lens where it forms the hyaloideocapsular ligament of Wieger. In the funnel, formed by these plicate membranes, is the primary vitreous, including such hyaloid artery remnants as Mittendorf's dot and Vogt's arc line. The plicate membranes are more easily seen during the ascension phenomenon and at times can be seen defining Cloquet's canal quite far posteriorly.

Syneresis. Syneresis, or liquefaction of the vitreous gel, is characterized by areas of decreased or absent Tyndall effect (Plate 3) in which thin curtains or sheets tend to aggregate in membranes or fiber bundles of increased opacity. High myopes may show an optically empty vitreous cavity, except for crisscrossing and rather thick trabeculae. The syneresis seen over some areas of lattice degeneration of the retina (Plate 4) corresponds to the cavitation described in histologic sections.

Vitreous detachment. The diagnosis of vitreous detachment is made by demonstrating a typical posterior hyaloid face with the slit beam (Plates 5 and 6). The optical section creates a characteristic stripe on the hyaloid face, in front of which is the Tyndall effect of the vitreous gel (Plates 5 and 6) and in back of which is an optically empty space containing fluid vitreous (Plates 5 and 6). In simple vitreous detachment (Plate 6), the stripe is a spherically curved marking because of the shape of the vitreous body. In detachment with collapse of the gel, the stripe is a sinuous ribbonlike marking because of the irregular manner in which vitreous collapses.

In both cases the hyaloid face is mobile unless thickened by pathologic organization. Blood, inflammatory cells, and flare may be visible in the usually optically empty space between the vitreous body and the retina. This condition must not be interpreted as representing the presence of vitreous gel behind the detached hyaloid. Blood or inflammatory deposits on the posterior hyaloid face may aid in identifying it.

At times gravity causes blood or exudates to collect in the sulcus between vitreous and retina, formed by the line of vitreoretinal adhesion, in the inferior part of the fundus. An irregular ring-shaped opacity that represents the former attachment of the vitreous to the optic disc usually is visible on the detached posterior hyaloid face (Plate 6). A less frequently seen but finer and more regular ringlike opacity on the hyaloid face corresponds to its former attachment to the macula. The closer the posterior hyaloid face is to the retina, the more difficult it is to detect. Detached vitreous is usually best detected superiorly because it collapses downward and anteriorly, moving the hyaloid face away from the retina. Minimal detachment of the vitreous at the posterior pole is best detected by a horizontal optical section. At times it is only by using the horizontal slit in combination with the ascension phenomenon that a detachment at the posterior pole can be demonstrated.

In the periphery, especially near the vitreous base, a condensation of fibers parallel and close to the retina may be seen (Plate 2).[8] It can be so definite as to be confused with the posterior hyaloid face of detached vitreous. This "pseudohyaloid face," however, is not so uniform as the true hyaloid face, and careful observation will reveal vitreous gel between it and the retina. It will also show branchings and

Text continued on p. 87.

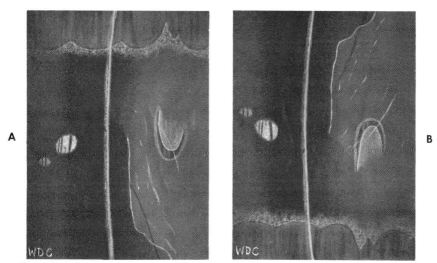

Plate 1. A, Real fundus at 12 o'clock; **B,** image seen in mirror is inverted with right side still right and left side still left.

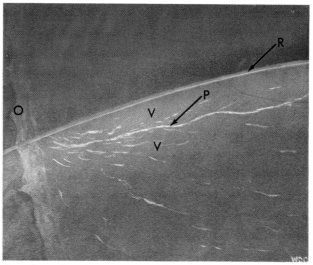

Plate 2. Optical section of undetached vitreous at 2 o'clock showing a pseudohyaloid face *(P); V,* vitreous gel; *R,* slit beam on retina; *O,* ora serrata.

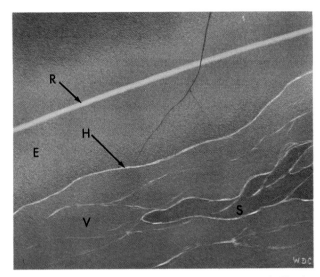

Plate 3. Area of syneresis or liquefaction *(S)* within the vitreous gel; *V,* vitreous gel; *H,* posterior hyaloid face; *E,* optically empty space; *R,* slit beam on retina.

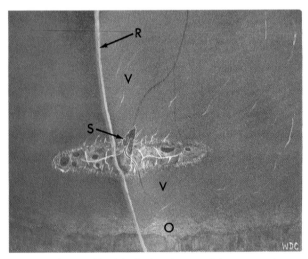

Plate 4. Lattice degeneration at 12 o'clock showing overlying syneresis or cavitation *(S); V,* vitreous gel; *R,* slit beam on retina; *O,* ora serrata.

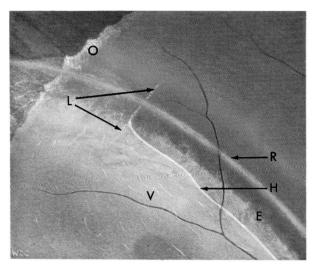

Plate 5. Posterior vitreous detachment at 4:30; *V*, vitreous gel; *H*, posterior hyaloid face; *E*, optically empty space filled with fluid vitreous; *R*, slit beam on retina; *O*, ora serrata; *L*, slight ridge along the posterior vitreous base.

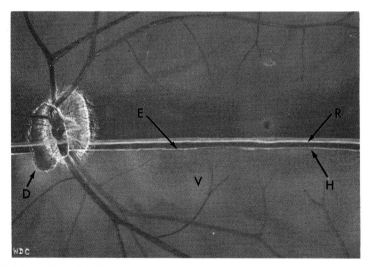

Plate 6. Minimal (simple) detachment of vitreous in the posterior pole of a young person; *V*, vitreous gel; *H*, posterior hyaloid face; *E*, optically empty space; *R*, slit beam on retina; *D*, ring opacity on posterior hyaloid face corresponding to normal attachment to the optic disc

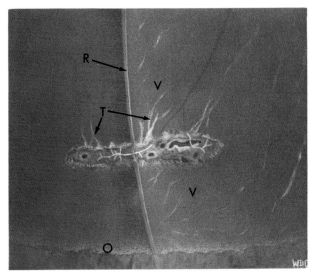

Plate 7. Lattice degeneration at 12 o'clock with strands *(T)* in the vitreous gel *(V)* exerting traction on the edges of the lesion; *R*, slit beam on retina; *O*, ora serrata. Several retinal breaks are present within the area of lattice degeneration; vitreous is not detached.

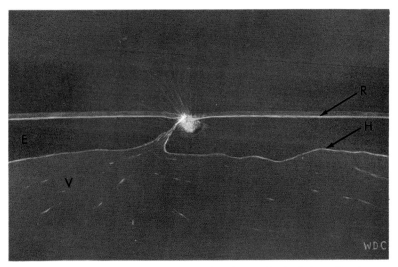

Plate 8. Vitreous attachment to the macula with a hemorrhagic lesion; *V*, vitreous; *H*, posterior hyaloid face; *E*, optically empty space; *R*, slit beam on the retina .

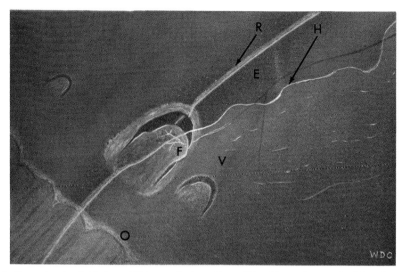

Plate 9. Posterior hyaloid face *(H)* attached to flap *(F)* of horseshoe retinal break at 1:30; *V*, vitreous gel; *E*, optically empty space; *R*, slit beam on the retina; *O*, ora serrata. Large break surrounded by subclinical retinal detachment outlined with a pigmented demarcation line; two smaller horseshoe retinal breaks are also seen.

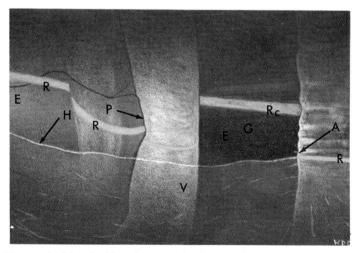

Plate 10. Giant retinal break *(G)* with posterior hyaloid face *(H)* attached to anterior edge of giant break *(A)*; *P*, posterior rolled edge of giant break; *V*, vitreous gel; *E*, optically empty space; *R*, slit beam on the retina; *Rc*, slit beam on the bare choroid.

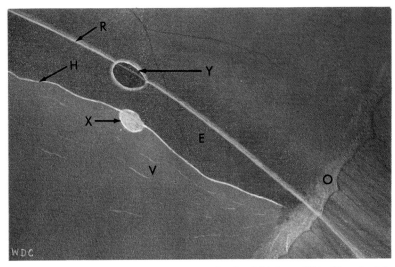

Plate 11. Free operculum *(X)* attached to posterior hyaloid face *(H)*; *Y*, retinal break; *V*, vitreous gel; *E*, optically empty space; *R*, slit beam on the retina; *O*, ora serrata.

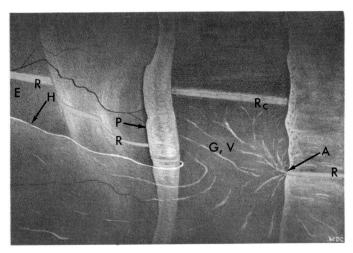

Plate 12. Giant retinal break *(G)* with vitreous gel *(V)* prolapsing into the break and under the retina; posterior hyaloid face (not visible) attached to anterior edge of break at *A*; *P*, posterior edge of break; *H*, posterior hyaloid face; *E*, optically empty space; *R*, slit beam on the retina; *Rc,* slit beam on the bare choroid.

anastomoses with lesser fibers, which are not typical of the posterior hyaloid face. A similar but less pronounced condensation is seen occasionally very near the retina at the posterior pole.

Early proliferation of new vessels and connective tissue in such conditions as diabetes mellitus may be present on the inner surface of the retina with no vitreous detachment present. Later the vitreous may be slightly detached, with new tissue growing on the posterior hyaloid face. Still later, a thick new-formed membrane on the posterior hyaloid face may exert enough traction to cause nonrhegmatogenous and even rhegmatogenous retinal detachment.

Occasionally an artifactitious ghost image of the slit beam will appear near the retina, simulating a very slightly detached posterior hyaloid face or other surface. Its homogeneous quality and disappearance when the angle of the beam is changed characteristically distinguish it from a true interface.

Adhesions between the retina and vitreous may be seen with biomicroscopy. Traction exerted by a vitreoretinal adhesion may be estimated by its size, density, and degree of tautness. The attachment of the posterior hyaloid face to the retina along the posterior border of the vitreous base may cause a slight but visible fold in the retina running in an equatorial direction and located between the ora serrata and the equator (Plate 5). At times this ridge can manifest the gliosis and pigment epithelium hypertrophy of *Ringschwiele* ("ring callus").

Retina and pigment epithelium. When one focuses on the retina, the parallelepiped formed by the optical section is useful in detecting certain clinical manifestations such as thickness, elevation, cyst formation, and location of deposits. Slight elevation of the retinal pigment epithelium is best seen with the slit lamp.

In lattice degeneration, visible strands of vitreous are often seen exerting traction on the margins of the area (Plate 7). The affected margins show irregular thickening, opacification, and slight elevation.

Attachments of the posterior hyaloid face to the macula (Plate 8) may play a role in the pathogenesis of certain lesions such as macular edema after cataract extraction, central serous retinopathy, and disciform degeneration. Macular attachments are best seen with a horizontal slit beam during the ascension phenomenon. Spontaneous macular pucker or that following intraocular surgery or retina surgery may be associated with a fine layer of preretinal new tissue.

Early preretinal organization is manifested by thickening and by increased visibility and decreased mobility of the posterior hyaloid face. Occasionally a barely visible grayish white film is seen on the retinal surface, and it may bridge retinal folds.

Massive preretinal retraction. In the condition of massive preretinal retraction, the retina is fixed and moves only with a slight tremor. Slit lamp microscopy invariably shows the preretinal organization to be much more extensive than it appears with indirect ophthalmoscopy. Extensive new-formed tissue may be visible on the retinal surface especially in front of the optic disc, gathering the retina into multiple high fixed folds. The vitreous gel is markedly retracted anteriorly and its posterior limit is thickened into an immobile equatorial membrane that bridges either portions of or the whole vitreous cavity. Dense bands of tissue may be visible in this new membrane or at times within the gel. The membrane pulls the retina into a high equatorial fixed fold. Cases of giant retinal break associated with massive preretinal retraction may show the posterior edge of the break fixed by the preretinal membrane.

Retinal breaks. The posterior hyaloid face invariably is attached to the flaps of horseshoe retinal tears (Plate 9) and to the anterior edge of giant retinal breaks (Plate 10). Free opercula from retinal holes (Plate 11) are always attached to the posterior hyaloid face, signifying cessation of vitreous traction at that site in the retina. Occasionally retinal breaks, not visible with indirect ophthalmoscopy, may be found by tracing along the attachment of the posterior hyaloid face to the retina.

Biomicroscopy is particularly useful under the following circumstances: (1) to detect retinal breaks on scleral buckles when the use of scleral depression is impossible; (2) to study an eye too tender after surgery for scleral depression; (3) to examine a suspected retinal break that is too posterior or too elevated for effective scleral depression; (4) to find retinal breaks when the choroidal background is atrophic, thus providing poor contrast; (5) to study very small breaks, as in the inner layer of a retinoschisis; and (6) to observe macular changes more accurately.

Aid in planning surgery

Biomicroscopy provides an estimate of the amount of fluid vitreous present that may pass through a retinal break at the stage of drainage of subretinal fluid. Continuing transfer of fluid vitreous from the vitreous cavity to the subretinal space via a retinal break can prevent adequate settling of the retina. Conversely, biomicroscopy also provides an estimate of the volume and configuration of the formed vitreous gel. Appropriate head positioning during surgery may place the vitreous gel so that it tamponades a retinal break, especially an inferior dialysis, and prevents such undesirable passage of fluid vitreous through the break.

The configuration of the vitreous body may determine whether it will prolapse into a giant retinal break (Plate 12), trapping the posterior edge of the tear in vitreous gel and preventing settling of the retina. Eyes with greatly shrunken vitreous gel have an excess of fluid vitreous in which the posterior edge of a giant break can float freely and invert (Plate 10). Biomicroscopy is mandatory for planning the most rational exercise, positioning, and type of surgery in cases of giant retinal break.[9]

Vitreoretinal relationships must be studied by biomicroscopy prior to vitreous surgery, such as cutting of vitreous membranes and bands,[10] injection of silicone oil, cryoprobe manipulation of the retina,[10] and forceps extraction of nonmagnetic foreign bodies.

REFERENCES

1. Schepens, C. L.: Un nouvel ophtalmoscope binoculaire pour l'examen du décollement de la rétine, Bull. Soc. Belg. Ophtal. 82:9, 1945.
2. Schepens, C. L.: Examination of the ora serrata region: its clinical significance, Acta XVI Concilium Ophthalmologicum (Britannia) 2:1384, 1950.
3. Schmidt, T.: Zur Theorie und Praxis der Spaltlampe, Acta XVIII Concilium Ophthalmologicum 2:1818, 1958.
4. Goldmann, H.: Einige Ergebnisse der Spaltlampenuntersuchungen des Kammerwinkels und des Augenhintergrundes, Ophthalmologica 117:253, 1949.
5. Rosen, E.: The ascension phenomenon of the anterior vitreous. Amer. J. Ophthal. 53:55, 1962.

6. Goldmann, H., and Schmidt, T.: Ein Kontaktglas zur Biomikroskopie der Ora Serrata und der Pars Plana, Ophthalmologica **149:**481, 1965.
7. Eisner, G.: Attachment for Goldmann three-mirror contact glass, Amer. J. Ophthal. **64:** 467, 1967.
8. Hruby, K.: Slit lamp examination of vitreous and retina, Baltimore, 1967, The Williams & Wilkins Co.
9. Schepens, C. L., Dobbie, J. G., and McMeel, J. W.: Retinal detachment with giant breaks; preliminary report, Trans. Amer. Acad. Ophthal. Otolaryng. **66:**471, 1962.
10. Freeman, H. M., and Schepens, C. L.: Vitreous surgery, Trans. Amer. Acad. Ophthal. Otolaryng. **72:**399, 1968.

6

Trophic degenerations of the peripheral retina

Robert Y. Foos
Louis M. Spencer
Bradley R. Straatsma

In evaluating the peripheral retina, one should supplement familiarity with normal topography and structure with information concerning the common developmental variations and degenerations of this region. Usually these lesions pose no threat to useful vision; however, the understanding of their morphologic features and pathogenesis will be helpful in separating them from the lesser number of harmful or potentially harmful conditions that must be recognized in this area. Many of the lesions to be discussed are causally related to the intimate association of the peripheral retina and the base of the vitreous body. Minor developmental variations of these structures cause functional derangements, which both predispose and exaggerate degenerative processes. Also, the vulnerability of the peripheral retina to degenerative change is undoubtedly related to its inherently marginal blood supply, which may be further compromised by senescence.

For clarity of communication, the descriptive terms to be used in these discussions will be defined. The term *developmental variation* encompasses minor degrees of topographic or structural deviations related to ocular development. *Degeneration* refers to an irreversible retrograde process. The degeneration is considered *trophic* when manifest as tissue loss related to local nutritional factors and *tractional* when the primary degenerative process is related to tugging or pulling from the vitreous body or zonule. The peripheral retina is considered as that portion of the sensory retina anterior to the equator, and this region will be divided into two equal circumferential zones: anterior and posterior. Subject to some biologic variation, the anterior zone corresponds to the retinal portion of the vitreous base. Recognizing the fallacy of implied cause in some categories where too little information is presently available, these discussions will include an orderly review of the major degenerative conditions that are categorized as trophic, tractional, or combined trophic and tractional.

In this discussion of trophic degenerations, the following various lesions are categorized according to their predilection for the inner, middle, or outer retinal layers:

Trophic degenerations of the peripheral retina
  I. Inner layers
     A. Excavations
        1. Vitreous base
        2. Other
     B. Holes
 II. Middle layers
     A. Cystoid degeneration
     B. Senile retinoschisis
III. Outer layers
     A. Paving-stone degeneration
     B. Senile peripheral tapetochoroidal degeneration

TROPHIC LESIONS OF INNER RETINA

The trophic lesions with a predilection for the inner retinal layers can be further categorized according to their appearance as excavations or complete retinal holes.

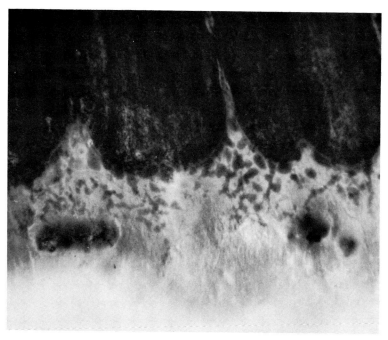

Fig. 6-1. Vitreous base excavations with sharply heaped margins and fine pigment dispersion in base of larger ovoid lesion *(left of center)*. Minimal cystoid degeneration, originating from base of dentate processes is also noted (×30).

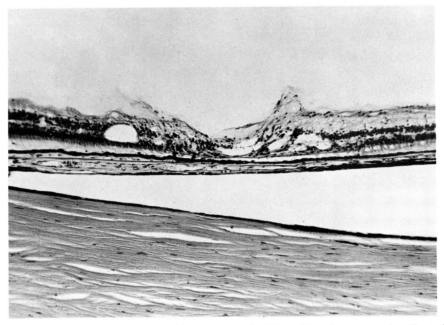

Fig. 6-2. Vitreous base excavation with traction and glial proliferation at margins. Centrally the retina is degenerated and exhibits microcystoid change; the pigment epithelium is reactive (H and E, ×125).

As will be discussed later, this distinction appears warranted since the two types of lesions appear to have different causes and rates of progression.

Vitreous base excavation is a trophic excavation of the inner retinal layers and is manifest as a solitary or, occasionally, multiple erosion, typically ovoid circumferentially and within the anterior zone (Fig. 6-1). Vascular change within the lesion is not conspicuous. The margins of this lesion are sharply heaped and pigment dispersion within its base is common. Occasionally the lesion is rounded or irregular in shape—a feature generally associated with multiple excavations. Rarely, a lesion may be exaggerated in length radially and may extend through 90 degrees of the oral circumference.

Histologically, these excavations within the vitreous base show varying degrees of tissue loss, predominantly of the inner layers (Fig. 6-2). Some lesions, however, may show extreme degrees of retinal thinning, and, in these instances or sometimes with lesser degrees of thinning, selective loss of the outer portions of the receptor cells is evident. Exaggerated attachments of vitreous fibers are evident at the elevated margins, and often the underlying pigment epithelium is in disarray, with accompanying dispersion within the lesion. The vessels within or about these excavations have no exaggerated pathologic features.

Studied in a series of 169 adult autopsy patients,[1] excluding five cases with concomitant lattice degeneration (see below), vitreous base excavations were present in 5% of the patients, were bilateral in none, and were found in 3% of the 312 eyes

Table 6-1. Degenerations of the peripheral retina

	Patients with lesions	Percent patients with lesions	Bilateral lesions	Percent bilateral lesions	Eyes with lesions	Percent eyes with lesions
Vitreous base excavation	8/169	5	0/8	0	8/312	3
Retinal hole	10/169	6	1/10	10	11/312	4
Cystoid degeneration	435/500*	87	435/435	100	870/1000	87
Senile retinoschisis	16/430	4	6/16	38	22/845	3
Paving-stone degeneration	134/614	22	51/134	38	185/1223	17
Peripheral tapetochoroidal degeneration	33/165	20	33/33	100	66/330	20
Noncystic retinal tuft	122/169	72	61/122	50	183/312	59
Cystic retinal tuft	100/169	59	39/100	39	139/312	45
Zonular traction tuft	27/169	16	3/27	11	30/312	10
Meridional fold	31/115†	26	15/31	48	46/230	20
Partial-thickness retinal tear:						
Paravascular	14/184‡	8	6/14	44	20/324	6
Posterior border of vitreous base	20/169	12	1/20	5	21/312	7
Full-thickness retinal tear	21/169	12	1/21	5	22/312	7
Lattice degeneration	12/202	6	6/12	50	18/404	4

*Over 8 years of age.
†Over 1 year of age.
‡Over 40 years of age.

examined (Table 6-1). There was no demonstrable meridional predilection. The lesions were all found within the anterior zone of the peripheral retina.

It was concluded from this study that the vitreous base excavation is probably a variant of lattice degeneration, modified by the special environment of the retinal portion of the vitreous base. Although no complicating holes were encountered in the above series, other experience in this laboratory indicates holes and localized retinal detachment do occur rarely as sequelae to vitreous base excavations (Foos, unpublished data).

Other trophic excavations of the peripheral retina have less distinctive gross features and are less easily categorized. As a rule, these excavations are found in the anterior zone of diffusely thinned retinas, and they may be focal or larger in size but without specific shape or without relationship to vessels (Fig. 6-3).

Microscopically, they present degenerative loss of the inner retinal layers and are of variable depth. Necrosis or proliferative features are lacking, and senescent vascular change is not noticeably exaggerated.

Statistical information on these lesions is lacking. Some of these nonspecific localized excavations may be antecedent to retinal holes, but apparently, with this exception, they are innocuous.

The *retinal hole,* a more advanced trophic lesion, is manifest grossly as a rounded complete retinal break without detectable flap or operculum (Fig. 6-4). These holes are found most commonly in the anterior zone, usually in an area of relatively normal retina rather than in an area involved with cystoid degeneration. The sloping margins of these holes usually show microcystic degeneration, but exaggerated

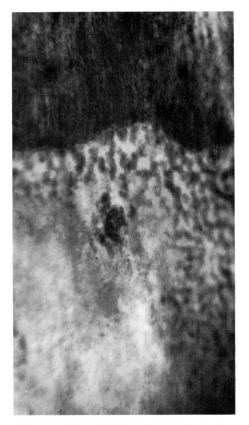

Fig. 6-3. Nonspecific trophic excavation with irregular nonelevated margins, behind and beside regions of cystoid degeneration (×30).

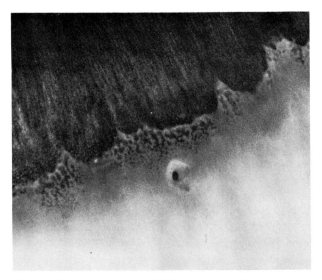

Fig. 6-4. Retinal hole behind focus of cystoid degeneration. Smooth margins slope sharply and exhibit microcystic change (×15).

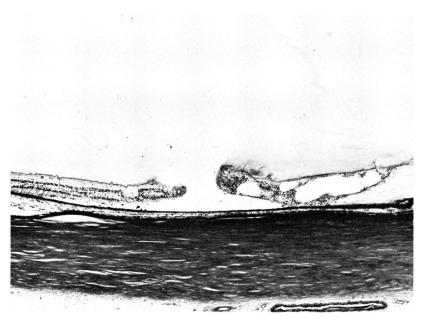

Fig. 6-5. Retinal hole showing complete loss of retinal tissue centrally, smooth margins, microcystic change with relatively wide loss of receptor cells, and reactive pigment epithelium (PAS, ×100).

vitreous attachments and proliferative reactions are distinctly absent. The underlying pigment epithelium ordinarily shows only minimal stippling.

Microsections of retinal holes demonstrate complete retinal discontinuity, with localized degeneration of all retinal elements but with minimal reactive gliosis and no inflammation (Fig. 6-5). In profile, the margins are generally smooth and rounded, and the pigment epithelium is mildly to moderately reactive.

In a series of 169 adult autopsy patients studied,[1] retinal holes were found in 6%, were bilateral in one case, and were present in 4% of the 312 eyes examined (Table 6-1). The holes were multiple in four eyes. They were slightly more prevalent in the lower and nasal quadrants, and 70% were in the anterior zone of the peripheral retina.

None of the retinal holes in this series was accompanied by significant localized retinal detachment, indicating that this lesion is a benign trophic process. From clinical and other laboratory experience, however, it becomes apparent that complete retinal breaks of this type, especially when they are posterior to the vitreous base, may occasionally be complicated by localized or even more extensive retinal detachment.

TROPHIC LESIONS OF THE MIDDLE RETINA

Cystoid degeneration, one of the trophic lesions of the middle retinal layers, is the most common peripheral retinal degeneration. It is characterized by intraretinal tissue loss and by formation of tiny blebs that coalesce as intercommunicating tunnels (Fig. 6-1). The process commences at the ora serrata, typically at the base of dentate processes, and extends by contiguity, posteriorly and circumferentially, on both the nasal and temporal sides (Fig. 6-6). Individual gross units may coalesce to form an extensive band of degeneration, partially or completely encircling the globe. The inner walls of advanced lesions may rupture, producing localized irregular excavations.

In routine microsections, cystoid degeneration typically involves the outer plexiform or inner nuclear layers and appears as rounded spaces (Fig. 6-7). Advanced lesions show virtually complete loss of parenchymal tissue between the radial supporting cells of Müller, although a recent study has demonstrated surprisingly long survival and even hypertrophy of the outer neuronal elements.[2]

In a series of 500 patients studied, peripheral cystoid degeneration was found in all patients over 8 years of age and even in a 10-month-old child.[3] With age, there was a linear increase in severity and usually a bilateral mirror symmetry. The superior and temporal quadrants were most extensively involved in adults. No relationship to eye size, chorioretinal lesions, or vitreal degeneration was found. The conclusion was that peripheral cystoid degeneration is innocuous.

Another trophic lesion affecting the middle layers is senile *retinoschisis*, characterized by splitting of the peripheral retina. In the laboratory specimen, the involved retinal area is rounded, is greater than 4 mm. in diameter, and occurs with varying degrees of ruptured radial supporting columns (Fig. 6-8). In the more advanced

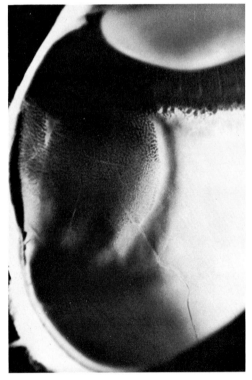

Fig. 6-6. Large circumscribed inferotemporal focus of cystoid degeneration showing typical preservation of supporting columns (×7).

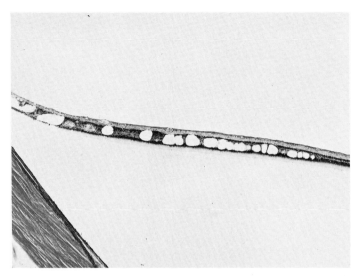

Fig. 6-7. Cystoid degeneration in microsection showing preservation of radial supporting columns despite coalescence of microcysts centrally and near ora serrata *(left)* (H and E, ×35).

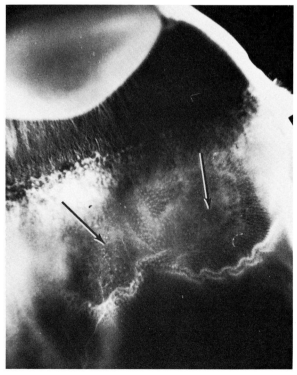

Fig. 6-8. Inferotemporal senile retinoschisis showing regions of ruptured radial supporting columns *(arrows)* and vessels within inner wall of posterior aspect of cavity on left (×10).

lesions, the degeneration may be found initially by the pocked appearance of the outer wall, which is related to partial or complete holes in this region. When examined with the stereomicroscope using oblique illumination, complete breaks in the membranous inner wall are rarely found. Breaks may rarely occur, however, in both the inner and outer walls of the cyst, and, in such instances, retinal detachment may ensue. Specimens with this lesion may have extensive cystoid degeneration or, conversely, there may be minimal cystoid degeneration in regions adjacent or remote to the retinoschisis.

Microscopically, there are exaggerated intraretinal cystoid cavities with only remnants of the radial supporting structures in evidence (Fig. 6-9). The thin inner wall usually contains the larger blood vessels. There is often surprising preservation of the outermost retinal layers. At the margins of the trophic lesion, cavitation of the outer plexiform layer is found, indistinguishable from common cystoid degeneration.

Studied in a series of 430 autopsy patients, 40 years of age or older (Foos, unpublished data), senile retinoschisis was found in 4%; it was bilateral in 38% of affected cases and was present in 3% of the 845 eyes examined. The lesions showed a definite predilection for the lower temporal quadrant; all other lesions were present in the upper temporal quadrant. Only five of the 25 eyes with retinoschisis had breaks of the outer wall of the lesion, and none had breaks of the inner wall; none had retinal detachment. Extension greater than 3 mm. behind the equator was not found.

There is substantial agreement of these data with those of Byer, who studied a series of 667 clinical patients 40 years old or older and found senile retinoschisis in 7%.[4] There was bilateral involvement in 82% of affected patients, and the mirror symmetry of this lesion was reaffirmed—occurring maximally in the lower temporal

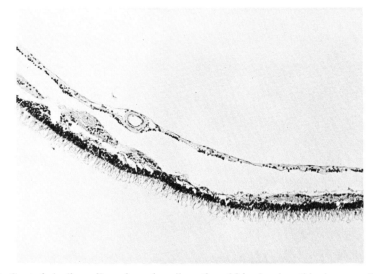

Fig. 6-9. Central (collapsed) region of senile retinoschisis showing thin inner wall with suspended vessel, complete loss of radial supporting columns, and partial holes in outer wall. Receptor cells are well preserved (×150).

quadrant. Significant association with hyperopia was noted. The findings in the above laboratory and clinical studies indicate that senile retinoschisis is an uncommon lesion that rarely leads to retinal detachment or to loss of central vision.

TROPHIC LESIONS OF OUTER RETINA

A trophic abnormality affecting the outer retinal layers is *paving-stone degeneration*. In its typical form, this disorder is characterized by one or more discrete, rounded foci of depigmentation and retinal thinning located between the ora serrata and the equator (Fig. 6-10). The lesions are yellow-white and often possess pigmented margins. The basic lesion of paving-stone degeneration is rounded in shape and ranges from 0.1 to 1.5 mm. in diameter. Clusters of these degenerations may merge to form larger lesions with scalloped margins and pigmented septa. Alternatively, coalescence may produce sharply demarcated circumferential bands in the anterior zone. This lesion has a remarkable predilection for the peripheral retina and only rarely violates the boundary imposed by the ora serrata and then, virtually always, within the limits of dentate extensions.

From a histological standpoint also, paving-stone degeneration is characteristic, with complete degeneration of the outermost retinal layers, including the pigment epithelium (Fig. 6-11). In the smallest unit lesion, almost complete fusion forms between the outer limiting and Bruch's membrane, with some attenuation or loss of the capillaries of the choriocapillaris. In the more advanced lesions, the middle retinal layers are degenerated and diminution in the choriocapillaris is more exaggerated. Inflammation and necrosis are significantly lacking in all instances. The adhesion between retina and inner choroid is as notable in the laboratory as in the clinical setting.

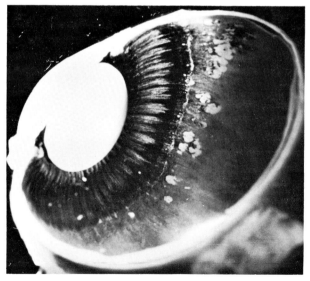

Fig. 6-10. Inferotemporal discrete and confluent depigmented paving-stone degenerations with hyperpigmented borders and septa. Hyperpigmented zone corresponding to anterior portion of vitreous base on the pars plana is also apparent (transillumination, ×4).

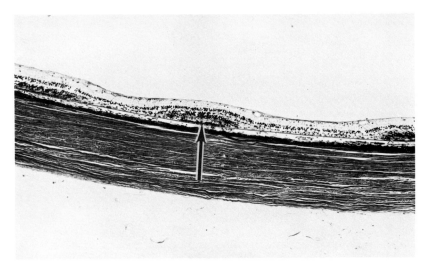

Fig. 6-11. Two foci of paving-stone degeneration with predominantly outer loss of retinal elements, including pigment epithelium. Central focus *(arrow)* with thickened pigment epithelium corresponds to pigmented septa noted grossly (H and E, ×55).

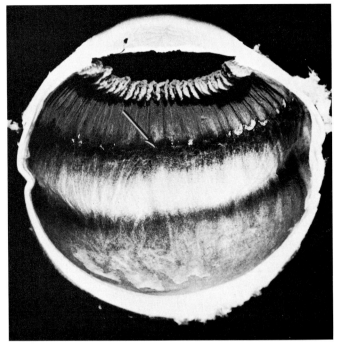

Fig. 6-12. Senile peripheral tapetochoroidal degeneration with retina removed to show exaggerated circumferential band of preequatorial depigmentation. Splotchy pigmentation corresponding to traction within posterior portion of vitreous base interrupts the band anteriorly *(arrow at ora serrata)* (×5).

In a series of 612 autopsy patients studied,[5] paving-stone degeneration was found in 27% of patients over 20 years old and it was bilateral in 70% of positive cases. In general, paving-stone lesions were most frequently located near the ora serrata, were less frequent at the equator, and were only rarely located farther posteriorly. Involvement was usually greater in the inferior and temporal quadrants.

Paving-stone degeneration does not predispose to retinal break nor to retinal detachment. However, if a retinal detachment from some other cause extends to involve an area of paving-stone degeneration, the retina may be torn at the marginal site of the chorioretinal adherence. The resultant retinal breaks are often small, irregular in shape, and inconspicuous.

In the older age groups, one often encounters another trophic lesion affecting the outer layers of the peripheral retina. This condition, categorized in our laboratory as *senile peripheral tapetochoroidal degeneration,* shows a diffusely depigmented circumferential band uniformly involving the peripheral fundus (Fig. 6-12). Typically, the posterior limit of this light-colored band terminates abruptly at the equator, but its uniformity may be interrupted by the splotchy depigmentation in the anterior zone, which corresponds to the region of vitreous base traction.

Histologically, there is significant diminution of the capillaries of the choriocapillaris and diffuse thickening of Bruch's membrane (Fig. 6-13). The pigment epithelium shows conspicuous degeneration, with loss of pigment granules and, usually, some loss of receptor cells.

In a study made on a series of 165 adult autopsy patients (Foos, unpublished data), senile peripheral tapetochoroidal degeneration was present in 20% of patients over 40 years of age and was bilateral in all cases. This diffuse degeneration appears age related and benign.

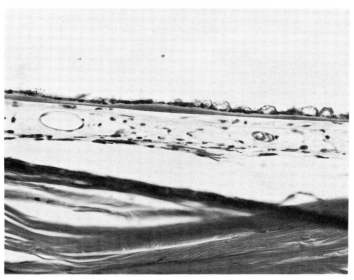

Fig. 6-13. Senile peripheral tapetochoroidal degeneration showing severe attenuation of choriocapillaris, thickening of Bruch's membrane, and degeneration of the pigment epithelium (H and E, ×125).

REFERENCES

1. Foos, R. Y., and Allen, R. A.: Retinal tears and lesser lesions of the peripheral retina in autopsy eyes, Amer. J. Ophthal. **64:**643, 1967.
2. Vrabec, F.: Neurohistology of cystoid degeneration of the peripheral human retina, Amer. J. Ophthal. **64:**90, 1967.
3. O'Malley, P. F., and Allen, R. A.: Peripheral cystoid degeneration of the retina, Arch. Ophthal. **77:**769, 1967.
4. Byer, N. E.: Clinical study of senile retinoschisis, Arch. Ophthal. **79:**36, 1968.
5. O'Malley, P. F., Allen, R. A., and Straatsma, B. R.: Paving-stone degeneration of the retina, Arch. Ophthal. **73:**169, 1965.

7

Tractional degenerations of the peripheral retina

Louis M. Spencer
Bradley R. Straatsma
Robert Y. Foos

In many important variations and degenerations of the peripheral retina, traction is a primary process. The traction may be of low magnitude and active over a prolonged period, for example, during ocular growth; or it may be of high magnitude and briefly operative, as during eye movements associated with visual acuity. The cumulative effect of those forces applied to vitreoretinal and zonuloretinal attachments that vary in distribution and strength is responsible for tractional lesions of the peripheral retina. For descriptive purposes, tractional lesions are classified as retinal tufts, folds, and tears as in the following outline:

Degenerations of the peripheral retina
  I. Tractional
    A. Tufts
      1. Noncystic
      2. Cystic
      3. Zonular
    B. Folds
      1. Meridional
      2. Other
    C. Tears
      1. Partial thickness
      2. Full thickness
  II. Trophic and tractional—lattice degeneration

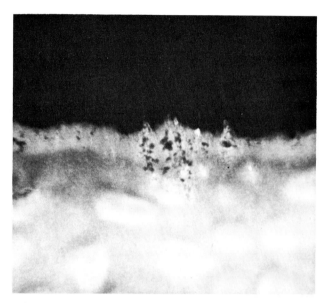

Fig. 7-1. Cluster of noncystic retinal tufts at ora serrata with surrounding slight cystoid degeneration (×15).

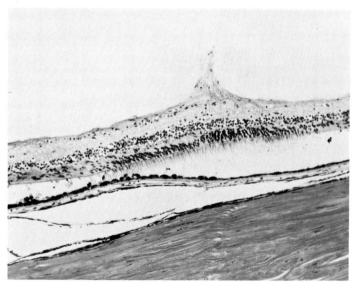

Fig. 7-2. Noncystic retinal traction tuft on inner retinal surface. The outer retinal layers are relatively well preserved (H and E, ×125).

TUFTS

Retinal tufts may be considered as cystic, noncystic, and zonular. A *noncystic retinal tuft* is a thin, short internal projection of retinal tissue that is almost invariably located within the posterior vitreous base and is often found in clusters (Fig. 7-1). From the vitreous attachment at the apex, the process extends to a base that is less than 0.1 mm. in diameter and unassociated with cystic retinal degeneration.

Histologically, a noncystic retinal tuft consists of a short strand of tissue that originates at a small base in the internal retina, projects into the vitreous, and terminates with an attachment to the vitreous body (Fig. 7-2). It is composed of altered retinal cells and proliferated glial tissue. The base is not surrounded by cystic retinal degeneration, and the underlying retinal pigment epithelium is not affected by the lesion.

A study of a series of 169 autopsy patients[1] showed that noncystic retinal tufts were present in 72%, were bilateral in 50% of affected cases, and were thus present in 59% of the 312 eyes examined (Table 7-1). Of the affected eyes, 36% had only one noncystic retinal tuft whereas the remainder contained from two to more than six. Noncystic retinal tufts were more common in the inferior than in the superior quadrants and more frequent nasally than temporally. In all but three eyes in the series, these tufts occurred in the zone of the peripheral retina corresponding to the vitreous base.

Although noncystic retinal tufts may be seen clinically, they are not associated with retinal breaks and can be considered innocuous.

The *cystic retinal tuft,* somewhat larger than the noncystic, is a nodule of tissue

Table 7-1. Degenerations of the peripheral retina

	Patients with lesions	Percent patients with lesions	Bilateral lesions	Percent bilateral lesions	Eyes with lesions	Percent eyes with lesions
Vitreous base excavation	8/169	5	0/8	0	8/312	3
Retinal hole	10/169	6	1/10	10	11/312	4
Cystoid degeneration	435/500*	87	435/435	100	870/1000	87
Senile retinoschisis	16/430	4	6/16	38	22/845	3
Paving-stone degeneration	134/614	22	51/134	38	185/1223	17
Peripheral tapetochoroidal degeneration	33/165	20	33/33	100	66/330	20
Noncystic retinal tuft	122/169	72	61/122	50	183/312	59
Cystic retinal tuft	100/169	59	39/100	39	139/312	45
Zonular traction tuft	27/169	16	3/27	11	30/312	10
Meridional fold	31/115†	26	15/31	48	46/230	20
Partial-thickness retinal tear:						
Paravascular	14/184‡	8	6/14	44	20/324	6
Posterior border of vitreous base	20/169	12	1/20	5	21/312	7
Full-thickness retinal tear	21/169	12	1/21	5	22/312	7
Lattice degeneration	12/202	6	6/12	50	18/404	4

*Over 8 years of age.
†Over 1 year of age.
‡Over 40 years of age.

that projects into the vitreous body from a base that is greater than 0.1 mm. in diameter (Fig. 7-3). This tuft is almost always located in the area corresponding to the vitreous base and may be single or multiple. The tuft and the area surrounding its origin are usually cystic and occasionally contain dispersed pigment granules. Condensed bands of vitreous are often visibly attached to the apex of the strand, and, frequently, the lesion is found posterior to a meridional fold.

In microscopic section, cystic retinal tuft is composed of degenerated, proliferated, cystic retinal tissue that projects from the retinal surface (Fig. 7-4). The pigmentation seen grossly can be identified in microscopic section, and exaggerated vitreous attachment to the apex of the tuft is often demonstrable.

In a series of 169 autopsy patients,[1] cystic retinal tufts were present in 59%, were bilateral in 39% of affected cases, and were present in 45% of the 312 eyes examined (Table 7-1). Thirty-five percent of the affected eyes had a single cystic retinal tuft, but the remainder contained from two to seven. In topographic distribution, cystic retinal tufts were equally prevalent in the superior and inferior quadrants but were more frequent nasally than temporally. Ninety-six percent of these lesions occurred in the zone of the retina corresponding to the vitreous base.

Though cystic retinal tuft is often a clinical finding, this alteration of the peripheral retina is only rarely associated with retinal breaks.

A *zonular traction tuft* is a projection of retina that extends anteriorly and is attached to one or more thickened zonular fibers, which, in autopsy eyes, are either visible or demonstrable by manipulation (Fig. 7-5). These tufts are generally small and originate immediately posterior to the ora serrata. Occasionally a much longer and thicker type of zonular traction tuft is seen. In this case, its base is usually situated somewhat more posteriorly, and it shows cystic change.

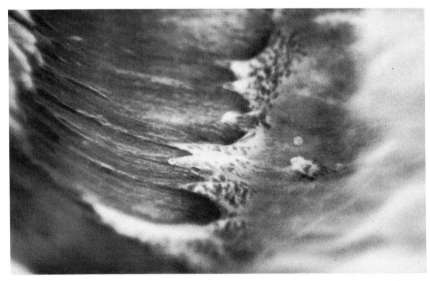

Fig. 7-3. Cystic retinal tuft behind small meridional fold and dentate process. Traction is demonstrated by avulsed retinal fragment in the overlying vitreous body and slight pigmentary reaction at its base (×15).

An occasional zonular traction tuft may be joined to the retinal base by only a thin strand of tissue, or it may be avulsed completely and be located adjacent to the anterior pars plana. These conditions may result in extreme retinal thinning or in a retinal break at the base of the tuft. Microsections through zonular retinal tufts reveal variable cystic degeneration, pigmentation, and retinal thinning at the base of

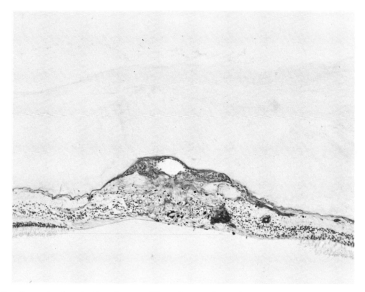

Fig. 7-4. Cystic retinal tuft showing proliferation and cystic degeneration of retinal tissue with dispersed pigment granules from underlying reactive pigment epithelium. Loss of retinal receptor cells is also seen (PAS, ×100).

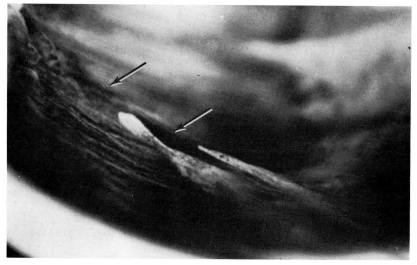

Fig. 7-5. Two large zonular traction tufts of ora serrata and peripheral retina in "piggyback" arrangement. Zonules *(arrows)* attached to tips of tufts are apparent (×20).

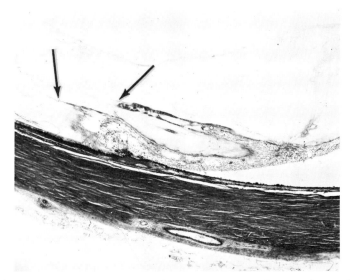

Fig. 7-6. Microsection through zonular traction tufts seen in Fig. 7-5, showing proliferative and cystic change of retinal tissue from traction exerted by zonule attached to tips *(arrows)* (PAS, ×25).

the strand, gliosis and cystoid alteration in the tissue projection, and characteristic zonular attachment at the apex of the tuft (Fig. 7-6).

In a series of 169 autopsy patients,[1] zonular traction tufts were present in 16%, were bilateral in 11% of affected cases, and were present in 10% of the 312 eyes examined (Table 7-1). In nearly two-thirds of the affected eyes, only a single zonular tuft was present and only one of the remaining eyes had more than three such lesions. In distribution, zonular traction tufts were slightly more common in the inferior than in the superior quadrants and were more frequent nasally than temporally. Lesions usually originated immediately posterior to the ora serrata and rarely from the region of the posterior border of the vitreous base.

The larger zonular traction tufts are greater in width and length than the noncystic and cystic retinal tufts related to vitreous traction. This increased dimension facilitates identification in clinical examination. Moreover, the larger zonular traction tufts are occasionally responsible for retinal breaks.

In addition to these three types of retinal tufts, which result from localized traction, there are often minute tags and fragments of retinal tissue at the ora serrata. Since these undoubtedly reflect a nonspecific degenerative change of the peripheral retina, they are of no clinical significance.

FOLDS

When traction occurs in a line, a retinal fold is formed. The most prevalent condition of this type is the *meridional fold* of the peripheral retina. The meridional fold is a radially oriented, linear elevation of the retina; it originates at the ora serrata and extends posteriorly for a distance of up to 3.5 mm. (Fig. 7-7). The fold may extend into the vitreous as much as 0.5 mm., and the edge of the fold may be

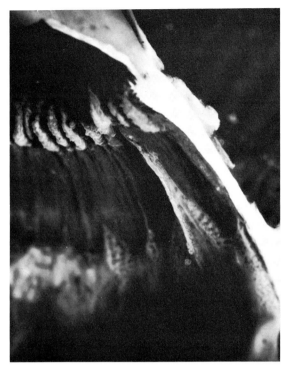

Fig. 7-7. Meridional fold associated with enlarged anomalous dentate and ciliary process. Traction is demonstrated by avulsed fragment of retinal tissue in the overlying vitreous body at its posterior margin (×15).

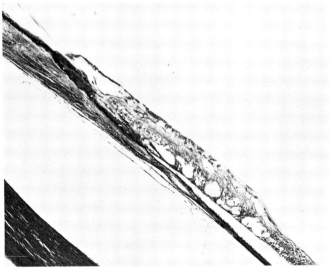

Fig. 7-8. Meridional retinal fold with prominent proliferative and cystic change (picroaniline blue, ×35).

rounded or knifelike. Most meridional folds coincide with a dentate process and, generally, are rather long. Often they are part of a meridionally aligned complex that may consist of an enlarged ciliary process, a large dentate process, and a meridional fold (Fig. 7-7).

Focal retinal thinning or, occasionally, hole formation is sometimes present posterior to a meridional fold or complex. Meridional folds may be aligned with an ora bay. They are generally rather short and are less frequently associated with a focal posterior retinal anomaly.

Histologic examination shows vitreous attached to the crest of the fold, with underlying cystoid degeneration and derangement of the retinal supportive structure (Fig. 7-8). Retinal thinning or a complete retinal break is sometimes seen at the posterior end of the fold or farther posteriorly.

In a series of 115 autopsy patients over 1 year of age, meridional folds were present in 26%, were bilateral in 48% of affected cases, and were present in 20% of the 230 eyes examined (Table 7-1) (Spencer, Straatsma, and Foos, unpublished data). Of the affected eyes, 68% contained one meridional fold each whereas each of the remaining eyes contained from two to six folds. In distribution, folds were most common nasally at or above the horizontal meridian. In fact, 86% of all folds occurred in the clock-hour positions from 1 to 4 o'clock in the right eye and in the corresponding positions from 8 to 11 o'clock in the left eye.

Seventy percent of meridional folds occurred with dentate processes, and 30% occurred posterior to ora bays. Of the former, 61% were associated with a meridional complex and 27% were associated with focal retinal thinning posterior to the fold.

Meridional folds are of clinical significance. These conspicuous features of the peripheral retina may be associated with retinal thinning and with retinal breaks in phakic and aphakic eyes, and they have been associated with retinal detachment.[2-5]

TEARS

Focal retinal tears are caused by traction from the detached vitreous body at sites of exaggerated or nonuniform vitreoretinal attachment. These tears may be considered as partial or full thickness. A *partial-thickness retinal tear* involves the inner layers of the retina and results in a thin flap or operculum. This lesion is usually multiple and its distribution allows classification into two types—one present in clusters adjacent to peripheral retinal vessels and the other aligned circumferentially along a segment of the posterior border of the vitreous base (Fig. 7-9). The former type is associated with an operculum and the latter with a flap attached to the face of the separated posterior hyaloid. Sometimes both types are seen in the same eye.

Microscopically, partial retinal tear appears on a focal inner retinal defect sometimes extending as deep as the inner nuclear layer. A flap or operculum is often identifiable, and the lesion is seen adjacent to an arteriole or just behind the posterior border of the vitreous base (Fig. 7-10).

In a series of 184 adult autopsy patients (Foos, unpublished data), partial tears of the paravascular type were found in 8%, were bilateral in 44% of positive cases, and were present in 6% of the 324 eyes examined. The lesions, when present, were multiple. Seventy-five percent occurred in the superior quadrants and predominated slightly on the temporal side; all were in the posterior zone of the peripheral retina.

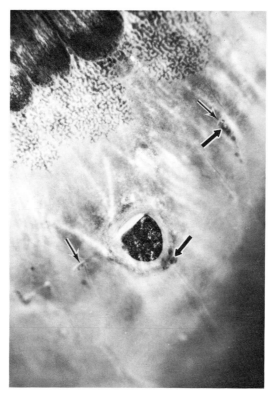

Fig. 7-9. Full-thickness retinal tear showing stippling of underlying pigment epithelium inside break and demarcation line of localized retinal detachment; partial-thickness tears along posterior edge of vitreous base (vitreous body detached) *(thin arrows)*; and paravascular partial-thickness tears *(thick arrows)* (×25).

Studied in a series of 169 autopsy patients,[1] partial tears at the posterior border of the vitreous base were present in 12%, were bilateral in one of the affected cases, and, of the 312 eyes examined, were present in 7%. Eight of these eyes had a single tear and up to 20 such lesions were noted in a single eye. Topographically, this lesion occurred almost equally in all quadrants and appeared in the posterior zone immediately adjacent to the posterior margin of the vitreous base.

The selective distribution of these partial tears and their invariable association with posterior vitreous separation suggest that they are causally related to exaggerated vitreoretinal attachments. Indeed, the presence of relatively firm vitreoretinal adherence at the site of peripheral retinal vessels has been suggested by others.[6-8] No evidence exists that partial retinal tears are progressive or that they lead to significant sequelae. Frequently, however, they are associated with full-thickness (Fig. 7-9) retinal tear—a lesion of greater clinical significance.

A *full-thickness retinal tear* is a complete break in the sensory retina. The tear is usually U- or V-shaped with a base directed anteriorly, with a flap extending into the vitreous, and with condensed strands of vitreous attached to the apex of this flap (Fig. 7-11). In some instances, part or all of the flap is avulsed and can be identified

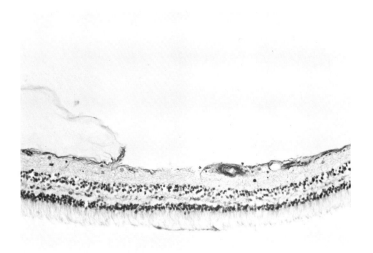

Fig. 7-10. Partial-thickness retinal tear at posterior border of vitreous base. Small flap is adherent to detached vitreous, and continuity of the internal limiting membrane is disrupted (H and E, ×125).

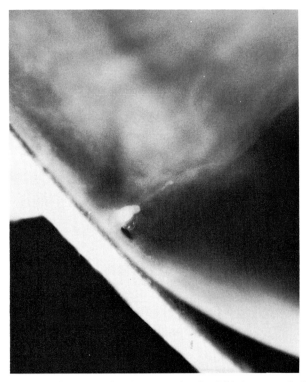

Fig. 7-11. Full-thickness retinal tear showing posterior hyaloid face attached to apex of flap (×20).

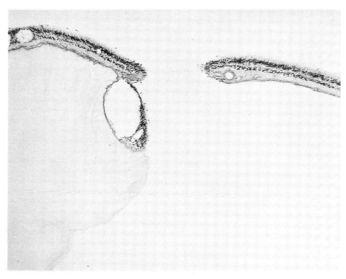

Fig. 7-12. Full-thickness retinal tear with cystic degenerated flap firmly adherent to detached vitreous body (Masson's trichrome, ×100.)

as an operculum in the overlying vitreous, almost always located anterior to the site of the retinal break. The flap or free operculum may be shrunken and degenerated, whereas the margin of the tear may be smooth and rounded (Fig. 7-9). Except when the tear occurs within the vitreous base, a localized or diffuse retinal detachment may occur. Seen through the retinal break, the pigment epithelium has a distinctive stippled appearance.

Histologically, the retinal tear demonstrates a flap or a free operculum firmly attached to condensed vitreous (Fig. 7-12). The flap or operculum demonstrates shrinkage and degeneration that may have conspicuous glial proliferation or cystoid characteristics. The margins of the retinal break, as a result of degeneration in the retina adjacent to the break, are smooth and rounded. Pigment epithelium degeneration and hyperplasia are variable features.

Excluding for statistical purposes retinal tears at the ora serrata or those related to a specific disease process, full-thickness retinal tears were noted in 12% of 169 autopsy patients.[1] One patient had bilateral retinal tears, so these lesions were present in 22 of the 312 eyes studied, or 7%. Of the affected eyes, 82% had a single tear whereas the remainder contained from two to four. These lesions were more prevalent in the inferior than in the superior quadrants and were slightly more frequent temporally. All tears occurred in the posterior zones of the peripheral retina. None were seen in the zone corresponding to the vitreous base.

Eleven of the 28 tears had a retinal flap and the other 17 presented a free operculum. Fifty-four percent of the tears were associated with local retinal detachment. Although peripheral retinal tears were somewhat more prevalent in the inferior than in the superior quadrants, they were more apt to be associated with localized retinal detachment when they occurred in the superior quadrants, particularly when they were present in the posterior zone of the preequatorial retina.

The clinical identification of these lesions is a major consideration in prevention and treatment of rhegmatogenous retinal detachment. From this study and from that of Okun,[9] however, it is clear that only a small percentage of retinal tears lead to clinically significant retinal detachment.

• • •

Trophic and tractional degenerations

In the foregoing review of trophic degenerations, there are conditions such as vitreous base excavation that are primarily trophic but that demonstrate some indication of traction. In like fashion, the discussion of tractional degenerations includes lesions such as zonular traction tuft, in which the primary process is tractional but in which a trophic element is also evident. Thus, these general processes of tissue loss and traction are not mutually exclusive. In fact, both trophic and tractional changes are present in a category of retinal degeneration that is of great significance. The principal abnormality in this category is lattice degeneration of the retina.

In its typical form, lattice degeneration is a sharply demarcated, circumferentially oriented lesion located at or somewhat anterior to the equator (Fig. 7-13). It is characterized by retinal thinning and abnormalities in the adjacent vitreous. Important additional distinguishing features include an arborizing network of fine white lines that are often continuous with blood vessels; alterations of retinal pigment, with frequent accumulations along the interlacing white lines (Fig. 7-14); round punched-out areas of retinal thinning or hole formation; small yellow-white particles on the surface of the lesion, at the margin, and in the adjacent vitreous; liquefaction of the

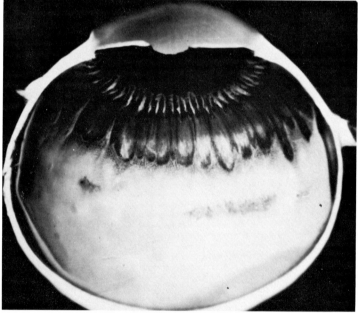

Fig. 7-13. Lattice degeneration illustrating sharp demarcation, circumferential orientation, and a typical location between equator and posterior margin of vitreous base.

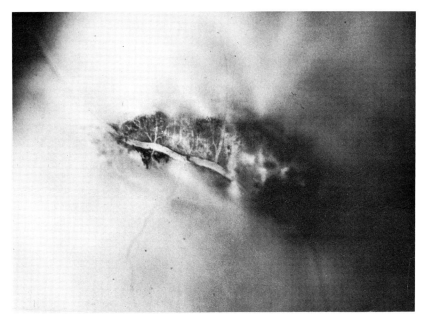

Fig. 7-14. Lattice degeneration demonstrating retinal thinning, abnormalities of overlying vitreous, arborizing network of white lines continuous with blood vessels and accumulations of retinal pigment along interlacing white lines.

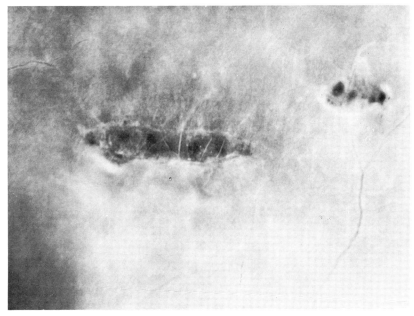

Fig. 7-15. Foci of lattice degeneration depicting round, punched-out areas of retinal thinning and small, discrete, white particles at margins of the lesions.

underlying vitreous; exaggerated vitreous attachments to the margin of the process; and a predilection for tears to develop along the posterior margin of the retinal thinning (Fig. 7-15).[10-12]

Though the general features of lattice degeneration are well recognized, precise evaluation of the condition necessitates consideration of variations related to (1) the degree or stage of the degeneration, (2) the extent of the process, and (3) the anteroposterior position of the lesion.

Early or mild stages of lattice degeneration appear grossly as elongated areas of retinal thinning and vitreous abnormality directed circumferentially and located at or somewhat anterior to the equator (Fig. 7-16). Within the discrete lesion, the internal retinal surface is eroded, thinned in a troughlike fashion, and often altered by the appearance of round, punched-out areas of extreme retinal thinning. A number of small yellow-white particles are attached to the retina within the lesion and at its margin (Fig. 7-17). Blood vessels within the process may be normal in appearance, and pigment alterations are minimal or absent (Fig. 7-18). The overlying vitreous is invariably liquified, and condensed vitreous bands are attached to the margin of the lesion.

When advanced in degree, lattice degeneration retains its distinctive shape and orientation. However, the lesions are somewhat wider, retinal thinning is generally more pronounced, arborizing white lines that are often continuous with blood vessels may ramify within the process, and pigment alterations are usually present (Fig. 7-19). In addition, round or oval areas of extreme retinal thinning are common, and retinal hole formation may be evident. Irregular white dots and tufts are often located along the margin of the lesion, the area of liquification in the overlying vitreous

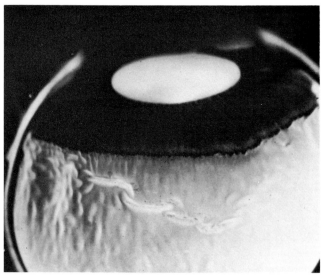

Fig. 7-16. Early or mild stage of lattice degeneration appearing as elongated areas of retinal thinning and associated vitreous abnormality.

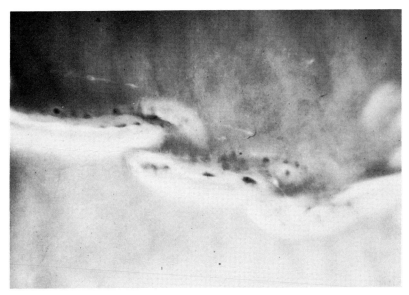

Fig. 7-17. Within and at margin of early lesions illustrated in Fig. 7-16, numerous small yellow-white particles attached to retina.

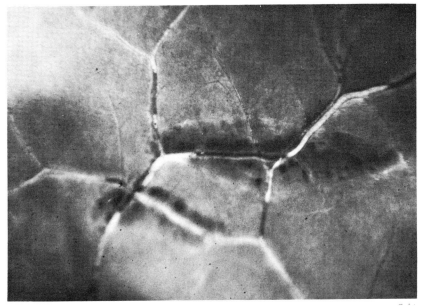

Fig. 7-18. Blood vessels within early lesions of lattice degeneration essentially normal in gross appearance.

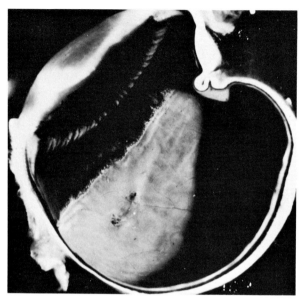

Fig. 7-19. Relatively wide, advanced lesion of lattice degeneration.

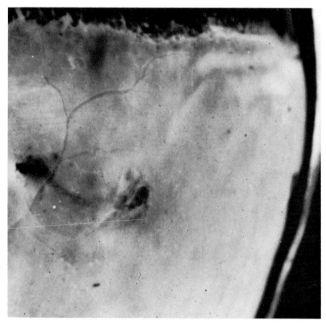

Fig. 7-20. Advanced lesion in Fig. 7-19 at greater magnification, illustrating round or oval areas of extreme retinal thinning and hole formation, and rather large zone of liquefaction in the overlying vitreous.

is usually greater, and the attachments of the vitreous to the margin of the lesion and the immediately adjacent retinal surface are more pronounced (Fig. 7-20).

Regardless of the degree of degeneration, the extent of the area of involvement varies according to the size and number of lesions. A single lesion may range in size from an island extending less than 30 degrees on the circumference of the globe to a band encompassing 120 degrees (Fig. 7-21). Twenty or more lesions may be present in an eye, and these may form two, three, or, rarely, four rows that are parallel to the equator and affect 270 or more degrees of the globe circumference (Figs. 7-22 and 7-23).

In addition to degree of degeneration and area of involvement, lattice degeneration varies with the anteroposterior location of the lesion. The typical form of lattice degeneration is generally located between the equator and the posterior margin of the vitreous base. When posterior to the equator, the lesion tends to be radial rather than circumferential in orientation and is often associated with postequatorial retinal vessels. The area of involvement is usually wider than the equatorial lesions, pigment alterations are almost invariably present, and vitreous attachments to the margin of the abnormality are more marked (Fig. 7-24).

Anteriorly, within the area corresponding to the vitreous base, patients with lattice degeneration frequently have lesions that possess all the characteristics of vitreous base excavation. These features include an oval or linear shape, a circumferential orientation, an absence of the inner retinal layers, and somewhat exaggerated vitreous attachments at the margin of the process (Fig. 7-25). Rarely, these excavations appear as a localized retinal hole and a localized retinal detachment. In all probability, vitreous base excavation represents a variant of lattice degeneration that is modified by location within the area of the vitreous base.

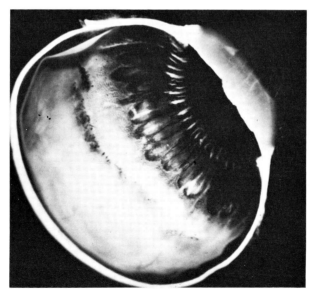

Fig. 7-21. Single lesion of lattice degeneration encompassing approximately 120 degrees of the equatorial circumference.

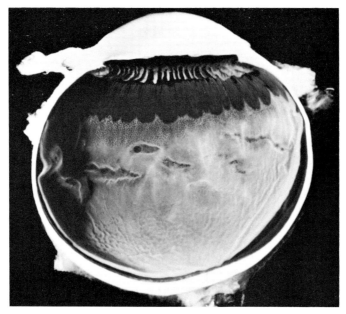

Fig. 7-22. At and somewhat anterior to the equator, numerous circumferentially oriented lesions of lattice degeneration.

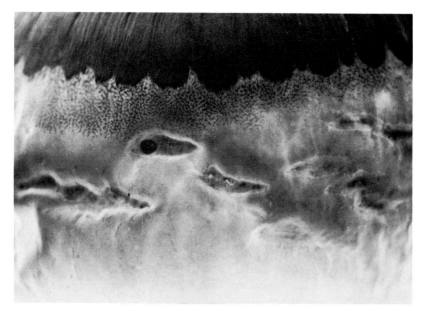

Fig. 7-23. Lesions in Fig. 7-22 at increased magnification, arranged in three or more rows parallel to equator. Conspicuous features are white particles at margins and areas of extreme retinal thinning and hole formation.

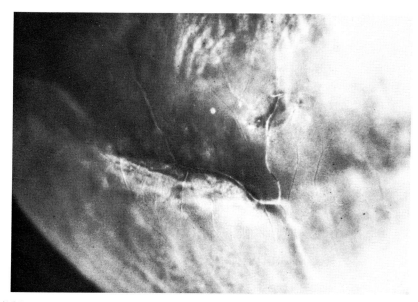

Fig. 7-24. Posterior to equator, focus of lattice degeneration somewhat radial in orientation and associated with retinal vessels. Lesion is relatively wide, with pronounced vitreous attachments at margins.

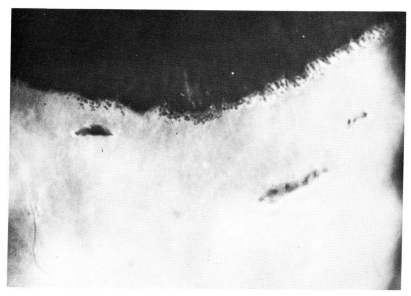

Fig. 7-25. Anterior to typical area of lattice degeneration, two linear circumferentially oriented lesions with all features of vitreous base excavations. Excavations are probably variants of lattice degeneration.

Related to the degree, extent, and anteroposterior position of the lattice degeneration is the tendency for tears to form along the posterior margin or end of the process. The tear assumes a U or horseshoe shape if there is anterior extension at each extremity (Fig. 7-26), an L shape if there is anterior extension at only one end, and a linear form if it is primarily along the posterior margin of the degeneration (Fig. 7-27). Tears may be single or multiple (Fig. 7-28) and small or very large in size (in clinical experience, extending over more than a quadrant). Even in eyes obtained at autopsy, retinal detachment of minimal or, occasionally, moderate extent may be associated with these tears.

Histologic features of lattice degeneration correlate well with the gross characteristics. At an early stage, the inner retinal layers are absent as if by erosion, a trough-like area of retinal thinning results, and areas of focal retinal thinning may also be present. Blood vessels within the lesion present mild thickening of the wall, and pigment changes are usually minimal or absent. Even when the process is minimal, changes in the adjacent vitreous body are always present (Fig. 7-29). These changes consist of a sharply circumscribed area in which all vitreous structure is lost, condensation of the vitreous body at the margin of the liquified area, and exaggerated attachments of the vitreous at the margin of the retinal lesion.

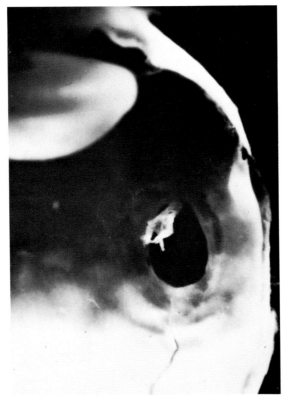

Fig. 7-26. Retinal rupture along posterior margin and both ends of a focus at lattice degeneration responsible for horseshoe-shaped retinal tear.

At an advanced stage, lattice degeneration presents a sharply circumscribed and rather broad area of retinal thinning. Within the thinned areas, the blood vessels are greatly thickened so that in some instances the lumen is completely obliterated. Pigment is often present in the paravascular spaces, and focal areas of extreme thinning or hole formation are not uncommon. Changes in the adjacent vitreous body correspond to alterations noted in the early lesions. In addition, however, vitreous attachments to the margin of the lesion are more pronounced, and glial extensions often extend from the retinal surface along the interface between liquid and formed vitreous (Fig. 7-30). In the pigment epithelium adjacent to the retinal degeneration, abnormalities are usually evident. Generally, these consist of an irregular degeneration and hyperplasia of the pigment epithelium.

In a series of 202 autopsy patients, lattice degeneration of the retina was present in 6% of the subjects, and in half of these cases, the degeneration was bilateral. Approximately 4% of the total number of eyes studied presented lattice degeneration.

Topographically, lattice degeneration is more common in the temporal than in the nasal quadrants and somewhat more frequent superiorly than inferiorly. In meridional distribution, it is most prevalent immediately adjacent to the superior and

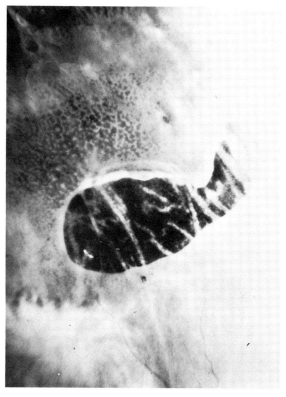

Fig. 7-27. Linear break in retinal continuity as result of retinal tear along posterior margin of a lesion of lattice degeneration.

inferior vertical meridians, less common in the temporal horizontal area, and least common in the vicinity of the nasal horizontal meridian. Usually, lattice degeneration occurs anterior to the equator and posterior to the vitreous base.

Of great clinical importance, lattice degeneration may be responsible for retinal detachment when round or oval holes within the areas of degeneration permit the passage of fluid or, more frequently, when retinal tears along the margin of the degeneration cause a retinal separation (Fig. 7-31).

Despite this clear relationship between lattice degeneration and retinal detachment, a comparison of the incidence of lattice degeneration, estimated at 6% to 7%,[10, 13] and the incidence of retinal detachment, reported as 0.005% per year,[14] makes it evident that the vast majority of patients with lattice degeneration do not develop retinal detachment.

Viewed, however, from the point of view of patients who do develop retinal detachment, lattice degeneration assumes major significance. Michaelson noted lattice degeneration in 20% of patients treated for retinal detachment[15]; Straatsma and Allen described lattice degeneration in 31% of patients operated upon for the prophylaxis or treatment of retinal detachment[10]; Colyear reported lattice degenera-

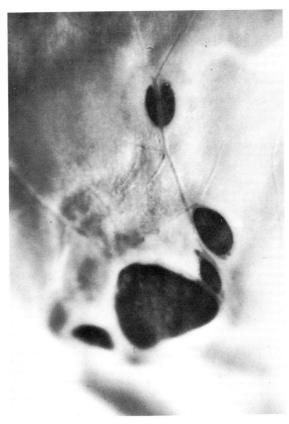

Fig. 7-28. Multiple retinal tears related to lesion of lattice degeneration located posterior to equator.

tion in 35% of patients on whom retinal surgery was performed[16]; and, more recently, Dumas and Schepens noted lattice degeneration in 30% of a series of patients with retinal detachment.[17]

On the basis of this evidence of clinical significance, it is essential to have an ap-

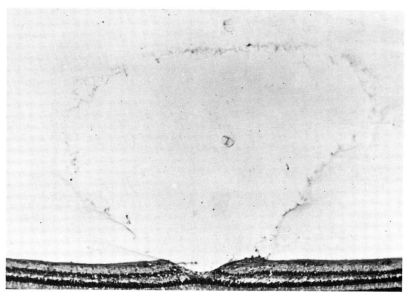

Fig. 7-29. Lattice degeneration in early stage, showing absence of inner retinal layers and liquefaction of overlying vitreous (Van Gieson, ×45).

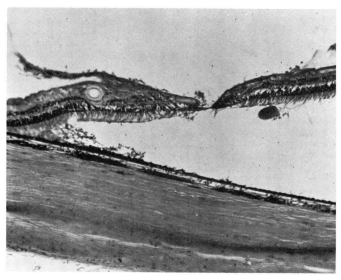

Fig. 7-30. Lattice degeneration in advanced stage, presenting profound retinal thinning, thickening of blood vessel walls, liquefaction of adjacent vitreous, and glial extensions along interface between liquified and formed vitreous (H and E, ×45).

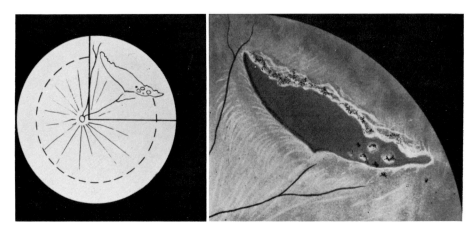

Fig. 7-31. Retinal tear along posterior margin of lattice degeneration, causing total retinal detachment.

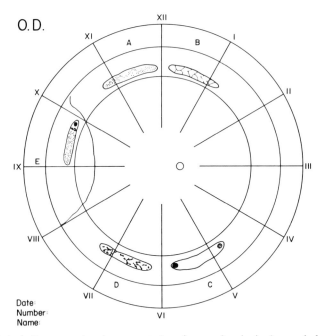

Fig. 7-32. Clinical diagrams showing extent, location, and principal morphologic features of lattice degeneration. In section *A,* blue dots portray tiny yellow-white particles at margin and on surface of lesion; in *B,* blue lines depict interlacing white lines that may be a conspicuous feature; in *C,* blue circle with oblique red lines records area of extreme retinal thinning; blue circle filled with red denotes retinal hole; in *D,* pigmentation is shown by black marks; and section *E* shows several features, including blue-colored section of retinal detachment.

preciation of the general features of lattice degeneration and a full awareness of the variations related to degree or stage of the degeneration, extent of the involvement, and the anteroposterior location of the process. In consideration of these factors, lesions predisposing to retinal detachment can in many instances be distinguished from more innocuous examples of lattice degeneration. To facilitate this determination, routine clinical diagrams of lattice degeneration should note (1) the principal morphologic features of the lesion, such as white dots, white lines, pigmentation, focal retinal thinning, and retinal holes, and (2) the extent and location of the process (Fig. 7-32).

In conclusion, the principal degenerations of the peripheral retina have been classified in this and the preceding chapters as trophic, tractional, and related to trophic and tractional factors. Each degeneration has been defined and further described to provide precise and rather detailed information regarding morphologic features, incidence, distribution, and clinical significance. This information forms the basis for the diagnosis of peripheral retinal degenerations and an assessment of the pathophysiologic implication of these retinal abnormalities.

REFERENCES

1. Foos, R. Y., and Allen, R. A.: Retinal tears and lesser lesions of the peripheral retina in autopsy eyes, Amer. J. Ophthal. **64:**643, 1967.
2. Schepens, C. L.: Subclinical retinal detachments, Arch. Ophthal. **47:**593, 1952.
3. Schepens, C. L.: Retinal detachment and aphakia, Arch. Ophthal. **45:**1, 1951.
4. Dumas, J., and Schepens, C. L.: Chorioretinal lesions predisposing to retinal breaks, Amer. J. Ophthal. **61:**620, 1966.
5. Rutnin, U., and Schepens, C. L.: Fundus appearance in normal eyes. II. The standard peripheral fundus and developmental variations, Amer. J. Ophthal. **64:**840, 1967.
6. Rieger, H.: Zur Histologie der Glaskörperabhebung. II. Ueber die Beziehungen des abgehobenen Glaskörpers zur Netzhaut, Graefe Arch. Ophthal. **146:**447, 1943.
7. Gärtner, J.: Histologische Beobachtungen über physiologische vitreovasculäre Adhärenzen, Klin. Mbl. Augenheilk. **141:**530, 1962.
8. Gärtner, J.: Ueber persistierende netzhautadhärente Glaskörperstränge und vitreoretinale Gefässanastomosen, Graefe Arch. Ophthal. **167:**103, 1964.
9. Okun, E.: Gross and microscope pathology in autopsy eyes. III. Retinal breaks without detachment, Amer. J. Ophthal. **51:**369, 1961.
10. Straatsma, B. R., and Allen, R. A.: Lattice degeneration of the retina, Trans. Amer. Acad. Ophthal. Otolaryng. **66:**600, Sept.-Oct. 1962.
11. Allen, R. A., and Straatsma, B. R.: Pathology of lattice degeneration of the retina. In: Surgery of retinal vascular diseases, Colloque (Amersfoort, 1963), Mod. Prob. Ophthal. **4:**49, 1966.
12. Straatsma, B. R.: Lattice degeneration: clinical description and course. In: Kimura, S. J., and Caygill, W. M., editors: Retinal diseases—symposium on differential diagnostic problems of posterior uveitis, Philadelphia, 1966, Lea & Febiger.
13. Byer, N. E.: Clinical study of lattice degeneration of the retina, Trans. Amer. Acad. Ophthal. Otolaryng. **69:**1064, Nov.-Dec. 1965.
14. Bohringer, H. R.: Statistisches zu Häufigkeit und Risiko der Netzhautablösung, Ophthalmologica **131:**331, April-May 1956.
15. Michaelson, I. C.: Retinal detachment: clinical evidence of the role of the choroid, Acta XVII Concilium Ophthalmologicum (Canada, United States of America) **1:**392, 1954.
16. Colyear, B. H.: Unpublished discussion of Straatsma and Allen, ref. 10.
17. Dumas, J., and Schepens, C. L.: Chorioretinal lesions predisposing to retinal breaks, Amer. J. Ophthal. **61:**620, 1966.

8

Photocoagulation with different light sources

Gerd R. E. Meyer-Schwickerath
K. J. Pesch

For more than 2 years we have had at our disposal different commercially available photocoagulators for experimental, histologic, and clinical comparative studies.

1. The ruby laser photocoagulator after Ingram from the Keeler Nelas Company
2. The ruby laser coagulator after Campbell[1] from the American Optical Company
3. The xenon flash photocoagulator after Comberg from the Optische Werke Jena
4. The xenon lamp photocoagulator from Zeiss-Oberkochen, West Germany
5. The xenon lamp photocoagulator with an automatic time-switch device

All of the apparatus has been placed in the surgical department of our eye clinic so that they could be used for routine photocoagulation as well as for operations.

I shall present here a short résumé of the clinical part of this study. A more detailed report is published by Pesch,[9] and one by Lund and Pesch is in preparation.

1. The *Ingram* or *Keeler Laser Ophthalmoscope* (Fig. 8-1) is a very handy instrument. For routine clinical work, however, we must complain about several points: The air cooling of this instrument is insufficient. After 40 to 50 laser shots, the ophthalmoscope gets so hot that one cannot hold it without gloves. More important is that this increase in heat is responsible for a loss of energy output of the laser beam. This heat might become dangerous, especially if one is not familiar with the apparatus. Because there is no reaction, one may speed up the machine with higher input energy. If the treatment is then interrupted and the ophthalmoscope has time to cool down and the next coagulation is performed with the same intensity, a heavy explosive reaction may occur, with a hemorrhage from the choroid. Besides this decrease of energy output as a function of heat, there is a certain

instability that seems to be present in all lasers we have tested. One may get a normal coagulation with a certain intensity, but the next coagulation with the same intensity may be explosive, with a hemorrhage. Shown in Fig. 8-2 is an example in which the coagulation in the middle was given with normal intensity from the clinical point of view. After 20 shots against the ceiling of our operation room, number 22 was given through the animal's pupil and led to an explosive reaction, with a small hemorrhage. After 20 further shots into the air, the next gave a very small, almost subclinical coagulation (left side of the photograph).

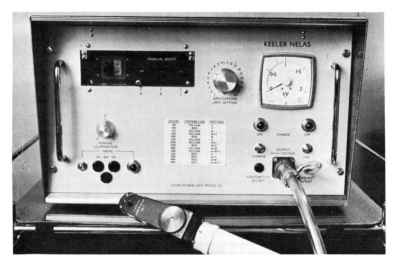

Fig. 8-1. The Keeler Nelas laser ophthalmoscope.

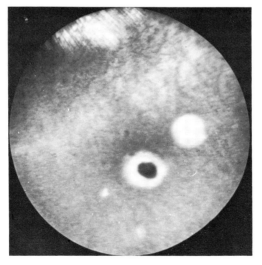

Fig. 8-2. Three coagulations with Keeler laser ophthalmoscope, all with the same intensity setting.

2. The *Campbell American Optical laser instrument* (Fig. 8-3) has a combined air and water cooling. This cooling is sufficient to prevent a sharp reduction of the output energy. In some cases we have produced more than 500 coagulations, one after the other without decrease of intensity. There is, however, an instability in the size of coagulations, without adjustment of the intensity switch (Fig. 8-4). There are some further differences of laser coagulation and conventional coagulation with the xenon lamp that seem to be true for all different types of lasers and that depend only on the very short exposure time of about 7/10,000 second. This short exposure time demands a very exact presetting of the output energy before the shot is released because the exposure time is constant. Compared with the xenon lamp coagulation, the laser coagulation is difficult to detect because the change of color of the retina does not occur in the same amount as in conventional photo-coagulation. This fact is especially true for the human eye in contrast to pigmented rabbit eyes. The reason is that during the short exposure time heat cannot be dissipated into the vicinity and the coagulation is more or less an explosion of the

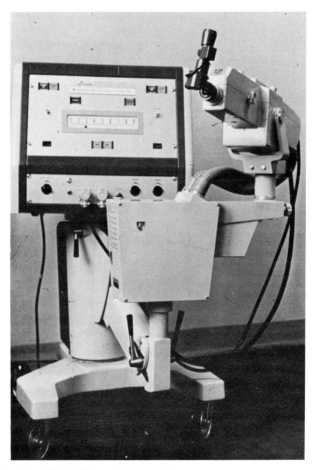

Fig. 8-3. The American Optical laser photocoagulator.

pigment epithelium.[4, 6, 7] Pieces of pigment are blown into the retina during this explosion, but Bruch's membrane usually remains intact because of its elasticity.

At the moment of explosion a small gas bubble typically occurs that leads to a hemispheric protrusion of the retina. The coagulation with the laser beam is therefore less visible than the conventional coagulation (Figs. 8-5 and 8-6). Visibility is especially difficult in cases of a fair fundus, whereas in a dark-pigmented eye the lesion is more visible. This fact makes it difficult to determine the correct dosage necessary to give an optimal lesion.

The great advantage of the laser coagulation is, however, that we do not need retrobulbar injection or general anesthesia to treat the patient. At the beginning we thought that this fact would make laser coagulation especially suitable for a postoperative coagulation. We are using postoperative coagulation a great deal since we think that what we call the two-step operation is a great advantage. This means that we first achieve only the reapplication of the retina and that after a short interval—which means some days—we occlude the hole by photocoagulation. We tried to do this also with laser coagulation and failed often, because the retina was not completely reattached in the area of the hole on the buckle of a volume-reducing operation. So we had to return to the conventional xenon lamp coagulator for this situation. To seal off nondetached retinal holes and equatorial degenerations, however, we have had good results with the American Optical laser coagulator.

There is another point to be mentioned that is due to the monochromatic nature of the laser beam. As you know, the wavelength of the ruby laser is 6943 Å. This limitation of the laser beam makes use of laser photocoagulation more or less impossible in coagulation of vascular structures of the fundus. About 94% of the laser light is not absorbed by the blood.[2] Therefore a direct coagulation of the blood is not possible. The laser beam, however, with higher intensity can occlude the retinal vessel by coagulating the surrounding tissue. On the other hand, the indifference of hemoglobin to the wavelength of the ruby laser is a help in coagulating the retina through more or less extensive hemorrhages. We have had good results in retinal holes that were due to perforating injuries and that were covered with blood.

Our experience in tumor treatment with laser instruments was disappointing. This was done mainly in the treatment of tumors that had to be enucleated. This mainly histologic study will be published later.

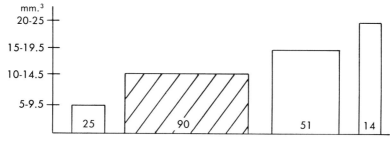

Fig. 8-4. Size of 180 laser lesions with constant intensity and field diaphragm 2.5. Planimetry of enlarged photographs in cubic millimeters.

There are several complications that seem to occur more often after laser coagulation than after conventional coagulation. Additionally, we have seen more contractions of pupils after laser coagulation than after conventional coagulation. In spite of good focusing of the beam in the patient's maximally dilated pupil, it seems that the iris is more sensitive to the laser beam or that the laser beam is smaller and therefore more intense in the level of the patient's pupil than is the conventional coagulation beam. In one case we saw a sort of iridoschisis after photocoagulation.

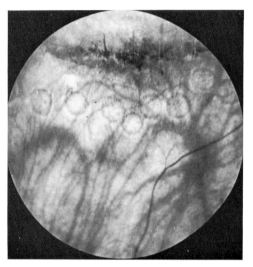

Fig. 8-5. Equatorial degenerations immediately after treatment with laser photocoagulation.

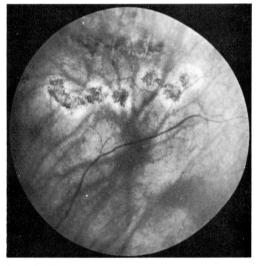

Fig. 8-6. Same as in Fig. 8-5. Two weeks later.

There has been a long discussion about the ultrasonic waves that are created when a laser beam is absorbed. These ultrasonic waves are, as far as we know, not dangerous to the eye.

3. The *xenon-flash coagulation* after Comberg from Optische Werke Jena (Fig. 8-7) lies between the laser coagulator and the conventional coagulator. The discharge time depends on the chosen intensity. With the switch on long-time coagulation, it ranges from 0.053 second (for intensity number 1) to 0.172 second (for intensity number 7). This is the half-intensity discharge time, which means that the curve of intensity has fallen down to half its maximum. It would be more suitable if we could have longer exposure times at low intensities and shorter at high intensities, but this cannot be changed because it depends on the nature of the flash. The great advantage of the Comberg instrument is the great visual field. The handling of the instrument, however, is not so easy as it seems to be at first. The flash head of the instrument turns around a point corresponding to the patient's pupil. If the patient's eye is moved, the pupil moves too and the instrument needs new adjustment. This is a time-consuming procedure and Comberg himself moves

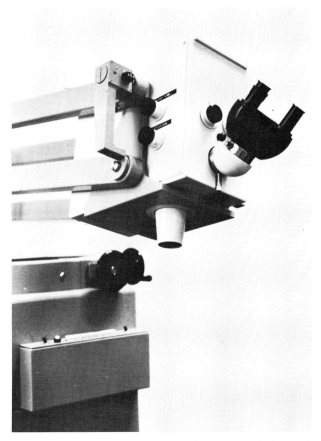

Fig. 8-7. The xenon flash coagulator after Comberg from the Optische Werke Jena.

the patient's head with one of his hands while looking through the instrument, a procedure that is an even greater handicap the farther out in the periphery the coagulations have to be performed.

The recharging of the condensers in the instrument needs some time, which also depends on the chosen intensity. Intensity switches III and IV need about 7 to 10 seconds for recharging. If we have many coagulations to perform, recharging can be a handicap because the whole procedure takes a long time.

There is a further definite disadvantage, in that the coagulation itself is not visible. The coagulated area is covered by a blind in order to protect the operator's eye, and one has to move the machine a little bit sideward in order to get the coagulation into view. Of course one can overcome all these difficulties with experience.

4 and 5. For 3 years we have been using clinically the old conventional *xenon*

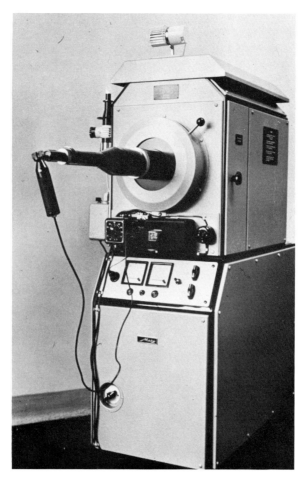

Fig. 8-8. The xenon lamp photocoagulator from Zeiss-Oberkochen with automatic time-switch device.

lamp photocoagulator (Fig. 8-8) with an electronic time switch, as was done by others too. The time can be regulated between 0.05 and 2 seconds, and therefore we were able to perform very short coagulations of very high intensity. I cannot go into detail about the different experiments we did with this machine. I would like to sum up by saying that we found no advantage in the very short coagulations over the conventional coagulation time of about half a second.

With some experience, one has a great advantage in being able to control the time factor according to the visible reaction of the retina. I think that this factor is so important that a photocoagulator with a constant burning light source will always be superior to one with a flash. It is interesting to remember that my first photocoagulator with the Beck arc was combined with an automatic shutter. I had used the shutter for quite a while, but I found that it was much more convenient to control the time with the fingertip, not automatically. Now we use the time switch only to limit the coagulation. The switch is especially helpful if somebody starts to learn photocoagulation. We usually set the time switch at 0.8 second so that the learner is not able to perform a coagulation longer than 0.8 second. He can, however, by releasing the push button, stop his coagulation before 0.8 second is reached.

I think that further experiments with constant-burning lasers as the helium-xenon laser are worthwhile. The only handicap at the moment is that they are still very clumsy and expensive.

SUMMARY

A comparative clinical study with different photocoagulators, including the ruby laser and xenon flash coagulators, has shown that the old method by timing the exposure with the fingertip according to the reaction on the fundus is still the safest and simplest method to perform photocoagulation.

REFERENCES

1. Campbell, C. J., Koester, C. J., Curtice, V., Noyori, K. S., and Rittler, M. C.: Clinical studies in laser photocoagulation, Arch. Ophthal. **74**:57, 1965.
2. L'Esperance, F. A.: Effect of laser radiation on retinal vascular anomalies. In Flocks, M., editor: Laser photocoagulation, Int. Ophthal. Clin. **6**(2):351, 1966.
3. Geeraets, W. J.: Laser-Strahlung und biologische Effekte, Bruns Beitr. Klin. Chir. **210**:259, 1965.
4. Geeraets, W. J., et al.: Laser versus light coagulator: a funduscopic and histologic study of chorioretinal injury as a function of exposure time, Fed. Proc. **24**:Suppl. 14:48, 1965.
5. Marshall, J., and Mellerio, J.: Histology of the formation of retinal laser lesions, Exp. Eye Res. **6**:4, 1967.
6. Mellerio, J.: The thermal nature of retinal laser photocoagulation, Exp. Eye Res. **5**:242, 1966.
7. Mellerio, J.: Is there a hazard in laser photocoagulation? Brit. Med. J. **1**:719, 1966.
8. Meyer-Schwickerath, G.: Lichtcoagulation, Ber. Deutsch. Ophth. Ges. **66**:313, 1964.
9. Pesch, K. J.: Ueber verschiedene Lichtkoagulatoren, Rhein. Westf. Augenärzte, p. 49, 1966.
10. Zaret, M. M.: Ocular hazards of laser radiation. In Flocks, M., editor: Laser photocoagulation, Int. Ophthal. Clin. **6**(2):285, 1966.

9

Cryotherapy in retinal detachment surgery

Edward W. D. Norton

Since the time of Gonin the following principles of detachment surgery have evolved:

1. Locate all retinal breaks.
2. Irritate the pigment epithelium in the area around the breaks.
3. Bring the retinal breaks into contact with the irritated pigment epithelium and keep them there long enough to form a firm union.
4. Accomplish this with the minimum damage to the vitreous and macula.

In 1948 Custodis, utilizing these principles, introduced the scleral buckling procedure with Polyviol as his implant material. He added the following innovations to Gonin's method:

1. Cover all retinal breaks with an implant.
2. Apply this implant to full-thickness sclera without scleral incision.
3. Do no fluid drainage.
4. Mobilize the patient early.

In 1962, with the reintroduction of cryosurgery by Lincoff and Kelman for the treatment of retinal detachments and the almost simultaneous development of silicone sponge as implant material, the Custodis procedure began to gain in popularity in the United States and, with certain variations, its use has become widespread.

It is important to emphasize that cryotherapy has *not* changed any of the principles of retinal detachment surgery. It has merely given the surgeon another modality with which to set up an irritation in the choroid and retina and a means of doing this without significantly damaging the sclera.

ADVANTAGES OF CRYOTHERAPY

The advantages of cryotherapy are set forth in the following list and most are discussed below:

1. Can be used transconjunctivally despite severe media haze
2. Scleral damage minimal
3. Unnecessary to incise scleral flaps

4. Eye softens with treatment rather than gets hard
5. Margin of safety greater
6. End point easily seen
7. Relocation of implants easier
8. Reduction in operating room time
9. Reduction in postoperative intraocular reaction
10. Reduction in postoperative infection
11. Reoperation easier and safer

Transconjunctival use

Transconjunctival use is certainly the most apparent advantage of cryotherapy. Patients with peripheral breaks that previously would be treated by photocoagulation are now more easily treated, under topical anesthesia, by scleral depression with the cryoprobe and freezing the desired area. In patients with recent tears and vitreous hemorrhage, this can be readily performed at a time when photocoagulation would be difficult if not impossible. In cases with lens opacities, similar advantages occur. At the present time, I prefer transconjunctival cryotherapy to photocoagulation, unless the break is too posterior to reach without a conjunctival incision.

Minimal scleral damage

Scleral damage from freezing is minimal. This fact, combined with ease of freezing the pigment epithelium and retina through full-thickness sclera, has eliminated the need for scleral undermining procedures. The principal reasons for combining scleral buckling procedures with scleral undermining were to avoid excessive coagulation of the sclera, with its accompanying shrinkage and necrosis, and to apply minimal heat to the choroid and retina in a uniform and predictable intensity by eliminating the variations in scleral thickness. Those disadvantages are no longer valid, since cryotherapy does not cause scleral necrosis and shrinkage and since variations in scleral thickness can readily and safely be adjusted for by experience in the use of the cryoprobe.

During the operation the most apparent evidence of lack of scleral damage is the softening of the globe that occurs in cryotherapy, in contrast to the increase in intraocular pressure accompanying the shrinkage of the sclera caused by diathermy. At the time of reoperations the apparent normalcy of the sclera that has been frozen is in marked contrast to the changes in the sclera that has been treated with diathermy.

Greater margin of safety

In some respects the margin of safety has to be a clinical judgment, since the intensity of application and the response of the eye to this therapy are also clinical judgments. There are some objective signs, however, that would appear to support this judgment.

When either photocoagulation or diathermy is applied to an attached retina, the loss in retinal transparency that results is much greater than that following cryotherapy. In fact, once the retina is allowed to thaw, it is difficult to determine the area of treatment unless green light and scleral depression are used. Cryotherapy does not appear to have the same damaging effect on large vessels as does diathermy and can therefore be applied to the sclera overlying the vortex ampullae and long ciliary vessels without the risks encountered with diathermy.

The intraocular reaction following cryotherapy, even when it is extensive, is usually minimal—so minimal, in fact, that the aqueous remains free of cells and the iris mobile even if it is not kept dilated. Although excess reaction may result from treatment with either modality, I have been impressed that the reaction is less with cryotherapy than with diathermy. This fact is particularly true with the more extensive operative procedures when large areas have required treatment.

The important question to be answered is: "Does cryotherapy damage the vitreous more or less than diathermy when each modality is properly used?" I do not believe this question can be answered at the present time. Certainly macular pucker and massive vitreous retraction occur after the use of either modality. The apparent tolerance in the laboratory of collagen fibers to cold, in contrast to heat, is suggestive evidence, but such is certainly not necessarily applicable to the clinical situation.

End point easily seen

When cryotherapy is applied to attached or minimally detached retina, the change in retinal transparency that occurs with freezing is obvious. Since this change indicates adequate treatment, applications in such situations should be made under direct observation. Because the thawed retina promptly regains its transparency, this method requires careful and continuous observation in order to avoid skipping areas needing treatment.

When cryotherapy is applied to highly detached retinas, the change in choroidal color from red to orange can be readily seen and is evidence of at least adequate treatment. In such cases, using the loss of retinal transparency as an end point will surely result in overtreatment.

Relocation of implants

Relocation of an implant that is on the surface of the sclera is considerably easier than relocation of the buried implant. If ophthalmoscopy shows the buckle to be too posterior or too anterior for the break, the sutures need only be relocated accordingly to obtain a proper position. There are no scleral flaps to extend, and it is not necessary to increase the size of the implant or the area of treatment.

Reduction in postoperative infections

Reduction in postoperative infections has been emphasized by Lincoff and certainly is consistent with our clinical experience.

Reoperation easier and safer

If the previous operation has included extensive surface diathermy, it is not necessary to expose down to sclera, but one can leave a layer of tissue overlying the necrotic sclera, and then merely freeze through it and apply a full-thickness buckle as desired. If the previous operation featured a buried implant, this may be left in place and cryotherapy applied anterior or posterior to it through the full-thickness sclera. If the implant was a silicone band, cryotherapy, by spreading through and around it, will give adequate reaction without reexposing the bed. This is not true with the larger silicone implants.

There is little doubt that the less trauma done to the eye, to get sufficient reaction around the retinal break and to get a buckle at the site of the break, the fewer the complications.

DISADVANTAGES OF CRYOTHERAPY

The disadvantages of cryotherapy are set forth in the following list:
1. Difficult to see area of treated sclera, retina, and choroid immediately post-treatment—therefore:
    a. Scleral marker required for topical localization of holes
    b. Care required to avoid "skip areas" in treatment
2. Must be careful moving cold probe
3. Dispersion of pigment of the pigment epithelium
4. Equipment

Difficulty in recognizing area of treated sclera and retina immediately posttreatment

In a sense, difficulty in recognizing the area of treated sclera represents one of the advantages of cryotherapy, since it indicates how little damage has been done

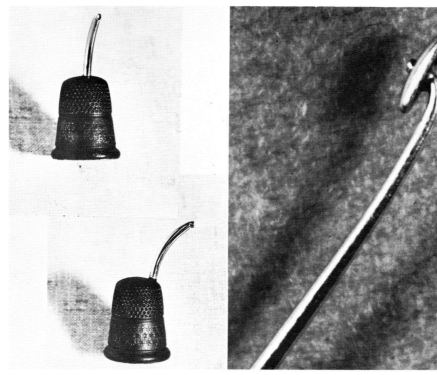

Fig. 9-1

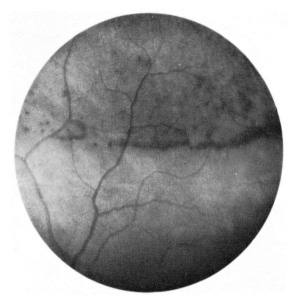

Fig. 9-2

to the globe. Once the surgeon learns to compensate for this difficulty, it rarely presents a problem. For a long time we have localized and marked the area of the retinal breaks on the sclera with some sort of dye, such as methylene blue, and more recently Scripto pencils, but it is even more essential now since cryotherapy does not recognizably change the sclera as diathermy does. We use either the sclera marker of Gass or the one of Linnen (Fig. 9-1) to locate the limits of the breaks (see Fig. 14-3.)

Danger from moving cold probe

Movement of the cold probe must be carefully avoided, since the probe is intimately joined to the ocular tissue by the "ice ball." I have not seen any ocular tissues "crack," but I have seen pieces of sclera avulsed by too rapid and forceful removal of the probe from the sclera. Serious complications can be imagined if this happens in thin sclera or when cryotherapy is applied to the bed of an undermined area. As long as the surgeon is aware of this complication, it should not be a serious risk.

Dispersion of pigment

Dispersal of pigment results from excessive freezing of the pigment epithelium cells, with subsequent rupture and release of pigment granules. The pigment floats free in the subretinal space, and if the detachment is limited and fluid is not drained, it may leave a pseudodemarcation line as the fluid is absorbed (Fig. 9-2). In other cases with total detachments, the pigment may settle in the posterior polar area, leaving large clumps (Fig. 9-3). The effect of these clumps on visual function remains to be determined. I used to see pigment dispersal almost routinely when

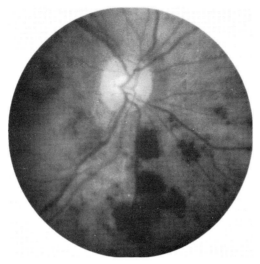

Fig. 9-3

I started using cryotherapy, but as I became more conscious of "overtreatment" and used minimal cryotherapy, this complication essentially disappeared.

Equipment

Probably the greatest deterrent to the acceptance of cryotherapy has been the deficiencies in the instrumentation. These instruments have been cumbersome and expensive, requiring special coolant materials and, most frustrating, having a high breakdown rate—so high that in the early days the operation started with cryotherapy but the surgeon was always prepared to shift to diathermy.

Although instrumentation remains a problem, tremendous progress has been made since 1963; and reliable, well-controlled, easily handled, and relatively inexpensive instruments are available.

Linde cryosurgical unit. The Linde cryosurgical unit was the original unit developed by Lincoff and the Linde Division of Union Carbide Company. It utilized liquid nitrogen as its coolant. Its advantages and disadvantages are listed below:

Advantages
1. Capacity for lower temperatures useful for:
    a. Eyes with thick sclera
    b. Reoperation in congested tissues
    c. Treatment through previously placed implants
    d. Elevated intraocular lesions
2. Larger probe available
3. Better temperature control

Disadvantages
1. Probe cumbersome
2. Frequent breakdown

3. Operating room technique more difficult
4. Handling of coolant more complicated
5. Not easy to use transconjunctivally

At present the company has not tried to further improve the development. It is not a practical instrument for the man in private practice because of its many problems. Its tremendous coolant capacity and its excellent temperature control have not been duplicated in the newer instruments, and, although I believe that more accurate temperature control would be desirable, it may not be essential.

Frigitronic cryosurgical unit. The Frigitronic unit has evolved through several instruments and continues to be improved. Its advantages and disadvantages, when compared to the Linde unit, are listed below:

Advantages
1. Probe easy to use
2. Easier and safer to use transconjunctivally
3. Greater reliability
4. Simple operating room technique
5. Packaged coolant almost instantly available
6. Rapid heating

Disadvantages
1. Prolonged freezing time required in presence of thick sclera, inflamed tissue, and elevated intraocular lesions
2. Occasional malfunctioning control valve
3. Occasional leakage of coolant from cord
4. Expense of coolant
5. Variable rate and extent of temperature drop

Amoils cryosurgical unit. The Amoils unit is the most recent addition to the available instruments and has received rapid and wide acceptance. It, too, continues to be improved. Its advantages and disadvantages are listed below:

Advantages
1. Coolant readily available to all operating rooms
2. Simplicity of operation; easy to use
3. Rapid cooling and reheating
4. Minimal breakdown

Disadvantages
1. Cools too rapidly and too cold, resulting in "overtreatment"

Not everyone is in agreement with my concern about the rapid and extensive cooling of the Amoils unit. I would prefer to be able to regulate the temperature drop more accurately, as with the Linde unit, so that the surgeon could select the degree of freezing obtained. This control may prove to be of small concern as I gain experience with the unit. It does reflect, however, my concern that we are probably still overtreating with cryotherapy. The presence of pigment dispersal indicates to me excessive treatment.

CRYOTHERAPY VERSUS DIATHERMY

In an effort to try to establish some comparison between cryotherapy and diathermy, Dr. George Hilton reviewed some of our case material, which was reported

Table 9-1. Preoperative findings

	Cryotherapy	*Diathermy*
Number of cases	150	150
Male	62%	67%
Average age	58	55
V.A. 20/50 or better	33%	27%
Duration greater than 1 month	28%	38%
Aphakia	41%	38%
Myopia—more than 6 diopters	9%	7%
Trauma	7%	5%
Secondary operation	9%	14%
Four quadrants	32%	31%
One quadrant	11%	14%
Macula off	68%	70%
One break	37%	43%
Fixed folds	40%	38%

Table 9-2. Retinal detachment surgery

	Cryosurgery	*Diathermy*
Scleral dissection	0%	80%
Drainage	77%	86%
Segmental buckle	43%	23%
Encircling buckle	55%	76%
Injection into vitreous	5%	7%
Operating time, average	106 min.	121 min.

at the A.M.A. meeting in June 1968. In this series he compared the last 150 consecutive cases treated by diathermy with the first 150 consecutive cases treated with cryotherapy. The similarity of the preoperative findings is indicated in Table 9-1.

It is to be emphasized that although these two groups are referred to as "diathermy group" and "cryosurgery group" these were *not* the only differences between the two groups even though that was the only basis for their selection. As can be seen from Table 9-2, the cryosurgery group differed, in addition, by an absence of scleral dissection, an increased use of segmental buckles with a reciprocal decrease in encircling buckles, and a decrease in fluid drainage.

Postoperative management was similar for the two groups. The number of postoperative days in the hospital was 1 week or less for 79% and 76% of the cryosurgical and diathermy series respectively. Supplemental postoperative photocoagulation was used in 12 cryosurgery patients and 10 diathermy patients.

A cure is defined as an anatomic reattachment for at least 6 months. The results of this study, shown in Table 9-3, indicate that the cure rate was similar for the two procedures. Although the number of eyes reattached in the cryosurgery group with one operation or overall is greater than in the diathermy group, in a series this size it is still not significant (p. < 0.2) and only suggestive, not indicative.

Table 9-3. Anatomic results

	Cryosurgery		Diathermy	
	No. of eyes	*%*	*No. of eyes*	*%*
Reattached with one operation	125	83	113	75
Reattached with two or three operations	16	11	20	14
Total	141	94	133	89

Table 9-4. Visual results of all reattached eyes

	Cryosurgery		Diathermy	
	No. of eyes	*%*	*No. of eyes*	*%*
20/15 to 20/50	79	56	62	47
20/70 to 20/200	41	29	31	23
Less than 20/200	21	15	40	30
Total	141	100	133	100

Table 9-5. Visual acuity in detachments involving the macula

	Preoperative				Postoperative—all reattached eyes			
	Cryosurgery		Diathermy		Cryosurgery		Diathermy	
	No. of eyes	*%*	*No. of eyes*	*%*	*No. of eyes*	*%*	*No. of eyes*	*%*
20/15 to 20/50	4	4	3	3	44	46	25	27
20/70 to 20/200	18	18	13	12	32	33	28	31
Less than 20/200	81	78	89	85	20	21	38	42
Total	103	100	105	100	96	100	91	100

The visual results of all reattached eyes, as recorded 6 or more months postoperatively, are tabulated in Table 9-4.

Although the results are better in the cryosurgery group, the difference for those who obtained 20/50 or better is not statistically significant (p. < 0.2). Of greater interest is the postoperative visual acuity in those eyes in which the macula was detached preoperatively. Table 9-5 indicates a marked difference in the postoperative visual acuity, although the preoperative visual acuity was similar in the two groups. In the cryosurgery group, 46% obtained 20/50 or better, whereas the diathermy group obtained this level of vision in 27% of the cases (p. < 0.02).

Table 9-6 portrays the effect of duration of the detachment. If the retina had been detached less than 2 weeks, 60% of the cryosurgery group obtained a vision 20/50 or better versus 33% of the diathermy group (p. < 0.02).

A similar difference was found when the case material was analyzed to differentiate those cases cured with one operation and those requiring two or more operations. In the single operative cases, 48% of the cryosurgery group and 29% of the

Table 9-6. Postoperative visual acuity—all reattached cases with preoperative detachment of the macula

Duration of detachment	*Cryosurgery*		*Diathermy*		*p.*
	No. of eyes	*% Va ≥ 20/50*	*No. of eyes*	*% Va ≥ 20/50*	
Less than 2 weeks	55	60	30	33	< 0.05
2 to 8 weeks	29	38	43	37	< 0.95
Over 2 months	12	25	18	0	< 0.02

Table 9-7. Number of operative complications

	Cryosurgery	*Diathermy*
Retinal incarceration	2	1
Hemorrhage—retinal, choroidal, vitreous	6	12
Vitreous loss	0	3
Rupture of globe	0	2

Table 9-8. Number of postoperative complications

	Cryosurgery	*Diathermy*
Choroidal detachment	27	22
Intraocular infection	0	2
Extraocular infection	2	9
Implant extrusion	0	5
Severe uveitis	0	6
Phthisis	0	2
Glaucoma	3	7
Massive vitreous retraction	4	4
Corneal changes	0	2

diathermy group obtained postoperative vision of 20/50 or better; in multiple operative cases, it was 30% for cryosurgery and 18% for diathermy that obtained 20/50 or better.

Tables 9-7 and 9-8 summarize the complications that occurred more than once in either series. Although the incidence of serious complications such as hemorrhage, vitreous loss, rupture of the globe, infection, severe uveitis, and phthisis is low, they all occurred more frequently in the diathermy group. There was no difference in the incidence of development of massive vitreous retraction. The series included 13 reoperations in eyes previously treated with cryosurgery. The only untoward feature was the unplanned drainage of subretinal fluid during the placement of an intra-scleral suture in one eye. In 71 reoperations on eyes previously treated with diathermy, serious complications of globe rupture, vitreous loss, or hemorrhage occurred in nine cases. Critical analysis of a series of cases such as this always poses problems, especially when they are chronologically separated. The three surgeons were more experienced in 1965, the cryosurgery period, than in 1963, the diathermy period. They were the same surgeons, however, and the case material was quite similar.

The evident contribution of this study is that the shift in operative techniques from scleral undermining and diathermy to full-thickness scleral buckles with cryotherapy has been accomplished without any decrease in the rate of successful reattachment. The overall reattachment rate, and especially the rate of reattachment with one operation in the cryosurgery group, should alleviate the concern regarding the strength of the chorioretinal adhesion.

The unexpected finding of superior postoperative visual acuity in the cryosurgery group, though suggestive, is not significant when compared with previously reported data.[1]

In a previous communication[1] it had been emphasized that final visual acuity was related to the presence and duration of macular detachment and evidence of preoperative vitreous traction. Since these factors are not under the control of the surgeon, one would not anticipate significant improvement in visual acuity by variation of surgical technique. This study negates that statement and suggests, as one would expect, that with fewer complications there will be less damage to macular function. Despite the suggestive evidence of these figures, impaired visual acuity postoperatively remains a very important and, as yet unresolved, problem in retinal detachment surgery.

This series indicates that the predicted benefits of cryosurgery, such as (1) reduced need for scleral dissection, (2) decreased operating time, (3) less postoperative complications, (4) safer reoperation, and (5) improved prognosis, have been realized.

This series fails to support the concern about the strength of the chorioretinal adhesions or about the increased incidence of bleeding at the drainage site.

It is evident that the prediction made in 1965[2] that "with the development of better instrumentation and more experience, cryotherapy will replace diathermy in retinal surgery" is close to realization. Only additional years can give the long-term comparison.

REFERENCES

1. Norton, E. W. D.: Retinal detachment in aphakia, Trans. Amer. Ophthal. Soc. **61:**770, 1963.
2. Norton, E. W. D.: Discussion of papers by Lincoff and McLean, Trans. Amer. Acad. Ophthal. Otolaryng. **70:**210, 1966.

10

Pathologic changes following retinal detachment surgery

Victor T. Curtin

Ocular changes following retinal detachment surgery encompass many pathologic conditions. In this review, I shall discuss four topics: a comparison of two eyes treated with cryotherapy and diathermy in the same patient, retinal membranes, choroid and suprachoroidea, and tissue reaction to synthetic implants and suture material. I shall correlate clinical findings and pathology to provide a better understanding of complications as well as their prevention and treatment.

Pathologists seldom have the opportunity to study eyes after successful retinal detachment surgery. Recently, a unique experience occurred when two eyes were sent to the pathology laboratory following the death of a patient who had been successfully treated for bilateral retinal detachments. The left eye had undergone two retinal detachment procedures that consisted of diathermy, scleral resection and encircling, and local silicone implants. The operations were 5 and 3 years prior to death. The right eye was treated with cryotherapy and with encircling silicone and local Silastic implants without scleral resection 8 months prior to death. Both eyes had attached retinas and retained good visual function. Figs. 10-1 and 10-2 compare the eyes externally, and Figs. 10-3 and 10-4 show relative thickness of walls of the eyes on cross section as well as chorioretinal adhesions at the sites of the retinal tears. Macroscopic sections (Figs. 10-5 and 10-6) emphasize those features apparent in the gross photographs. Thin, scarred sclera in the resected bed treated with diathermy can be compared with sclera of normal thickness in the eye treated with cryotherapy. Chorioretinal adhesion in each eye is firm enough to prevent separation of retina from underlying choroid by artifactitious detachment (Figs. 10-5 and 10-6). No significant inflammatory reaction is present within either eye or its wall. The area of scleral resection and diathermy beneath the retinal tear is seen in Fig. 10-7, and sclera treated with diathermy posterior to this is seen in Fig. 10-8. Scleral scarring represented by increased cellularity and haphazard nuclear arrange-

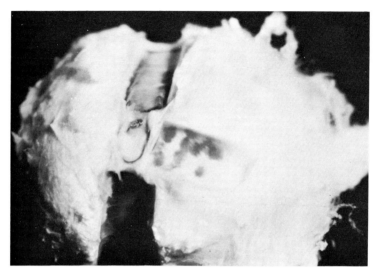

Fig. 10-1. (OS) Diathermized area of equatorial and radial scleral resection. Implants removed. Suture of radial implant remains.

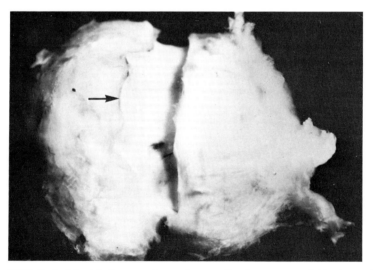

Fig. 10-2. (OD) Bed of buckle in area of cryotherapy. Implants removed. Dark scar in middle of bed is the fluid drainage site. Indentation of eye produces dark shadow on the posterior side of the buckle. Note connective tissue sheath *(arrow)* along anterior edge of buckle and how it is folded forward.

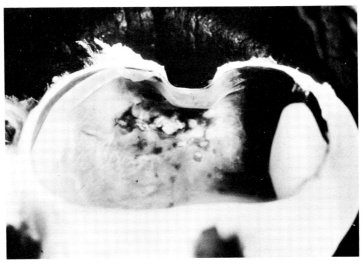

Fig. 10-3. (OS) Cross section of eye treated with diathermy. Thin sclera at site of resection. Pigmented scar from diathermy at site of original retinal tear. Posterior detachment is artifactitious.

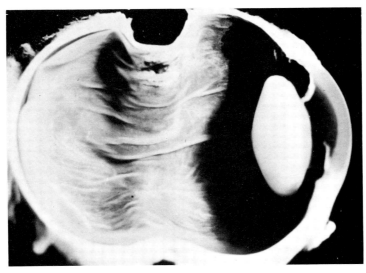

Fig. 10-4. (OD) Cross section of eye treated with cryotherapy. Normal scleral thickness. Pigmented scar from cryotherapy about the superior nasal retinal tear. Retinal folds represent postmortem change.

ment presents a significant change when compared to the sclera treated with cryotherapy in Fig. 10-9. Here, nuclei and collagen fibers retain their normal orientation with little, if any, alteration from adjacent untreated sclera. Chorioretinal adhesions in each eye (Figs. 10-8 and 10-9) appear firm and similar, except that choroidal atrophy secondary to cryotherapy is more pronounced. Retinal atrophy in each eye is quite similar.

The preceding photographs demonstrate that cryotherapy produces a firm chorio-

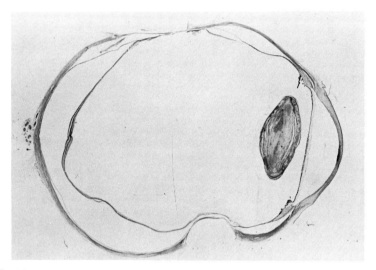

Fig. 10-5. (OS) Thin, attenuated sclera in area of resection and diathermy. Artifactitious retinal detachment. (H and E, ×6.)

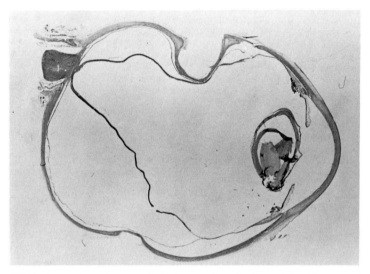

Fig. 10-6. (OD) Approximately normal-thickness sclera in bed of buckle treated with cryotherapy. Artifactitious retinal detachment. (H and E, ×6.)

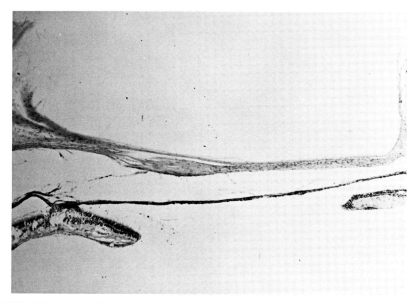

Fig. 10-7. (OS) Area of scleral resection and diathermy. Round margins of retina represent edges of retinal tear. Thin, scarred sclera in area of diathermy. (H and E, ×44.)

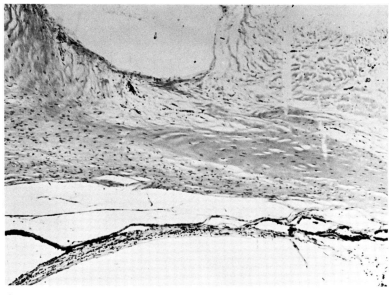

Fig. 10-8. (OS) Area posterior to Fig. 10-7. Scar secondary to diathermy through thicker sclera. Firm chorioretinal adhesion. (H and E, ×70.)

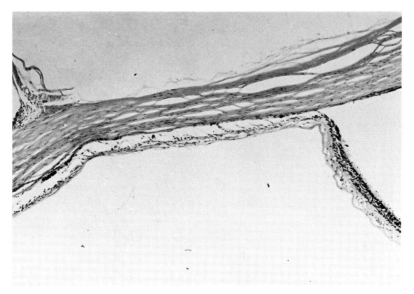

Fig. 10-9. (OD) Area of cryotherapy through full-thickness sclera. Scleral nuclei and fibers show little alteration from adjacent untreated sclera. Firm chorioretinal adhesion. (H and E, ×70.)

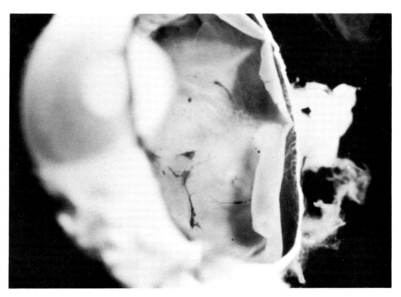

Fig. 10-10. (OS) Same eye as in Fig. 10-3. Pigmented scars extend along the surface of the retina.

retinal adhesion, with neither scleral necrosis nor scarring. The ancillary benefits of this feature to retinal surgeons are manifold. In primary retinal detachment surgery, scleral undermining or resection is unnecessary since transscleral cryotherapy can be applied without scleral damage. Intrascleral sutures position implant material on the scleral surface. Relocation of sutures may simply move the implant, if desired. Additional implant may be incorporated into initial buckle with supplemental sutures. The fact that there is little scarring and that the strength of the scleral wall is about the same as in an untreated eye[1] provides even greater dividends at reoperation. Less scarring facilitates exposure of the previous operative area, and a stronger wall decreases the risk of rupturing the globe. Muscles need not be detached from the globe even in areas of previous cryotherapy. Treatment with cryotherapy may proceed with the same precautions as in primary cases, with no greater fear of perforation. Thus cryotherapy has facilitated retinal detachment surgery technically and, at the same time, produces satisfactory chorioretinal adhesion.

Retinal and vitreous membranes provide interesting ocular pathology, but to the patient and ophthalmologist they may cause great concern. Fig. 10-10 demonstrates another view of the same eye as Fig. 10-3 does. Linear pigmented scars course along the inner retina. Photomicrographs reveal these scars to be cellular membranes lying on the retinal surface containing pigment. One membrane extends from the posterior aspect of the retinal tear (Fig. 10-11) to the disc across the macula (Fig. 10-12). Here the membrane can be seen distinct and detached from the plicated internal limiting membrane. In spite of these changes on the internal retinal surface and a detached macula prior to operation, visual function remained at 20/50. Similar preretinal membrane formation was observed clinically in a 61-year-old man who had a large superonasal retinal tear. Photocoagulation was placed about the

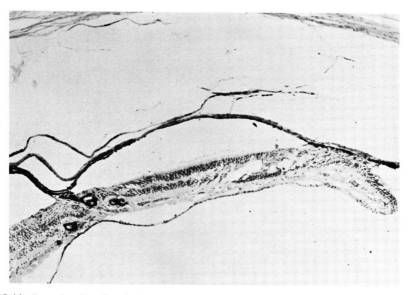

Fig. 10-11. Posterior lip of retinal tear with preretinal membrane extending toward the disc. (H and E, ×70.)

tear, but its nasal margins became elevated after treatment. Twelve days later, surgery was performed with Silastic sponge implanted beneath the tear, which was treated with cryotherapy. Fig. 10-13 shows the macula 2½ weeks after surgery when vision had decreased from 20/20 in the first postoperative week to 20/80. At this time, the macula had a slight grayish cast. There was a retinal traction fold extending from the posterior aspect of the tear with adherent vitreous. Two weeks

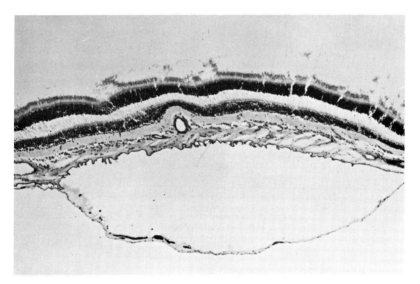

Fig. 10-12. Preretinal membrane containing pigment in the macular region and detached from the folded internal limiting membrane. (PAS, ×70.)

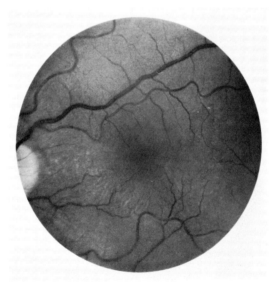

Fig. 10-13. Fundus photograph of slight macular graying in patient with 20/80 vision 1 month after retinal detachment surgery.

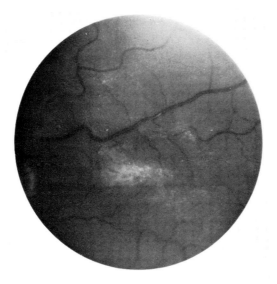

Fig. 10-14. Fundus photograph 2 weeks after that of Fig. 10-13. Macular pucker evident. Vision 20/300.

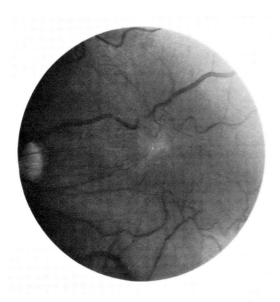

Fig. 10-15. Fundus photograph 1 month after that of Fig. 10-14. Macular folds more discrete. Vision 20/200. Note the increased tortuosity of the blood vessels when compared to those in Fig. 10-13.

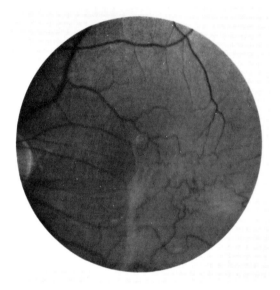

Fig. 10-16. Fundus photograph of macular pucker and increased tortuosity of retinal blood vessels.

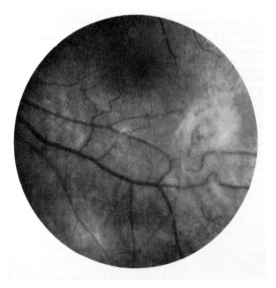

Fig. 10-17. Fundus photograph of same eye as in Fig. 10-16 six months later. Wrinkles in macula are gone, with decreased vascular tortuosity. Traction folds are now inferotemporal to macula. Tortuosity of retinal blood vessels is primarily in area of traction.

later, macular puckering reduced vision to 20/300 (Fig. 10-14). In 4 more weeks, macular traction became consolidated (Fig. 10-15). The retinal folds were more discrete and tortuosity of retinal vessels increased when compared with Fig. 10-13. Vision stabilized to 20/200 where it has remained for the past year. These photographs record the acute phase of preretinal membrane formation beginning 1 month after symptoms and photocoagulation and 2½ weeks after surgery.

Another case of preretinal membrane formation causing macular pucker (Fig. 10-16) comparable to the previous case occurred in a 63-year-old woman who had noted visual distortion 2 months previously. However, she had received no treatment of any kind. Examination demonstrated characteristic wrinkling of the internal retinal layers with adherent vitreous and vision decreased to 20/70. Ophthalmoscopy of the peripheral fundus revealed three retinal tears. Six months later (Fig. 10-17), the area of traction had moved inferotemporally from the macula, which now appeared smooth with less vascular tortuosity. Vitreous was still attached to wrinkled gray retina and was in continuity with a band that extended from the flap of the horseshoe tear at 6 o'clock. Retinal blood vessel tortuosity is primarily associated with the new area of traction. With this shift in retinal traction, vision improved to 20/30.

These three cases illustrate many features of preretinal membrane formation in its less severe degree. The involved area has retinal graying with tortuosity of retinal blood vessels. Examination of the retina with a contact or Hruby lens reveals folds of the internal retinal layers. Vitreous can usually be traced to peripheral retinal folds but not necessarily to the macula since vitreous may have been detached previously from this area. These cases point out that preretinal membrane may occur not only after diathermy, photocoagulation, and cryotherapy but also spontaneously. The

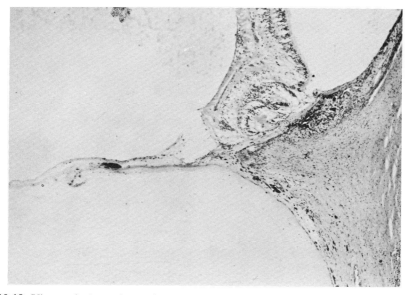

Fig. 10-18. Vitreoretinal membrane formation at site of penetrating diathermy scar. (H and E, ×70.)

onset after the initiating episode so frequently ranges from 4 to 6 weeks that we recognize it as the "6-week syndrome" at the Bascom Palmer Eye Institute. Vision may be affected to varying degrees, but, following detachment surgery once the acute phase is over, there is relative visual stability. In a similar fashion, the retina usually does not detach later if it does not do so in the acute phase. The etiology and origin of inner retinal membranes have not been determined. The membrane stains blue with the Masson trichrome stain. A mesodermal rather than a neural origin seems more likely, and vitreocytes probably play a major role in its formation. Predisposing conditions include large horseshoe tears, multiple horseshoe tears, tears with vitreous bleeding, inflammation in the vitreous, penetrating trauma of the posterior segment, retinal perforation when treating with diathermy (Fig. 10-18) or when draining subretinal fluid, and overzealous use of diathermy, cryotherapy, or photocoagulation. Diseased or damaged vitreous is prevalent in all these conditions. An appealing concept is that the cell begins to lay down its membrane after the initiating episode and contraction of this membrane occurs during the next 4 weeks.

Preretinal membrane formation of a more malignant degree, frequently called "massive vitreous retraction," is demonstrated in an eye of a 46-year-old man whose symptoms dated 3 weeks prior to surgery. Although extensive surgery was required to close at least 10 horseshoe tears, the retina was reattached 1 week postoperatively. However, at the time of examination 10 days later and about 5 weeks from onset of his detachment, his retina was nearly totally detached in many rigid folds and so remained for the next 4 months (Fig. 10-19). Because of extensive vitreous membrane formation, surgery was performed to incise these bands under direct microscopic examination after removal of the lens. This procedure was considered preparatory to

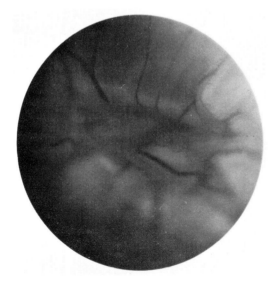

Fig. 10-19. Fundus photograph 4 months after unsuccessful retinal detachment surgery. Nearly total detachment with extensive retinal folds obscuring the disc. Small area of attachment to the buckle above.

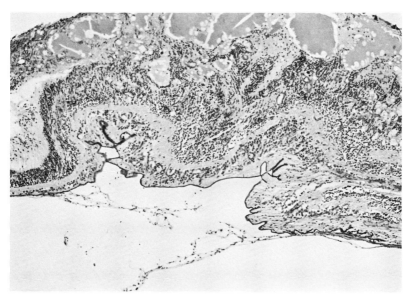

Fig. 10-20. Preretinal and vitreous membrane formation. Note the cellular membrane connecting the retinal folds and extension of the membrane into the vitreous. (PAS, ×70.)

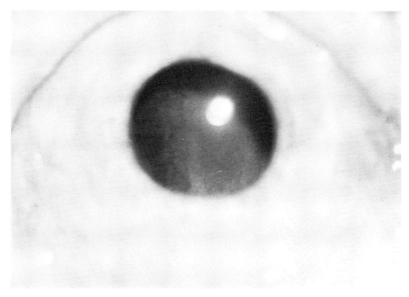

Fig. 10-21. Massive choroidal detachment in an aphakic eye. Dome-shaped area extending from below and occupying most of the pupillary area is the choroidal detachment. The dark band on the left side of the mound is the pars plana ciliaris.

another scleral buckling procedure. When the patient returned 6 weeks postoperatively, the retina was attached throughout except for extensive traction folds over and posterior to the buckle. This case emphasizes again the relation in time of this condition to the symptoms and surgery. It also demonstrates more extensive membrane formation. The fact that the retina has changed little in 2 years again indicates relative stability after initial shrinkage of the membrane. A pathologic illustration of extensive preretinal formation and rigid retinal folds after unsuccessful retinal detachment surgery is seen in Fig. 10-20. Long-standing retinal degenerative changes and exudation are particularly apparent in the outer retinal layers. Cellular membranes unite the folds of internal retinal layers and extend into the vitreous. This photomicrograph illustrates the membranes that retinal surgeons attack when performing intravitreal surgery and indicates how formidable a task the cure of this disease is.

Passing from preretinal membrane formation, I wish to discuss choroid and suprachoroidal space following detachment surgery. Expansion of suprachoroidea occurs to some degree after all retinal detachment surgery and is recognized as a smooth, round, grayish brown elevation on ophthalmoscopic examination. This expansion of the suprachoroidal space is commonly known as choroidal detachment or "choroidals." In ordinary circumstances, it regresses without difficulty, but, on occasion, the suprachoroidal space can enlarge so much that choroidal detachment is visible on examination with a hand light and prevents viewing of part or all of the fundus. The photograph (Fig. 10-21) illustrates such a case in the early postoperative period of a 76-year-old aphakic woman. The dome-shaped elevation occupying the inferior three fourths of the pupil is a choroidal detachment. This patient had a transient period of elevated intraocular pressure that abated as the choroidal regressed. Elevation of the choroid and ciliary body by expansion of the suprachoroidal space pushes forward the head of the ciliary body and iris root. If severe enough, this process occludes the filtration angle. Fig. 10-22 illustrates a choroidal detachment extending over the ciliary body and rotating it forward to compromise the angle. Clinical examination confirms this impression since the anterior chamber is very shallow peripherally and the angle is closed on gonioscopy. Occasionally, uncontrolled pressure requires surgical drainage of the choroidal detachment, but the vast majority of cases respond to medical therapy in the acute period and require no further medication.

Trauma and hypotony are two of the components in formation of choroidal detachment. The use of cryotherapy during surgery enhances hypotony because there is no shrinkage of collagen as with diathermy. On the other hand, cryotherapy decreases manipulation of the globe because scleral undermining is eliminated. My initial impression was that the incidence of choroidal detachment was higher following cryotherapy. In comparison of 150 cases using diathermy and 150 cases using cryotherapy,* choroidal detachment was recorded 22 and 27 times, respectively. This figure indicates no significant statistical difference in the incidence of choroidal detachments in either group. Surprisingly, choroidal detachment did not influence the success of the operation or the visual result. Twenty-five of 27 eyes (93%) with cho-

---

*I wish to thank Dr. George F. Hilton for providing the data in these cases.

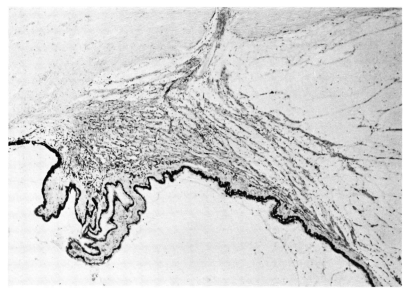

Fig. 10-22. Choroidal detachment extending over the ciliary body and rotating it forward to occlude the angle. (H and E, ×44.)

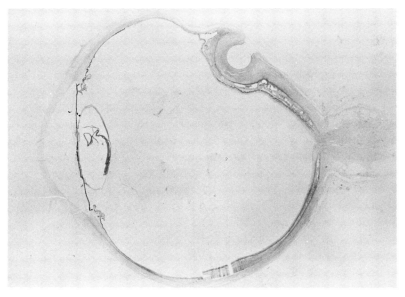

Fig. 10-23. Photomacrograph 3 days after successful scleral buckling. Retina is attached. Engorgement of choroid. Empty circular space outside sclera represents site of polyethylene implant. (H and E, ×5.) (Courtesy of the Pathology Laboratory of the Massachusetts Eye and Ear Infirmary.)

roidal detachment and 116 of 123 eyes (94%) without choroidal detachment had successful reattachments. In each group, 56% attained visual acuity of 20/50 or better in 6 months or more. Choroidal detachment does bear a relationship to postoperative glaucoma since two of three eyes with glaucoma were among the 27 eyes with choroidal detachment. Surgical drainage of the choroidal detachment was not performed in any of these eyes. In all three cases, medical management satisfactorily controlled the glaucoma. Perhaps surgical drainage in selected cases would reduce postoperative glaucoma, but this series cannot statistically evaluate this hypothesis.

Dilatation and engorgement of the choroidal vessels occur during and following detachment surgery. The photomacrograph (Fig. 10-23) illustrates an eye of a patient who died 3 days following uncomplicated retinal detachment surgery. The retina is attached throughout and the eye is apparently on its way to an uneventful recovery. The choroidal engorgement and dilated vessels overlie the buckle (Fig. 10-24). Pigment epithelium and inner choroid are thrown into shallow folds. On the opposite side of the eye, in addition to choroidal engorgement, suprachoroidal hemorrhage has separated its fibers and expanded its space (Fig. 10-25). And so, even in well-executed retinal detachment surgery, there is secondary dilatation of choroidal vessels and, at times, a small amount of bleeding into the suprachoroidal space. Following cryotherapy, there is also engorgement of the choroidal vessels. Fig. 10-26 demonstrates a lesion 30 minutes after application of transscleral cryotherapy in a rabbit eye. Increased choroidal thickness readily demarcates the area of treatment. The clinical importance of this observation is that meticulous care should be used to avoid rupturing choroidal blood vessels during drainage of subretinal fluid. Subretinal dissection of blood into the macula may convert an eye with good visual prognosis

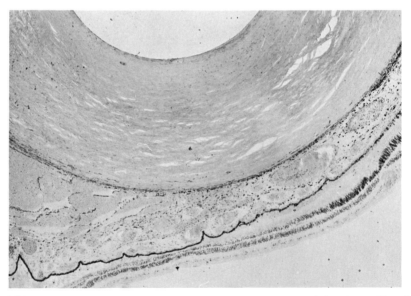

Fig. 10-24. Retina and choroid overlying buckle of eye in Fig. 10-21. Note dilatation of choroidal vessels and folds of pigment epithelium and inner choroid. No inflammatory reaction about site of polyethylene tube. (H and E, ×44.)

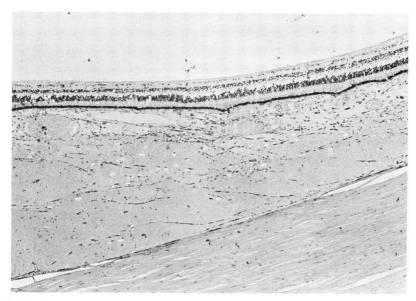

Fig. 10-25. Opposite side of eye in Fig. 10-22. Note expansion of suprachoroidal space by blood. (H and E, ×44.)

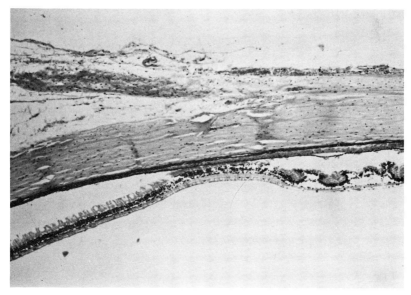

Fig. 10-26. Area of transscleral cryotherapy 30 minutes after treatment in a rabbit. Note dilatation of the choroidal vasculature in the area of treatment on the right side compared to the untreated left side. (H and E, ×44.)

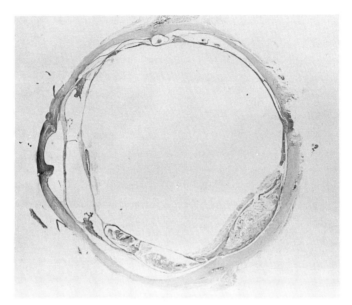

Fig. 10-27. Photomacrograph of blood in the subretinal space long after retinal detachment surgery. (H and E, ×5.)

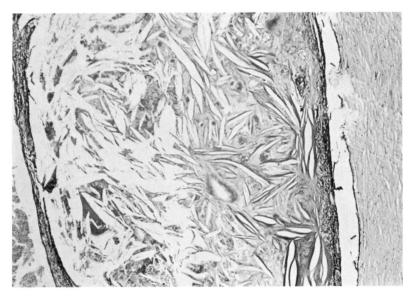

Fig. 10-28. Thin, atrophic, degenerated retina overlying blood and cholesterol in subretinal space. Blood is in the vitreous to the left of the retina. (H and E, ×44.)

to one with poor prognosis in spite of successful reattachment. The photomacrograph (Fig. 10-27) and photomicrograph (Fig. 10-28) demonstrate blood in the subretinal space. Retinal degeneration overlying the residual blood and cholesterol destroys visual function in this area. Choroidal hemorrhage may extend into and expand the suprachoroidal space so that the hemorrhagic choroidal detachment may cause problems previously described with serous choroidal detachment. At operation, the globe becomes firm and operative management more difficult. Postoperatively, if glaucoma ensues, it may be more refractory to management than glaucoma following serous choroidal detachment, especially since the choroidal detachment may last longer. Blood usually dissects into the vitreous with large hemorrhagic choroidal detachments and may obscure the fundus for a prolonged period of time. Since hemorrhage at the drainage site has so many serious consequences, careful inspection of the puncture site to avoid rupture of a choroidal vessel cannot be overemphasized. If the retinal detachment can be managed without subretinal fluid drainage, according to Custodis' technique,[2] this is the operation of choice.

The possibility of confusion of choroidal detachment with malignant melanoma bears mention. Recent surgery and opportunity to observe regression of the choroidal detachment should temper any hasty decision to make the diagnosis of malignant melanoma. The frequently circumferential distribution of the choroidal detachment favors its diagnosis, as well as the lack of a transillumination defect, if the fluid is serous. However, blood may produce a defect on transillumination and interference with transillumination does not in itself indicate a tumor.

The final aspect of pathologic changes following surgery that I wish to discuss is

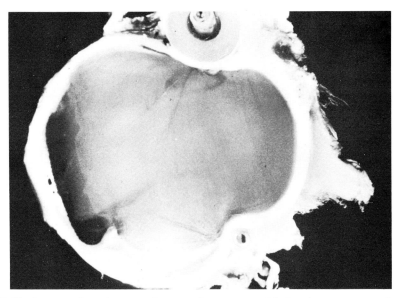

Fig. 10-29. Cross section of an eye 4 years after unsuccessful detachment surgery. Large silicone tube encompasses two polyethylene tubes. Total retinal detachment. No scleral reaction about implant.

tissue tolerance to the implant material and suture. After reviewing microscopic slides in which polyethylene and silicone implant material has been used, I have been impressed by the remarkable lack of reaction about polyethylene and silicone implants. Photomacrographs in Figs. 10-5, 10-6, and 10-23 and photomicrographs in Figs. 10-7 to 10-9, and 10-24 confirm this observation. Usually, if any inflammatory reaction is seen, even in eyes that are abject failures, it is about suture material and not about implants. The gross pathologic specimen (Fig. 10-29) demonstrates an eye removed 4 years after unsuccessful detachment surgery. A large silicone tube envelops two polyethylene implants. Grossly, no inflammatory reaction encompasses the implant material. Microscopically, no inflammation surrounds the implant site and only a small linear area of chronic inflammatory reaction, perhaps along a suture tract, is seen (Fig. 10-30). Another case in point is a piece of Silastic sponge material that was implanted anterior to the superior rectus muscle 2 years previously in a 58-year-old man. This implant has been tolerated well, with no evidence of reaction (Fig. 10-31). Likewise, reaction to suture is minimal in uncomplicated cases. The tissue about a piece of 5-0 monofilament nylon suture in the next photomicrograph (Fig. 10-32) contains a few chronic inflammatory cells and is very minimal. This suture was in place 8 months and the section is from the same eye as in Fig. 10-2. The thin hyaline band immediately beneath the site of the implant and external to the sclera represents a thin connective tissue sheath that forms about silicone implants. The external aspect of the sheath, which overlays the silicone implant (Fig. 10-2) can be seen at the anterior edge of buckle and folded forward after it was cut. Usually, minimal inflammatory reaction occurs about the suture and none about the implant.

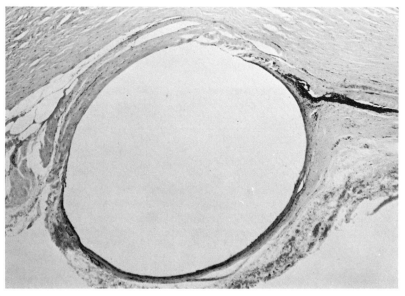

Fig. 10-30. Same eye as in Fig. 10-29. Site of silicone tube. No inflammatory reaction about the implant. Dark band on right represents focal area of chronic inflammation. (H and E, ×44.)

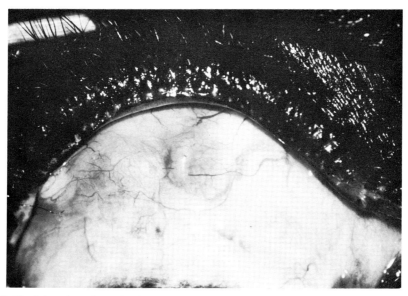

Fig. 10-31. Subconjunctival Silastic sponge implant anterior to superior rectus muscle in place for 2 years.

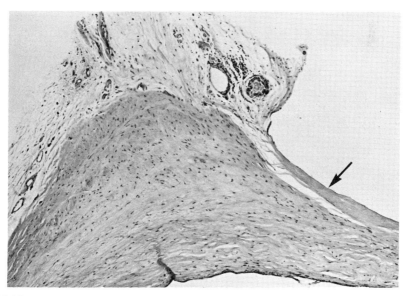

Fig. 10-32. Suture in episclera at margin of site of silicone implant. Minimal collection of chronic inflammatory cells. Thin hyaline band *(arrow)* on scleral surface is a connective tissue sheath. (H and E, ×70.)

More significant reaction may occur, as demonstrated in an eye in which scleral resection had been performed a year previously. Extensive granulomatous inflammatory reaction, including foreign-body giant cells, surrounds the suture (Fig. 10-33). Suture material may evoke formation of granulation tissue, as illustrated in Fig. 10-34. Invariably, a fistulous tract adjacent to the granulation tissue will lead to a suture. Reaction may be localized. If so, excision of suture and adjacent implant material may heal this area without removing the whole implant. Persistent postoperative pain should alert the ophthalmologist to infection about the implant, as illustrated in the case of a 60-year-old diabetic woman who presented diffuse redness and tenderness over the buckle 1 month after retinal detachment surgery (Fig. 10-35). At the time of removal of the silicone implant, there was a drop of pus at the 12 o'clock position. Internally, the eye was not affected, and the retina remained attached after removal of the implant.

In our cases, *Staphylococcus aureus* has been the most commonly isolated organism. Even *Staphylococcus albus* may be a pathogen in the presence of foreign material and should not be regarded as merely laboratory contaminant if there is significant growth on culture. In most eyes, if the retina is completely attached with a secure chorioretinal scar about the retinal break, implant material can be removed without compromising the surgical result. If infection extends into the eye, intensive antibiotic therapy must begin and the implant be removed. The seriousness of this complication cannot be overestimated since the eye may be lost. Postoperative pain without other obvious explanation must always remind the ophthalmologist of infection. Redness and tenderness help confirm this suspicion. If reaction is local, both antibiotic therapy and the patient's defense mechanism may suffice. If not, local or com-

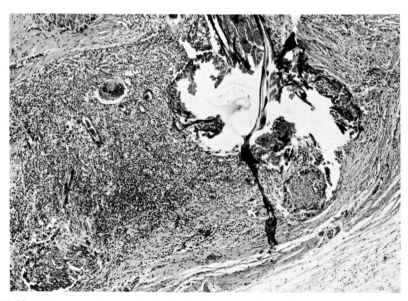

Fig. 10-33. Suture granuloma with foreign-body giant-cell reaction at the site of a scleral resection 1 year previously. (H and E, ×70.)

plete removal of the suture and implant is based upon the conditions. On ophthalmoscopic examination a white glob of exudate overlying the buckle, especially in the area of subretinal fluid drainage, signals the presence of infectious endophthalmitis. This demands rigorous antibiotic therapy and removal of the implant posthaste.

Cryotherapy has dramatically reduced inflammatory problems in our retinal detachment cases. No case of endophthalmitis has occurred in more than 750 cases in which cryotherapy has been the only physical agent used. In comparative series of

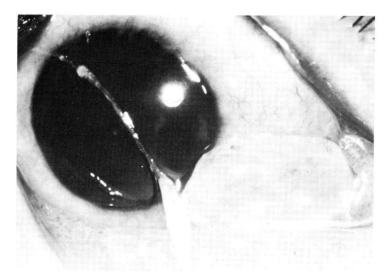

Fig. 10-34. Granulation tissue in postoperative scleral buckling.

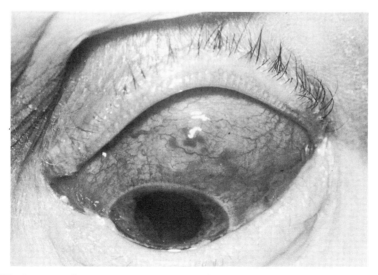

Fig. 10-35. Postoperative scleral buckling procedure with diffuse redness and local scleral abscess at 12 o'clock.

150 cases of diathermy and cryotherapy, there were two cases of endophthalmitis with diathermy versus none with cryotherapy. There were nine cases of external infection after diathermy and two cases after cryotherapy. No implant extrusion occurred with cryotherapy and five cases occurred with diathermy. These clinical results correlate well with experimental work of Langston,[3] who concluded that the necrosis of connective tissue by diathermy played a significant role in infection.

The advances in retinal detachment surgery in the past 20 years rank with the finest achievements in all surgery. The intent of this pathologic review is to help the ophthalmologist understand the ocular reaction to detachment surgery so that complications will be fewer, be recognized earlier, and be more amenable to treatment.

REFERENCES

1. Hall, G. A., and Schlegel, W. A.: Relative bursting strength of rabbit sclera after cryosurgery and diathermy, Arch. Ophthal. **78:**521, 1967.
2. Custodis, E.: Bedeutet die Plombenaufnähung auf die Sklera einen Fortschritt in der operativen Behandlung der Netzhautablösung? Ber. Deutsch. Ophth. Ges. **58:**102, 1953.
3. Langston, R., Lincoff, H. A., and McLean, J. M.: Scleral abscess. II. The experimental production in animals, Arch. Ophthal. **74:**665, 1965.

11

Current management of giant retinal breaks*

H. MacKenzie Freeman

Giant retinal breaks (Fig. 11-1) extend 90 degrees or more around the circumference of the ocular globe. Not all giant breaks carry a poor prognosis; the treatment of favorable cases such as giant retinal dialysis does not necessarily pose unusual difficulties. This presentation discusses preoperative management, surgical technique, and results in a series of 42 patients examined at the Retina Service of the Massachusetts Eye and Ear Infirmary and at the office of Retina Associates during 1967. In addition to the management of favorable cases, this report discusses the surgical treatment of more difficult ones: those complicated by inversion of the posterior retinal flap, an inverted retinal flap fixed to the underlying retina, and a posterior retinal flap immobilized by preretinal and vitreous membranes of massive preretinal retraction.

PREOPERATIVE MANAGEMENT

Preoperative management includes a study of both fundi with the binocular indirect ophthalmoscope and scleral depression. Examination of the deep vitreous with the contact lens and biomicroscope is indispensable to determine the presence of vitreous membranes or vitreous gel that would interfere with closure of the giant break. The patient is given a binocular bandage and put to complete bed rest. His head is so positioned that the anterior edge of the giant break is placed dependent. For example, a patient with a temporal giant break in the right eye lies with his head turned to the right. For a patient with a superior giant retinal break, the foot of the bed is raised.

Many cases are complicated by a partial or complete inversion of the posterior retinal flap (Fig. 11-2). The aim of preoperative management is to determine to

*This work was supported by U. S. Public Health Service research grants NB-03489 and NB-05691-03 from the National Institute of Neurological Diseases and Blindness.

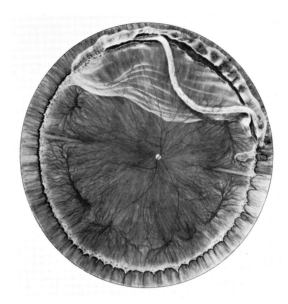

Fig. 11-1. Traumatic giant retinal dialysis. Vitreous base with torn strip of retina hanging into vitreous cavity.

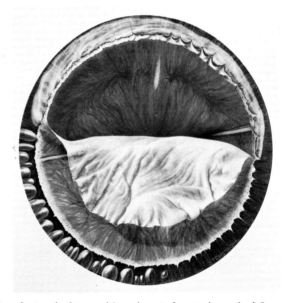

Fig. 11-2. Superior giant retinal tear with an inverted posterior retinal flap.

what extent the flap can be unfolded.[3] In such cases, supine positioning of the patient usually produces little or no improvement. In some cases, the flap can be made to unfold by prone positioning of the patient. In order to fully utilize the effects of gravity in unfolding the flap, a special power-driven operating table[4] is used (Fig. 11-3). After the patient has been secured to the table, it is rotated around a horizontal axis to a position that will unfold the flap. Best results are usually obtained when the patient is placed in the prone position because gravity moves the vitreous gel away from the inverted flap, allowing it to unfold (Fig. 11-4). The head and body are positioned at the angle that places the anterior edge of the giant break dependent. Gravity will then tend to bring together the two edges of the break. For instance, in a superior giant break the posterior retinal flap is inverted in an inferior direction toward the optic disc. Therefore, the patient is placed in the prone position with the head lowered at 45 degrees (Fig. 11-5, *B*). In order to place the anterior edge of a temporal giant break dependent, the patient must turn his head toward the shoulder opposite the affected eye (Fig. 11-5, *A*).

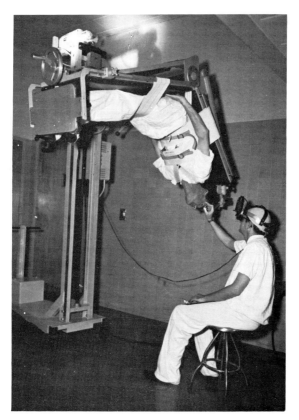

Fig. 11-3. Preoperative ophthalmoscopic examination is performed with the patient on the table. By rotating the table into various positions, it is possible to determine which position will unroll the inverted flap of a giant retinal break. For retinal incarceration, the patient is placed in this position.

In some cases in which the retinal flap cannot be unfolded by positioning, head movements or exercises are used. These movements consist of a fast component, a pause, and a slow component performed with the patient in the prone position. The fast component is made in the direction in which the flap is folded. For instance, in a superior giant break with a retinal flap folded downward, the fast movement is a rapid flexing of the neck downward (Fig. 11-6, *A*). In an inferior giant

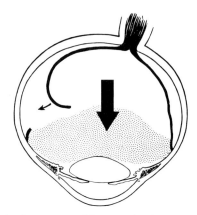

Fig. 11-4. With the patient in the prone position, gravity has moved the vitreous gel anteriorly, allowing the inverted posterior retinal flap to unfold.

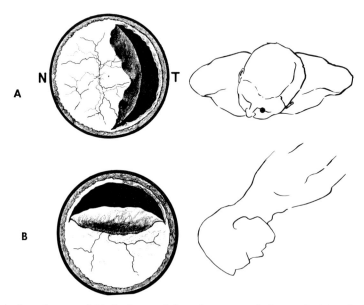

Fig. 11-5. A, In order to unfold the inverted flap of a temporal giant retinal break, the patient is prone positioned and his head is turned to the shoulder opposite the affected eye. (*N*, nasal; *T*, temporal.) **B,** In order to unfold the inverted flap of a superior giant retinal break, the patient is prone positioned and his head is lowered 45 degrees.

break the fast component is made in the opposite direction by starting with the chin on the chest and rapidly extending the neck. At the end of the fast component a pause is made to a slow count of three. During this pause the fluid vitreous continues to move in a circular path within the globe and impinges on the retinal flap to unfold it (Figs. 11-6, *B* and 11-7, *B*). Then the head is slowly moved in the reverse direction to the starting position of the next fast component. With temporal giant breaks, the flap is folded nasally; therefore, the fast component is made by rotating the head toward the shoulder opposite the affected eye (Fig. 11-7, *A*). These exercises are carried out under ophthalmoscopic control. After the exercises have been repeated five times, the fundus is carefully examined.

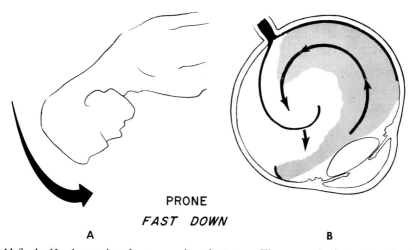

PRONE
FAST DOWN

A   B

Fig. 11-6. A, Head exercises for a superior giant tear. The arrow indicates the direction of the fast component. **B,** Movements of fluid vitreous within the eye at the end of the fast component.

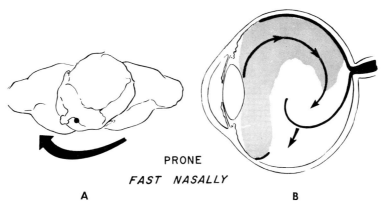

PRONE
FAST NASALLY

A   B

Fig. 11-7. A, Head exercises for a temporal giant retinal break. Arrow indicates the direction of the fast component. **B,** Movements of fluid vitreous at the cessation of the fast component.

For reference during surgery a notation is made of the position of the head that maintains the posterior retinal flap unfolded and of the direction of the fast component that unfolds an inverted retinal flap. With the patient in the prone position, a fundus drawing is made to show the extent to which the flap can be unfolded. In cases in which the posterior flap does not unfold completely, vessels of the exposed choroidal vasculature can mark the extent to which the flap unfolds.

The patient is returned to his bed and placed in the position that will keep the flap unfolded. Complete bed rest with both eyes covered is continued until surgery. Surgery should not be delayed because the unfolded retina may rapidly return to its original position and become immobile.

SURGICAL TECHNIQUE

The surgical technique in four types of cases will be considered: (1) a relatively favorable case such as a giant retinal dialysis with a posterior retinal flap that is not inverted when the patient is supine and that has no tendency to invert when the eye moves into different positions of gaze, (2) a case in which the posterior flap of a giant tear inverts when the patient is supine, (3) a giant tear with a posterior retinal flap that is inverted and adherent to the underlying retina, and (4) an eye in which shrinkage of the preretinal and equatorial membranes of massive preretinal retraction results in immobilization or retraction toward the disc of the posterior edge of the tear.

Posterior retinal flap remains unfolded with the patient supine (Fig. 11-1)

In relatively favorable cases such as a giant retinal dialysis in which the posterior retinal flap remains unfolded and shows no tendency to invert with the patient supine, a localizing mark is made about two disc diameters posterior to the lateral ends of the dialysis and in the meridian midway between these two. The incision for the scleral undermining joins these localizing marks. A lamellar scleral undermining 10 mm. wide is made to extend 5 mm. beyond the lateral ends of the giant break. The posterior scleral flap is made 6 mm. wide and the anterior flap is 4 mm. wide. An effort is made to preserve vortex veins by splitting the flaps of the scleral resection on each side of them. Sparse but strong diathermy is applied in the scleral undermining. A silicone rubber implant is inserted in the bed of the scleral resection, an encircling band is placed around the globe, and subretinal fluid is drained. If ophthalmoscopy reveals that the retinal break is situated well anterior on the scleral buckle and there are no meridional folds extending posteriorly over the crest of the buckle, no retinal incarcerations are attempted. The operation is completed as in the usual scleral buckling procedure. If meridional folds are present, the buckle is lowered by loosening the sutures of the scleral resection and by the intraocular injection of saline. If the posterior edge of the giant tear becomes partially inverted during release of subretinal fluid, retinal incarcerations as described in the following paragraph are attempted.

Posterior retinal flap that inverts with patient supine (Fig. 11-2)

In cases with an inverted posterior retinal flap, the operation is begun with the patient supine. Localizing marks are made two disc diameters posterior to the

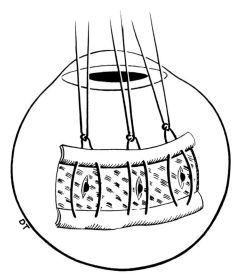

Fig. 11-8. A scleral resection with three sclerotomy sites. A knuckle of choroid is seen protruding through the sclerotomies.

lateral ends of the giant retinal break. Attempts are made to unfold the retinal flap using forced ductions of the globe in the direction in which the flap is inverted. In rare cases in which forced ductions performed with the patient in the supine position will unfold the retinal flap, a localizing mark is made two disc diameters posterior to the posterior edge of the giant break, midway between the marks that localize the lateral ends of the giant break. In most cases, however, the posterior retinal flap cannot be adequately unfolded with the patient supine because of the effect of gravity on the vitreous gel that rests on the retinal flap. After reference to the preoperative drawings, a localizing mark is made three disc diameters posterior to the choroidal vessels that mark the extent to which the tear unfolded preoperatively. The incision for a 10 mm. lamellar scleral undermining is made by joining these localizing marks and extending 5 mm. beyond the lateral ends of the giant retinal break. Meridional sclerotomy sites for retinal incarcerations are localized 45 degrees apart in the posterior half of the lamellar scleral undermining (Fig. 11-8).[5] They must be located to avoid large vessels during perforation of the choroid. The choroidal vasculature is revealed by transillumination through the cornea with a compact and powerful transilluminator built for this purpose. A 3 mm. scleral incision is made in a meridional direction at each incarceration site. A mattress suture is placed in the scleral flaps over each sclerotomy, and a small implant of silicone 6 mm. wide and 8 mm. long is placed under each mattress suture (Fig. 11-9). The knuckle of choroid exposed through the incision is treated with very light surface diathermy by use of a blunt electrode to lessen the chance of hemorrhage during perforation.

The patient is rotated to the prone position, which places the anterior edge of the giant break dependent, and ophthalmoscopy is performed to check that the posterior retinal flap is unfolded and remains draped over the incarceration sites. If the retinal flap is not adequately unfolded, forced ductions of the globe are done in the direction it is folded. When it has been unfolded as far as possible, the most easily accessible incarceration site is perforated and a substantial amount of fluid is drained to make room for injection of air into the vitreous cavity. The 6×8 mm. silicone implant is placed over the perforation site to prevent further drainage from the eye.

The injection of air into the vitreous cavity can be a useful adjunct in the treatment of giant breaks that have a mobile posterior retinal flap. It may further unfold an inverted retinal flap in cases in which insufficient improvement is obtained with positioning and exercises. An air bubble can be utilized to prevent the posterior retinal flap from inverting during attempts to incarcerate the retina. By proper postoperative positioning of the patient, the air bubble can be made to tampon the posterior retinal flap against the treated area. Injection of air is made through the pars plana on the side of the globe opposite the giant break. This injection is made under indirect ophthalmoscopic control to be sure that the air is not injected behind the flap. The patient's head is rotated in such a way that the bubble migrates across the posterior pole and then against the flap, which it tends to flatten against the choroid (Fig. 11-10).

The silicone implant is removed and a retinal incarceration is made by gently pressing a lens loop against the sclera over the area adjacent to the exposed choroidal perforation. Moderately rapid evacuation of fluid by gentle pressure of the lens loop helps to achieve incarceration. A sudden stoppage of flow suggests that incarceration has been achieved. Occasionally, incarcerated retina will appear grossly as a tiny gelatinous knuckle in the choroidal perforation. This appears ophthalmoscopically as a tiny star-shaped figure or a dimple in the retina. As soon as a small incarceration is obtained, the area is covered again with the 6×8 mm. silicone implant and the mattress suture is pulled up and temporarily tied. Then incarcerations are attempted at the remaining sites. A very oblique perforation of the choroid is made to avoid

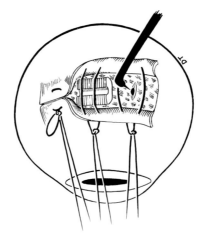

Fig. 11-9. Technique of retinal incarceration. Needle electrode is used to perforate the choroid of the sclerotomy. Retinal incarcerations have been made in the middle and right sclerotomy, which has been closed using a silicone implant.

perforating the posterior flap of the giant retinal break. If the eye becomes soft during attempts at incarceration, additional air is injected into the vitreous cavity.

When all the intended incarcerations are obtained, the patient is returned to the supine position and the silicone implants covering the incarcerations are replaced with a single implant beneath an encircling silicone band. It is important that the buckle be relatively low, because a high buckle may produce a purse-string effect on the retinal flap and cause meridional retinal folds. A double row of cryoapplications is applied over the untreated circumference of the globe. A narrower silicone implant is placed over the sclera and beneath the encircling band to produce a buckle that extends 360 degrees around the eye.

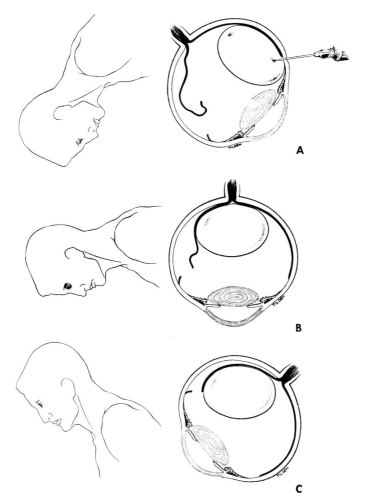

Fig. 11-10. **A,** Injection of air into the vitreous cavity in a superior giant break. In order to prevent the air from passing through the giant break, the patient's head is lowered and the injection is made through the pars plana opposite the tear. **B,** As the patient is rotated horizontally, the air bubble moves over the optic disc. **C,** When the head is raised, the air bubble passes over to the posterior retinal flap to tampon it against the choroid.

Postoperatively, the patient's head is positioned so that the air bubble will tampon the posterior retinal flap against the treated area. The patient is kept prone in bed 2 to 3 days with his head positioned to maintain the bubble against the flap. Maintaining the prone position is especially important in aphakic eyes to prevent the bubble from moving anteriorly to produce closure of the chamber angle and the formation of anterior synechiae. On the third or fourth day the patient is allowed to sit up, and, in order to maintain the bubble posteriorly against the retinal flap, his head is allowed to rest on an overbed table. The bubble is usually absorbed within 5 to 10 days.

Posterior retinal flap inverted and fixed to the underlying retina (Fig. 11-11)

In some cases the inverted retinal flap may adhere to the underlying retina so that it cannot be unfolded by positioning, head exercises, or an intravitreous air bubble. In such cases we have employed a vitreous cryoprobe, cooled by carbon dioxide, to mobilize it. The part of the probe that enters the eye is 1.4 mm. in diameter and 2 cm. in length. It is introduced into the vitreous cavity through a sclerotomy over the pars plana in the meridian opposite the middle of the giant tear. The tip of the probe is guided under indirect ophthalmoscopic control to the posterior edge of the giant break. A small iceball is produced at the probe tip so that the free edge of the giant tear will adhere to it. Gentle and slow traction may free the flap from the underlying retina. The probe tip is reapplied to the edge of the flap in meridians where it appears to remain fixed. The incidence of vitreous hemorrhage has been high in our hands. To lessen the chance of hemorrhage, care should be taken to keep the tip of the probe in sight at all times to prevent the iceball from coming in contact with bare choroid or large retinal vessels. Once the posterior retinal flap has been freed from the underlying retina, the surgical technique is as described under part 2 for cases with an inverted retinal flap.

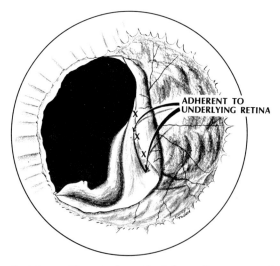

Fig. 11-11. Giant retinal tear with posterior retinal flap adherent to underlying retina.

Giant tear complicated by massive preretinal retraction (Fig. 11-12)

Preoperative and postoperative massive preretinal retraction is one of the commonest causes of failure in the treatment of giant retinal breaks. Shrinkage of the preretinal membrane produces immobilization or retraction toward the disc of the posterior flap of the giant break so that it cannot be unfolded by prone positioning, exercises, or an intravitreous air bubble. We have previously reported the injection of silicone oil into the vitreous cavity as a last resort in the treatment of these desperate cases.[1, 6, 7]

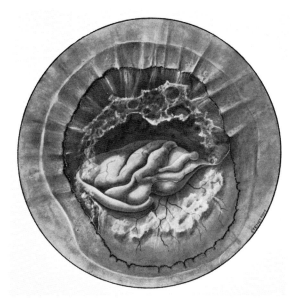

Fig. 11-12. Superior giant retinal tear complicated by massive preretinal retraction that results in immobilization of the inverted posterior retinal flap.

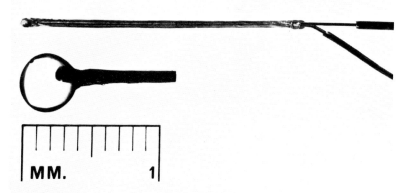

Fig. 11-13. The intraocular balloon used to manipulate a fixed inverted posterior retinal flap. The inset shows the balloon inflated.

Recently we have been evaluating the use of an intraocular balloon to unfold a fixed posterior retinal flap. The instrument consists of an inflatable balloon mounted on the end of one barrel of a double-barreled steel cannula (Fig. 11-13).[8] One cannula is used to inflate the balloon and the other to inject air or saline into the vitreous cavity while the balloon is being deflated. The globe is moderately softened by the release of subretinal fluid. The cannula is introduced into the vitreous cavity through a sclerotomy in the pars plana, and its tip is guided under indirect ophthalmoscopic control beneath the inverted retinal flap. The balloon is slowly inflated to a diameter of 3 mm. and used as a soft-tipped probe to break adhesions between the preretinal membranes of the inverted retinal flap and the underlying retina. Once these adhesions have been broken, the posterior retinal flap becomes mobile. The patient is rotated to the prone position, and an air bubble is injected under indirect ophthalmoscopic control beneath the flap to unfold it. The operation is completed as described in part 2.

In some eyes the dense vitreous membranes or bands may attach to the posterior retinal flap and prevent it from unfolding. These membranes or bands may be cut with special scissors[9] introduced through the pars plana ciliaris. Prior to operation, slit lamp examination of the vitreous cavity is indispensable to determine the extent of the structures that require cutting. Sectioning of the vitreous bands is done as a first step in the operation according to a technique already described. If this step is successful, the other surgical steps are executed as described in part 2.

RESULTS

Results are based on 42 eyes with giant retinal breaks operated on during 1967. It is significant that 100% of the eyes examined were operated on. Thus we are now attempting surgery in a greater number of unfavorable cases. Nine eyes (19%) had had from one to four procedures prior to referral. The retina was reattached in 22 of 42 eyes (52%). A 6-month follow-up is available on 11 of these 22 eyes.

Intraocular injection of silicone was used as a last resort in 12 eyes that developed severe massive preretinal retraction. The retina was reattached in 6 of these 12 eyes.

Too few operations using the vitreous cryoprobe or intraocular balloon have been done to warrant a significant comment on results. However, we have learned that the posterior retinal flap can be manipulated gently without serious complications and that adhesions immobilizing a retinal flap can be broken by use of the balloon or cryoprobe. It has been our experience that manipulation of the retina with these instruments can produce an extension of the giant break or serious hemorrhage into the vitreous cavity. The vitreous cryoprobe was used in six desperate cases. The retina was successfully attached in one eye, severe vitreous hemorrhage occurred in four eyes, and extension of the giant tear was produced in one eye. The intraocular balloon was used in three eyes. In one of these the retina was reattached. In another, the flap was successfully manipulated onto the buckle but surgery could not be completed because of vitreous hemorrhage. In the third eye, manipulation of the balloon resulted in the extension of a 300-degree giant tear to 360 degrees. In one eye, the retina reattached itself spontaneously, following the cutting of a vitreous membrane that developed after giant tear surgery.

Surgery failed in 20 eyes. Massive preretinal retraction resulted in 13 failures;

rupture of the globe occurred in one eye that had previously been ruptured by trauma; perforation of the globe occurred in one eye; severe vitreous hemorrhage complicated surgery in three eyes; and the giant tears were extended during surgery in two eyes.

SUMMARY

This report is based on the management of 42 cases of giant retinal break seen during 1967. The preoperative management includes careful binocular indirect ophthalmoscopy with the patient in both the prone and supine positions, biomicroscopy of the vitreous, and a study of the effects of positioning and exercises upon the inverted flap of the giant break. Present surgical techniques involve wide scleral undermining, intense but sparse diathermy applications in the undermined area, and small intentional incarcerations of the retina into the choroid in unfavorable cases. The injection of air into the vitreous cavity is an important and useful adjunct to unfold an inverted retinal flap and maintain it against the choroid during and following surgery. Preliminary work on desperate cases has been done with utilization of a vitreous cryoprobe, an intraocular balloon, or vitreous scissors to mobilize a fixed posterior retinal flap. One hundred percent of 42 eyes with giant breaks were operated on—nine eyes (19%) had had from one to four retinal detachment procedures prior to referral, and the retina was reattached in 22 eyes (52%). Massive preretinal retraction continues to be the most common cause of failure in these cases.

REFERENCES

1. Schepens, C. L., and Freeman, H. M.: Current management of giant retinal breaks, Trans. Amer. Acad. Ophthal. Otolaryng. **71:**474, May-June 1967.
2. Tolentino, F. I., Schepens, C. L., and Freeman, H. M.: Massive preretinal retraction, Arch. Ophthal. **78:**16, July 1967.
3. Freeman, H. M.: Treatment of giant retinal tears. In McPherson, A., editor: New and controversial aspects of retinal detachment, New York, 1967, Harper & Row, Publishers.
4. Schepens, C. L., Freeman, H. M., and Thompson, R. F.: A power-driven multipositional operating table, Arch. Ophthal. **73:**671, May 1965.
5. Schepens, C. L., and Freeman, H. M.: Surgery of retinal detachment. In Sorsby, A., editor: Modern trends in ophthalmology, ed. 4, London, 1967, Butterworth & Co., Ltd.
6. Dohlman, C. H., and Freeman, H. M.: Recent advances in the use of alloplastic materials in ocular surgery, Docum. Ophthal. **25:**1-20, 1968.
7. Freeman, H. M., and Cockerham, W. S.: Proceedings of the Fifth Symposium of the Gonin Club, 1968. (In press.)
8. Couvillion, G., Freeman, H. M., and Schepens, C. L.: Intraocular balloon. (In preparation.)
9. Freeman, H. M., Schepens, C. L., and Anastopoulou, A.: Vitreous surgery. II. Instrumentation and technique, Arch. Ophthal. **77:**681, May 1967.
10. Freeman, H. M., and Schepens, C. L.: Vitreous surgery, Mod. Prob. Ophthal. **7:**311, 1968.
11. Freeman, H. M., and Schepens, C. L.: Vitreous surgery, Trans. Amer. Acad. Ophthal. Otolaryng. **72:**399-409, May-June 1968.

12

Lamellar undermining, diathermy, and tissue transplantation versus cryotherapy and full-thickness scleral buckling*

Edward Okun

INTRODUCTION

Retinal detachment surgery and techniques have changed so rapidly over the past several years that one hardly has a chance to evaluate a particular procedure or material before a new one becomes available and receives enthusiastic support. Before all the old techniques are given up completely, it would be well to evaluate them critically and compare them to the new. Five years ago tissue transplantation as an adjunct to retinal detachment surgery was first subjected to intensive trial. It has given such excellent results that I feel this report is indicated. It is the purpose of this paper not only to report on our results with the use of preserved human sclera and autogenous plantaris tendon but also to compare these techniques to more recent methods of retinal detachment surgery utilizing full-thickness scleral buckling plus cryotherapy.[1]

The various techniques of scleral buckling with preserved human sclera and plantaris tendon have been adequately reported.[2-11] For the past several years we have used preserved human sclera primarily as a lining material to be placed between the encircling silicone band and the undermined, diathermized scleral bed. In this way, the implanted sclera acts both as padding to close the retina breaks and as protection against intrusion of the plastic element. A strip of sclera approximately 4 mm. wider than the undermined bed and of equal length is cut from a scleral shell that has been preserved in absolute alcohol (Fig. 12-1). The edges are serrated (Fig. 12-2), and the strip is then rinsed in three separate jars of saline to assure complete removal of all the alcohol. A running 5-0 Supramid suture is used

*This investigation was supported in part by research grant NB-01789, from the National Institute of Neurological Diseases and Blindness, National Institutes of Health, Bethesda, Maryland.

to close the bed, taking occasional bites in the anterior and posterior edges of the scleral implant (Fig. 12-3). In this way, the sclera is wrapped around the silicone implant, preventing direct contact between the synthetic material and the treated bed.

The second most popular use for preserved human sclera has been to stuff out

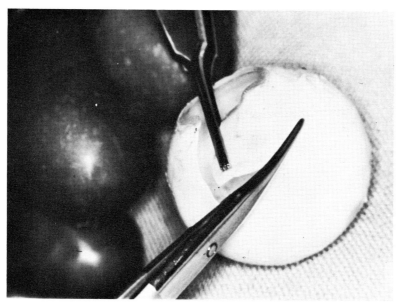

Fig. 12-1. Scleral strip being cut from scleral shell.

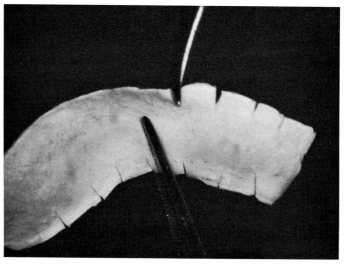

Fig. 12-2. Edges of strip of preserved sclera being serrated to insure smooth coverage of the silicone band.

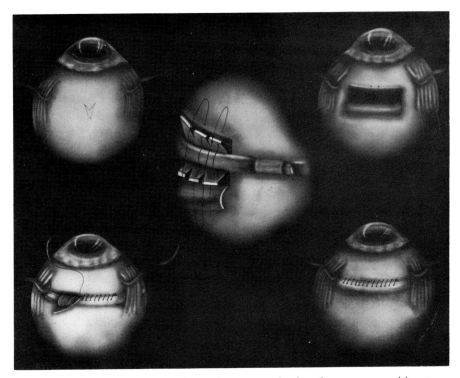

Fig. 12-3. Drawing shows method of suturing preserved sclera into proper position to serve both as lining of diathermized bed and as additional padding to help close the retinal break.

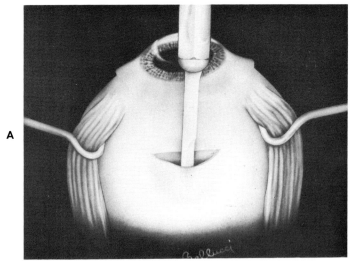

Fig. 12-4, A to **E.** Drawings illustrating the formation and stuffing of an intrascleral pocket with strips of preserved human sclera.

intrascleral pockets, the choroidal sides of which have been treated by either diathermy or cryosurgical applications. This procedure requires sclera of moderate thickness and usually entails drainage of subretinal fluid, sometimes combined with an intravitreal saline injection. The pocket is first lined by a piece of sclera that approximates the size of the pocket. One half of the pocket is then closed with a running 5-0 Supramid suture and scleral strips are pushed in between the outer wall of the pocket and the conforming piece of sclera. If this does not close or almost close the break, subretinal fluid is drained in the area of highest elevation, as far away from the break as possible. Following this, enough of the scleral strip is intro-

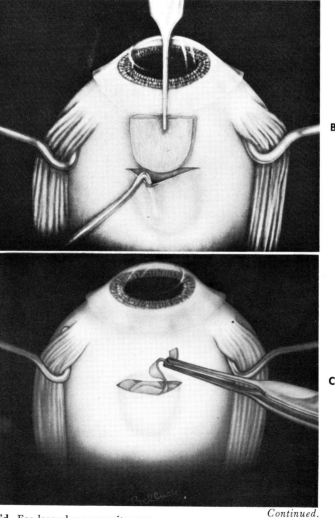

Fig. 12-4, cont'd. For legend see opposite page.

Continued.

duced into the pocket to form a smooth closure of the break. The opening to the pocket is then closed (Fig. 12-4).

Our favorite procedure for disinsertions of 2 to 5 hours has been the use of an intrascleral segmental buckle utilizing twisted or folded preserved sclera. A running 5-0 Supramid suture is used to loosely enclose the strip of sclera, and as the subretinal fluid is being drained, the preserved sclera is twisted and the running suture is gradually pulled tight from both ends. This procedure eliminates a period of marked hypotony and blocks the disinsertion before meridional folds have had a chance to form, thus producing a smooth, high buckle (Fig. 12-5).

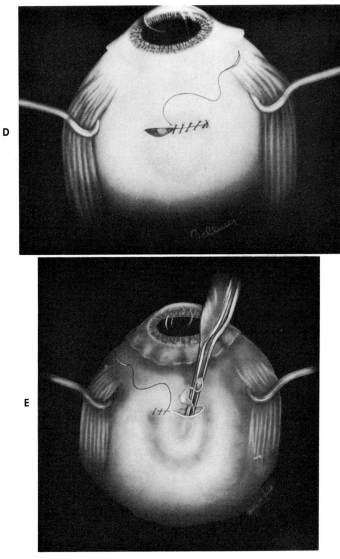

Fig. 12-4, cont'd. For legend see p. 186.

The autogenous plantaris tendon has been used in young people primarily as an encircling element. Padding can be provided either by the formation of a fusil as advocated by Crock[11] or by adding preserved human sclera under the implant. Since a more permanent buckle results from the latter technique, this has been our procedure of choice. The tendon has very little elasticity, necessitating evacuation of a moderate amount of subretinal fluid for the creation of a permanent buckle. It is anchored in each quadrant by a scleral tunnel and the ends secured by the first throw of a surgeon's knot in the tendon itself, plus one encircling and two transfixing 4-0 Supramid sutures (Fig. 12-6). The technique of tendon removal has been reported elsewhere.[11, 12]

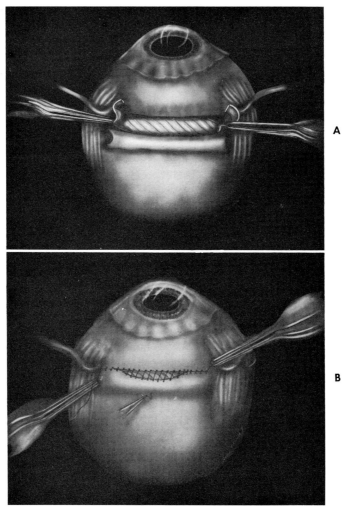

A

B

Fig. 12-5. Drawings illustrating the use of intrascleral, twisted, preserved sclera in the formation of a segmental buckle.

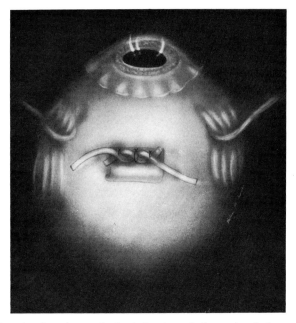

Fig. 12-6. Drawing showing the method of fixation of the ends of the encircling plantaris tendon. One 4-0 Supramid suture is tied around the first throw of a surgeon's knot created by the ends of the tendon itself. At either side of this knot, the tendon ends are transfixed with 4-0 Supramid.

RESULTS

The eyes in which sclera has been used as a lining for the undermined bed have displayed very smooth, healthy-appearing buckles (Fig. 12-7). There has been very little inflammatory activity in these eyes and the functional results have been most gratifying. Since only 5 years have elapsed since the earliest of these procedures, it is still too early to know whether intrusion will become a later problem. There have been no instances of choroidal hemorrhage, although in some cases the band has become prominent, mainly over staphylomatous areas where the band was left episcleral. In all the eyes in which preserved sclera has been used, smooth transitions are seen between the buried and nonburied areas of the band. Of 883 encircling procedures utilizing preserved human sclera, eight eyes remained irritated enough to warrant removal of the implant. There were three cases of endophthalmitis. Seventy-nine percent have remained successful without later complications. In contrast to this experience, intrusion of the silicone band with vitreous hemorrhage has occurred in several cases that were performed with scleral undermining and an encircling no. 40 silicone element without padding of any type.

In over 100 of these cases reoperation was required. These reoperations were much less hazardous than those in which plastic elements were allowed to remain in contact with the resected bed. In those reoperations occurring 3 or more months after the original scleral transplant, it appeared as if an episcleral procedure had

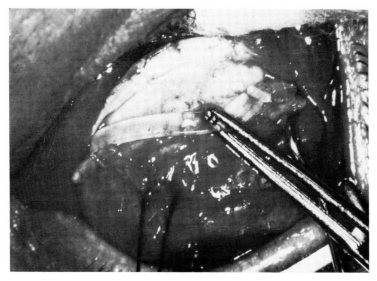

Fig. 12-7. Appearance of area of lamellar undermining, with overlying scleral graft 2 years postoperative. It appears as though a full-thickness scleral buckling has been performed.

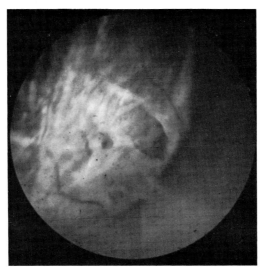

Fig. 12-8. Ophthalmoscopic appearance of intrascleral pocket plombage, 2 months postoperative.

been originally performed. The sclera appeared thicker in the previously diathermized zone and no signs of diathermy necrosis were visible (Fig. 12-7). In only three of the reoperated cases was the bed obviously weakened. A review of each of these cases revealed that there was a history of early postoperative inflammation that had apparently led to a certain degree of autolysis of the scleral graft. Reoperation was carried out without complication in each of these instances.

The localized pocket procedure results in a smooth, dome-shaped choroidal elevation that fills out and closes even the most dangerous-appearing retinal breaks (Fig. 12-8), effectively preventing "fish mouthing." Most of these pocket procedures lose their indenting effect after about 3 months. One year after surgery, these eyes appear as though they have been subjected to a straight diathermy procedure. Two recurrences have been attributed to this flattening effect. Of 197 of these procedures that have been followed longer than 6 months, 84% remain successfully reattached. One scleral implant had to be removed because of infection. The retina has remained well attached and this eye has maintained 20/25 visual acuity for the past 2 years.

The intrascleral segmental buckles consisting of twisted scleral implants have remained much longer. However, after 2 years, many of these buckles have also greatly diminished in height. Of 93 buckles, 79% have remained successfully reattached after 6 months.

Of 58 cases of scleral buckling procedures utilizing plantaris tendon as the encircling material, 88% have remained successful. The buckle created by this procedure is very smooth and has a tendency to gradually decrease with time. Two recurrences of aphakic detachments were attributed to this gradual loss of the buckle. Some eyes have retained excellent buckles 2½ years after surgery (Fig. 12-9).

Table 12-1 compares the 6-month reattachment rates achieved in comparable procedures since 1965. Procedures utilizing lamellar undermining, diathermy, and preserved sclera are compared to similar procedures utilizing cryocoagulation and full-thickness buckling. The slightly higher success rates achieved by the latter technique reflect, at least in part, the fact that initially these were more favorable cases. Whereas in 1965 cryocoagulation and full-thickness buckling made up only 10%

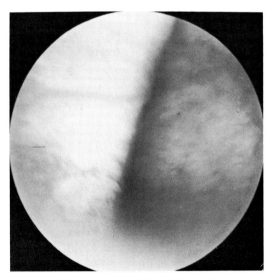

Fig. 12-9. Appearance of a 360-degree scleral buckling with autogenous plantaris tendon, 2½ years postoperative.

of our cases, in 1967 they made up 40%. In 1967, scleral undermining with tissue transplantation was used most frequently in young patients and in those with complicated retinal detachments.

COMMENTS

Scleral transplantation in the scleral buckling procedures allows the use of controlled diathermy in a thinned bed, with the advantage of full-thickness scleral protection. Since cryotherapy with full-thickness scleral buckling also provides full-thickness scleral protection, comparison must be between the permanency of the scars produced by diathermy and cryocoagulation, the relative tolerances of the materials used, and the operative risks of the procedures performed (Tables 12-2 and 12-3).

Diathermy has the distinct advantage of having weathered the test of time. When properly applied, it produces excellent, long-lasting, watertight chorioretinal seals. The cryogenic scars have done well thus far. However, there are certain differences in their clinical behavior and appearance. The early reaction from cryonecrosis does not seem to produce the sticky exudate that one sees with slightly excessive diathermy. Such an early reaction is advantageous in the therapy of very

Table 12-1. Anatomic reattachments after 6 months (January 1965—July 1967)

Lamellar undermining with diathermy and sclera			*vs.*	*Full-thickness buckling with silicone and cryocoagulation*	
*Number of cases**		*Percent success*			*Number of cases†*
82	Paufique pocket	84	93	Local (80% s̄ drainage)	116
93	Segmental buckle	79	85	Segmental buckle (56% s̄ dr.)	42
573	Encircling buckle	79	85	Encircling buckle (30% s̄ dr.)	115

*75% primary
†89% primary

Table 12-2. Diathermy vs. cryocoagulation

	Diathermy	*Cryocoagulation*
Long-term follow-up	+ + + +	+ +
Early sticky exudate	+ + + +	
Ideal chorioretinal scar	+ + +	+ +
Ophthalmoscopic control	+	+ + + +
Vitreous effect (overtreatment)	– – –	– –
Scleral necrosis	– – –	–
Elevation of I.O.T.	– – –	–
Thrombosis vortex veins	– – –	–

+ = Desirable quality
– = Undesirable quality

Table 12-3. Sclera vs. silicone

	Sclera	*Silicone*
General tolerance	++++	++++
Tolerance to large implants	++++	++
Effectiveness—intrascleral	++++	++++
episcleral	+	++++
Intrusion protection	++++	++
Intrusion		– –
Extrusion		– –
Safety of reoperation, previous diathermy	+++	++
Safety of reoperation, previous cryocoagulation	++++	++++
Effectiveness without drainage SRF	++	++++

+ = Desirable quality
– = Undesirable quality

large disinsertions. In general, cryotherapy produces greater retinal necrosis and subsequent atrophy with more abrupt margins. When the retina in these eyes redetaches, large ragged holes are sometimes produced. Both diathermy and cryocoagulation can produce good chorioretinal scars with very little evidence of vitreous damage. On the other hand, overtreatment with either modality can cause severe irreversible vitreous damage. Vitreous haze and subsequent band and strand formation as well as massive fibroplasia have been seen with excessive diathermy. Excessive cryocoagulation has also resulted in increased vitreous haze, with massive amounts of pigment released into the vitreous, and subsequent band and strand formation, with fibroplasia.

Our main indication for scleral lamellar undermining with diathermy and encirclage has been in aphakic and myopic retinal detachments associated with multiple small retinal breaks at various levels between the equator and ora, and associated with marked equatorial vitreous traction. These eyes have also been treated with episcleral encircling bands, plus full-thickness cryocoagulation. Our experience to date reveals a higher initial success rate in those cases that received the diathermy blockade. Several of the episcleral cases have either pulled away from the cryo scars or leaked between scars, leading to recurrences that have then responded to lamellar undermining with diathermy chorioretinal scarring. Regardless of the type of buckling procedure, full-thickness cryocoagulation has been applied to all areas of suspected leakage anterior to the buckle.

Intrascleral buckling with inclusion of preserved sclera generally produces a less irritated eye than does intrascleral buckling with episcleral silicone sponges and long sutures. Some of the more anteriorly placed sponges have become quite prominent and will probably have to be removed in the years to come. Interestingly enough, removal of the these sponges has not yet resulted in a recurrence of the detachment. Thus far, infection has not been a problem; however, as more sponges begin to extrude, this will most likely become more of a problem.

As long as the sutures remain in place, the indenting effect also remains. Some of our patients still show large internal plombages 3 years after surgery. The indentation produced by an episcleral technique is not as smooth as that produced by an intrascleral pocket, and the cryogenic chorioretinal scarring does not cover the area of push as evenly as in an intrascleral pocket procedure. Treatment that has been placed beyond the area of the episcleral push has led to secondary retinal breaks in two instances. Placement of therapy outside of the zone of choroidal push cannot occur in intrascleral procedures since, in these cases, the therapy is limited to the base of the pocket, with the possible exception of some anterior cryocoagulation.

One of the greatest advantages of cryotherapy over diathermy lies in the fact that cryocoagulation can be applied under opththalmoscopic control, assuring perfect placement of the lesions. Diathermy can also be applied in this way, but it results in excessive scleral necrosis, extensive retinal necrosis, and, in some instances, premature drainage of subretinal fluid.

It is technically easier to develop a very posterior intrascleral pocket than it is to place very posterior sutures for full-thickness scleral buckling. On the other hand, vortex veins can more easily be avoided by cryotherapy combined with full-thickness buckling.

In skilled hands, I do not believe that there is any greater operative risk to a primary scleral undermining than there is to a primary full-thickness scleral buckling. Inadvertent perforation, hemorrhage, and even vitreous loss and retinal incarceration can occur with either technique. Undermining is contraindicated in eyes with very thin scleras. Reoperations during the first 3 months are technically more dangerous in those eyes that have had scleral undermining plus diathermy. After 3 months, the reoperative risk is about the same, regardless of whether scleral undermining with scleral transplantation or full-thickness scleral buckling had been performed as the primary procedure.

Drainage of subretinal fluid can frequently be avoided by cryotherapy and full-thickness scleral buckling. This is a distinct advantage and avoids the occasional complication that can occur with drainage of subretinal fluid. However, if these cases end up with a higher long-term recurrence rate, we might wish that we had used diathermy and tissue transplantation and taken the operative risk of drainage of subretinal fluid during the primary procedure.

There are many different techniques available to reattach a detached retina. The best method is that which is least traumatic to the eye and at the same time yields the best long-term functional results. If two or more techniques are shown to give the same short-term results, repeated critical follow-up evaluations are required. Until one method of therapy is shown to be superior, we shall continue to use both lamellar undermining with diathermy and full-thickness buckling with cryocoagulation, favoring the use of tissue transplantation in young people.

REFERENCES

1. Lincoff, H. A., Baras, I., and McLean, J.: Modifications to the Custodis procedure for retinal detachment, Arch. Ophthal. 73:160, Feb. 1965.
2. Rodriguez-Vasquez, F.: New implant material for retinal detachment surgery, Amer. J. Ophthal. 53:937, 1962.
3. Paufique, L.: Rapport sur "inclusion sclérale." Presented before Club Jules Gonin, Lausanne, Switzerland, 1961.
4. Wilson, F. M.: Homografts of preserved sclera in retinal detachment surgery, Arch. Ophthal. 72:212, 1964.

5. Cibis, P. A., and Knobloch, W. H.: Scleral implants with preserved human sclera, Mod. Prob. Ophthal. **5:**293, 1967.
6. Knobloch, W. H., and Cibis, P. A.: Retinal detachment surgery with preserved human sclera, Amer. J. Ophthal. **60**(2):191, 1965.
7. Cibis, P. A., and Knobloch, W. H.: Scleral buckling procedures with preserved human sclera. In McPherson, A., editor: New and controversial aspects of retinal detachment, New York, 1967, Harper & Row, Publishers.
8. Spira, W.: Rapport sur deux ans d'inclusion sclérale. Presented at the third meeting of the Club Jules Gonin, Utrecht, Holland, 1963.
9. Sachsenweger, R.: Die Verwendung von lyophilisierten Gewebe als Plombenmaterial bei Ablatiooperation, Klin. Mbl. Augenheilk. **141:**431, 1962.
10. Miller, H. A., and Laroche, M.: Les techniques du bourrelet scléral dans le décollement de la rétine, Bull. Soc. Ophtal. Franc. **9:**946, 1961.
11. Crock, G. W., and Galbraith, J. E. K.: Autogenous biological polymers in retinal detachment surgery. I. The plantaris fusil, Brit. J. Ophthal. **50:**517, Sept. 1966.
12. Boniuk, I., and Okun, E.: An evaluation of the use of plantaris tendon in retinal detachment surgery. In Becker, B., and Drews, R., editors: Current concepts of ophthalmology, St. Louis, 1967, The C. V. Mosby Co.

13

Management of complex cases*

Charles L. Schepens

Complex cases of retinal detachment show infinite variety, and it is impossible to describe in detail how to handle each specific instance. In this presentation I will limit myself to a discussion of examples in which problems occur preoperatively or during surgery and to a description of the management of two types of problem cases.

PREOPERATIVE PROBLEMS

The two most frequent preoperative problems are interference with fundus observation and glaucoma. Other less frequent problems[1] such as the presence of active uveitis, choroidal detachment preceding retina surgery, external infection, medical disorders, and emotional instability will not be discussed here.

Interference with fundus observation

In all instances when ophthalmoscopy is rendered difficult by either a small pupil or opacities in the transparent media, the small-pupil ophthalmoscope,[2] designed according to Pomerantzeff's findings, is invaluable. This instrument is described in Chapter 3, "Techniques of Examination of the Fundus Periphery." Difficult ophthalmoscopy may be caused by vitreous hemorrhage, corneal or lens opacities, capsular remnants, and a small fixed pupil.

Vitreous hemorrhage. If the hemorrhage is so severe that the retinal breaks cannot be located, it is best to wait for it to clear. When the bleeding is recent, strict bed rest with a binocular bandage often hastens settling of the blood and minimizes the risk of further bleeding. It is helpful to place the bleeding site in a dependent position, if this site can be identified. If the vitreous has not cleared satisfactorily after 4 to 7 days of complete bed rest, it is better to postpone surgery until it does, the patient being allowed to return to his normal activities and examined in the office at intervals of 1 week or more. In some cases it is useful to perform

*This work was supported by U. S. Public Health Service research grant NB-03489.

ophthalmoscopy by using as a light source a powerful transilluminator whose tip is placed over the sclera (see Chapter 3). Attempts to aspirate a vitreous hemorrhage prior to retina surgery are not recommended.

In most cases in which a vitreous hemorrhage is caused by retinal detachment, bleeding occurs from a retinal vessel bridging a retinal break, generally a horseshoe-shaped tear. If the blood vessel is completely torn, a sudden large hemorrhage may follow. If it is only partly torn, chronic bleeding ensues that may continue for months or years. As soon as the retinal break responsible for the hemorrhage is found, it must be treated. The method of choice is a scleral buckling with fairly strong diathermy around the site of the break in an attempt to close the offending retinal vessel. If no buckling is effected, the retina may become reattached but bleeding may continue and a recurrence of retinal detachment is likely. In rare cases, the retina becomes reattached following a scleral buckling, but bleeding continues. An attempt is then made to occlude the offending vessel with photocoagulation, provided that the media are sufficiently clear and the retina is in contact with the buckle.

Lens or corneal opacities. In some instances of immature cataract or of corneal opacities with retinal detachment, retinal breaks cannot be found. If the retinal detachment is localized to one half the fundus or less and ophthalmoscopy is sufficiently clear so that the surgeon is confident that no retinal breaks are present posterior to the equator, it is best to perform a buckling procedure at the equator over the area of the detachment.

If the retinal detachment is total and the surgeon is fairly certain that no retinal breaks are present posterior to the equator, he may consider operating around 360 degrees in one session, placing the buckle at the equator. If this is done, three precautions must be taken: first, no more than two extraocular muscles should be detached; second, the long ciliary arteries and nerves should be spared from diathermy or cryoapplications; and, third, relatively light applications should be made. Even with cryoapplications, I have observed occasional damage to the long ciliary arteries, and this damage may lead to anterior segment ischemia or necrosis, particularly in old patients. If weak applications are made in a total detachment, the retina may fail to reattach and the whole operation may have to be repeated. For this reason I prefer to operate around 360 degrees in two stages: at the first operation three fifths of the circle are treated with fairly strong applications. Then, if the balance of the circle requires treatment, the buckle is completed 3 or 4 weeks later.

In all cases of total retinal detachment in which the fundus anterior to the equator cannot be adequately viewed because of cataract, one may prefer to perform a cataract extraction prior to retina surgery. This method becomes imperative in all retinal detachments, either partial or total, in which the fundus view is so impaired that breaks posterior to the equator cannot be ruled out. In these cases the lens should be removed in the capsule, with a full iridectomy. Personally, I routinely perform a sphincterotomy at the 6-o'clock position in order to ensure adequate viewing of the lower fundus even if the pupil becomes dragged toward the wound.

If a cataract is so dense that the fundus is not visible and a retinal detachment is known to exist, important elements of the examination are as follows: a careful history may help determine when the retinal detachment occurred and in what portion of the fundus it began, how many times it was operated on, and whether vitreous hemorrhage occurred. The existence by history of vitreous hemorrhage is of bad prognosis as it is often followed by massive preretinal retraction. A determination of light projection may help decide whether the retinal sensitivity is gravely damaged over part or all of the retina. It should be noted that light projection has a relative value only and its presence should never be taken as evidence that the retina is attached in that area. Gonioscopy reveals whether the angle is open or closed. In cases of reoperation, the angle may be totally closed and the eye soft. As a rule, it has been found that a cataract extraction was worthwhile, provided that the following conditions were met: (1) the filtration angle is not completely closed, (2) there is no evidence of large vitreous hemorrhage, (3) the retina has been totally detached for less than 2 years by history, (4) projection of a strong light is accurate in at least one quadrant, and (5) no other complicating factors are present such as corneal damage or glaucoma. A retina operation can be performed 6 weeks after an uncomplicated cataract extraction.

Capsular remnants after an extracapsular cataract extraction. Capsular remnants are frequently a serious handicap to clear ophthalmoscopy. In many cases diligent, prolonged study of the fundus will reveal findings that permit the surgeon to go ahead with the retina procedure. If retinal breaks cannot be located, the problem is treated as outlined under the discussion on immature cataracts. When necessary, excision of the pupillary membrane is performed through a generous corneoscleral incision, with use of corneoscleral sutures. A full iridectomy is done above and a sphincterotomy at 6 o'clock.

Small pupil. Failure of the pupil to dilate well is seen (a) in Marfan's syndrome, (b) iris atrophy, (c) dislocated lens, (d) following cataract surgery with a round-pupil extraction, and (e) as a result of posterior synechiae. The handicap of a small pupil for complete ophthalmoscopic examination of the fundus has been decreased considerably by the availability of the small-pupil ophthalmoscope. However, this in-

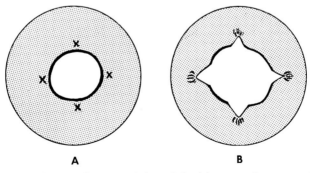

A   **B**

Fig. 13-1. In an aphakic eye, photocoagulation of the iris may enlarge a small pupil that fails to dilate with mydriatics. **A,** The photocoagulating beam is focused on the iris just outside the pupil in four locations. **B,** This causes the iris to shrink immediately, with a resultant increase in the size of the pupil. (From Okamura, I. D., et al.: Arch. Ophthal. **74:**792, 1965.)

strument is new and its full usefulness must be established by long experience. If after the use of intensive mydriatics the fundus cannot be fully evaluated, even with the small-pupil ophthalmoscope, the following steps are taken: In a phakic eye, a full iridectomy is performed 2 weeks prior to retina surgery. Posterior synechiae should be lysed at the same time. In an aphakic eye, an attempt is made at opening the pupil with photocoagulation. Several precautions must be taken in this case: a water bath is used to cool the cornea; if the anterior chamber is shallow, it must be deepened with a saline injection; the image of the photocoagulating source on the iris must be small; and care should be taken not to explode iris tissue. As a rule, enough shrinkage of the iris occurs by simply burning the area of the pupillary sphincter in four locations (Fig. 13-1).

Occasionally a pupil that was well dilated at the beginning of an operation becomes constricted during surgery. An important cause of pupillary constriction is hypotony. Such an eye does not respond to mydriatics even when injected subconjunctivally. This problem can be overcome to a degree by increasing the ocular pressure, by injecting 0.1 ml. of 0.1% Adrenalin solution into the anterior chamber, or, even better, by using a sterile small-pupil ophthalmoscope.

Presence of glaucoma

When a retinal detachment affects more than one quadrant, the intraocular pressure is generally below normal. With reattachment of the retina, the pressure usually rises toward normal levels. However, in some cases, the preoperative intraocular pressure is below normal but the pressure rises into the glaucomatous range as a result of surgical reattachment of the retina. In other cases, dilating drops cause a moderate elevation of the ocular pressure although the filtration angle remains open. The association of glaucoma with retinal detachment is frequent enough to make tonometry, gonioscopy, and perimetry of both eyes part of the routine for all patients with retinal detachment. Tonography should be performed whenever there is any suspicion of glaucoma.

Because chronic open-angle glaucoma is not rare in eyes with retinal detachment, the disc should always be checked for the presence of cupping. Even in the absence of cupping or of elevated tension, the outflow coefficient may be pathologically low, but the intraocular pressure may also be low because of the presence of retinal detachment. In some patients the pressure is normal in the eye with retinal detachment but elevated in the fellow eye, a finding that should arouse suspicion about the existence of bilateral open-angle glaucoma. In an eye with a retinal detachment affecting more than one quadrant, chronic open-angle glaucoma must be suspected either when the ocular pressure is higher in this eye than in the fellow eye or when the pressure is 18 mm. of mercury or more in the eye with retinal detachment. In these cases the intraocular pressure often tends to rise above normal following reattachment of the retina.

A special type of chronic open-angle glaucoma may result from contusion of the globe. As a rule, the vitreous base becomes partly torn from its attachment, and a retinal dialysis is produced, generally in the upper nasal quadrant.* At the

*See Chapter 20, "Traumatic Retinal Detachment."

same time, the filtration meshwork may be partly torn from the scleral spur, causing an abnormally large recess to appear in the angle, and this finding is often accompanied by chronic open-angle glaucoma.

Another type of glaucoma sometimes associated with retinal detachment is that accompanied by the formation of peripheral anterior synechiae. It is most frequent in longstanding cases of retinal detachment with secondary uveitis, in eyes that have been submitted to repeated retina operations, and in retinal detachment that follows surgical aphakia. In many of these cases extensive peripheral anterior synechiae result from a choroidal detachment that followed a previous eye operation.

A fourth type of ocular hypertension occurs in eyes with retinal detachment and acute uveitis with fibrin and cells in the aqueous and posterior synechia formation. The angle is open by gonioscopy, but inflammatory products impair the aqueous outflow.

The preoperative management of these four different types of glaucoma consists in controlling any elevation of pressure by the use of acetazolamide in doses of 125 to 500 mg. every 6 hours, depending on the severity of the case, and 1% epinephrine bitartrate drops 3 or 4 times a day. In addition, active inflammation is treated with mydriatics and with drops of 0.4% prednisolone every hour. If the inflammatory process fails to respond to this treatment, systemic steroid therapy is advised, such as prednisone 60 to 100 mg. daily by mouth for a few days.

An acute glaucoma may be precipitated by instillation of mydriatic drops for fundus examination prior to the retina operation. Generally, this occurs in patients with narrow angles. Acetazolamide should be given prophylactically in patients whose angles are suspected of being narrow, and mydriasis is then obtained by using successively 1% cyclopentolate hydrochloride and 10% phenylephrine hydrochloride. Such mydriatics can be overcome by strong miotics such as 4% pilocarpine hydrochloride in the event of a sudden rise in tension. Fortunately, few cases are encountered in which the use of acetazolamide and the preceding mydriatics bring about an alarming rise in tension. If glaucoma occurs in spite of these precautions, a full iridectomy should be performed prior to the retina procedure, allowing 1 to 2 weeks between the operations.

PROBLEMS DURING SURGERY

In this section, two types of problems will be discussed: first, those in which reattachment is difficult because of marked fixed retinal folds or massive preretinal retraction; and, second, eyes with extremely thin sclera.

Fixed folds and massive preretinal retraction
Clinical description

One of the most frequent and discouraging difficulties in retina surgery is the presence of fixed retinal folds. Fixed folds do not change in shape or position with movements of the eye or with changes in position of the body. Any movement in fixed retinal folds is no more than a slight tremor, as if they were imprisoned in jelly. Sometimes, visible vitreous bands are attached to them. Fixed folds may be star shaped, in which case they occur with predilection in the inferior half of the fundus and not infrequently at or near the macula. Another type is a sharp fixed fold that runs more or less parallel to the equator; generally it appears below first and may run around 360 degrees. Sometimes it forms a spiral, one end of the fold running much closer to the disc than the other.

The fundus of an eye that is going to develop massive preretinal retraction shows no ophthalmoscopic signs indicating the impending problem. However, slit lamp examination reveals that the vitreous gel is extensively liquefied, forming a huge optically empty cavity between the posterior cortical layer of the vitreous and the anterior vitreous gel. The posterior cortical layer and the posterior layer of the vitreous that has retracted anteriorly have an increased optical density.

In the early stages of massive preretinal retraction, the color of the fundus reflex changes from orange to pale gray and the fundus details become hazy, due to an increase in vitreous opacities and in the Tyndall effect of the gel. Intraretinal hemorrhages develop along the equator, and the retinal vessels become dilated and tortuous. Fixed retinal folds appear posterior to the equator, initially involving one or more quadrants and eventually appearing in all quadrants. Any retinal breaks that were closed surgically become reopened, or new breaks form.

In established massive preretinal retraction, the retina is totally detached and fixed and takes the shape of a corrugated cone with its apex at the disc. Later the cone narrows into a funnel. Fixed radial folds are present in all quadrants and extend from disc to equator like the spokes of a wheel. Near the disc, the ends of

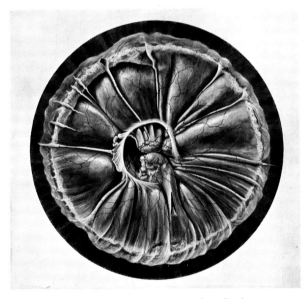

Fig. 13-2. Fundus painting of massive preretinal retraction. Retina, ora serrata, and posterior part of pars plana ciliaris are detached. The retinal detachment contains numerous fixed radial folds and retinal breaks at 5:30 and 11 o'clock. The posterior portion of the retinal detachment is a narrow funnel at the bottom of which the optic nerve head is hidden by retinal folds. Preretinal tissue forms a circular traction band that extends clockwise from 6 to 3 o'clock. (From Tolentino, F. I., et al.: Arch. Ophthal. **78:**16, 1967.)

the retinal folds are rounded. In particularly severe cases retinal folds obscure the optic disc. Sedimented blood is frequently seen along the course of the equatorial fold inferiorly. Gradually, the equatorial fold shrinks into a progressively smaller circle and moves nearer the optical axis of the globe (Fig. 13-2).

In an established case, the most important changes in the vitreous are a generalized shrinkage of the vitreous gel with increased Tyndall effect in the gel, condensation of vitreous fibers into bands and membranes that later contract, and a condensation of the preretinal layer of vitreous. Two kinds of vitreous membranes are constantly found—equatorial and preretinal. Fixed retinal folds occur where the preretinal membrane is adherent to the retina.

Surgical management

Before the advent of scleral buckling procedures, eyes with marked fixed folds and eyes with massive preretinal retraction were often incurable. It is the scleral buckling with a circling element that has substantially increased the percentage of reattachment in such unfavorable cases. Since its first description,[3] in 1957, the technique of scleral buckling has been improved, thereby decreasing the incidence of complications. The most important improvement was the use of soft silicone as implant material.[4] This is a synthetic rubberlike substance that can be autoclaved or heat sterilized many times and stored for long periods with little or no hardening. It is translucent, colorless, and easy to cut with scissors or knife and will not support bacterial growth.

The general technique of scleral buckling with a circling element will be described first, and special techniques used for cases of marked fixed folds and massive preretinal retraction will be discussed next.

General surgical technique[4]

After the sclera is exposed, the fundus is examined with an indirect ophthalmoscope while the assistant applies pressure on the sclera with a flat electrode, being careful to avoid traumatizing a vortex vein. When the rounded elevation produced by the electrode on the choroid coincides with the posterior edge of a retinal break, the surgeon directs that the diathermy current be turned on. If the retinal detachment is shallow, this generally produces a white diathermy mark in the retina; if the retina is elevated, no mark will show in the fundus but there will be a mark on the sclera. All retinal breaks are localized in this fashion.

A lamellar scleral undermining is performed, with use of a Desmarres scarifier, on both sides of a single scleral incision that is parallel to the limbus and located near the disc edge of the retinal breaks (Fig. 13-3). The undermining should extend at least 2 mm. beyond the retinal breaks on the side of the optic disc and, whenever possible, on the side of the ora serrata. The length of the undermining should extend 3 to 4 mm., in an equatorial direction, beyond any retinal breaks. Mattress sutures of 5-0 braided polyester fiber are passed in the scleral flaps.

Diathermy is applied in the area undermined. Light surface applications are made with a very small applicator, such as a blunt conical electrode, which is applied gently against the thin sclera without perforating it. Applications should not be confluent, their borders being about 2 mm. apart. The long ciliary arteries and

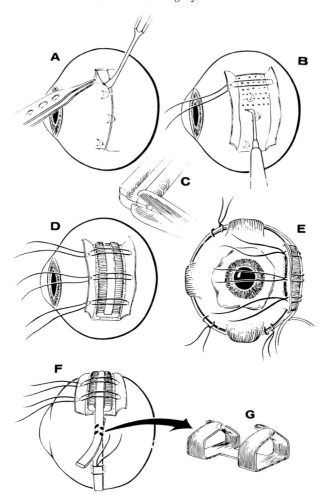

Fig. 13-3. Essential steps of scleral buckling operation with silicone implant and circling band. **A,** After localization of retinal breaks, sclera is undermined. **B,** Light diathermy is applied with small electrode, and mattress sutures are passed in scleral flaps. **C,** Sharp edges of silicone implant are carefully trimmed. **D,** Implant in place. **E,** Circling band is anchored in each quadrant where sclera was not undermined. **F,** and **G,** Ends of band fitted into tantalum clip. (From Schepens, C. L., and Freeman, H. M.: Mod. Trends Ophthal. **4:**209, 1967.)

nerves and the large choroidal vessels in the area of each vortex ampulla should be avoided. Their exact location may be determined by transillumination of the thinned sclera through the pupil (Figs. 13-4 and 13-5).

Silicone has been molded in shapes* best adapted to scleral buckling operations (Fig. 13-6) and grooved to fit under a circling band. The narrow grooved pieces are straight, and the wide pieces curved to fit the globe. The implant used should have no sharp edges that, at a later date, may possibly erode thinned sclera or Tenon's capsule. These edges must be rounded off with scissors.

*Available from **M.I.R.A.**, 150 Causeway Street, Boston, Massachusetts, U. S. A.

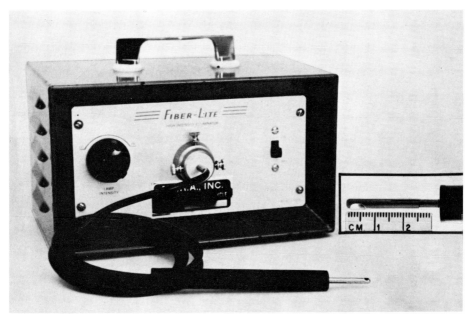

Fig. 13-4. Transilluminator used to reveal choroidal vasculature. Inset at right shows enlargement of transilluminator tip. (From Schepens, C. L., and Freeman, H. M.: Trans. Amer. Acad. Ophthal. Otolaryng. **71:**474, 1967.)

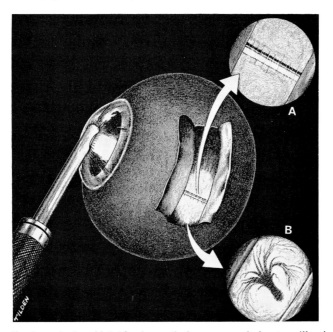

Fig. 13-5. Localization of choroidal blood vessels by means of the transilluminator. **A,** The long posterior ciliary artery and its accompanying nerve are transilluminated during diathermy application so that they can be avoided. **B,** By a similar technique the outline of a vortex ampulla and tributaries can be exposed.

The choice of the silicone implant depends on the width and height of the buckle that one desires to obtain. If the undermined area is 7 mm. wide or less, a straight grooved shape is advisable (nos. 219 or 220). If it is 8 mm. wide or over, a curved implant or tire trimmed to fit the case is used (no. 276, 277, or 279). For a very high and localized buckling effect or for a buckling wider than 12 mm., it is advisable to use an implant cut from the large tire (no. 281). After the implant is in place, the mattress sutures are pulled up and temporarily tied and a circling silicone band is carried around the globe, beneath the attached muscles and in the groove of the implant. It has been found advantageous to widen the circling band from 2 mm.—originally recommended—to 2.5 mm. and to make it slightly flatter. The groove of all the implants has been widened accordingly. The location of the

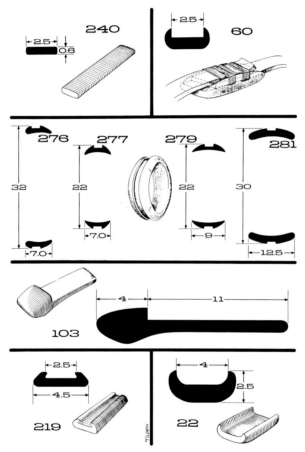

Fig. 13-6. Silicone shapes currently used. No. 240 circling band; no. 60 (boat) fits under tantalum clip holding ends of circling band. Tires: asymmetrical no. 276 (7 mm. wide), and symmetrical no. 277 (7 mm. wide), no. 279 (9 mm. wide), and no. 281 (12.5 mm. wide). Meridional pieces: no. 103 (4 mm. wide) and no. 106 (6 mm. wide). Straight grooved pieces: no. 219 (4.5 mm. wide) and no. 220 (6 mm. wide); no. 22 is additional piece fitting under no. 219.

resection determines whether the circling band must follow either the globe's equator or another great circle around the eye. At this point, anchoring sutures are placed over the circling band, one in each quadrant not containing scleral flaps with mattress sutures. Anchoring sutures of the mattress type, tied snugly enough to hold the band in place without indenting it, will allow the band to move under the sutures so that the final tension will be distributed equally throughout the elastic band. The ends of the band are pulled to eliminate slack and fitted between the flattened prongs of a tantalum clip (Fig. 13-3). The flattened prongs should cause sufficient friction to hold the ends of the band in place but still allow enough motion so that the band can be shortened by pulling its ends without releasing the prongs of the clip. The excess of silicone band beyond 10 mm. from the clip is trimmed.

Release of subretinal fluid is generally performed through a single perforation, suitably placed, posterior to the undermined area itself. The perforation must be in a location where subretinal fluid is abundant, away from the retinal breaks, the vortex veins, and the long ciliary arteries. The preferred locations are on either side of the horizontal meridian and near 12 or 6 o'clock. A meridional scratch incision is made in the sclera, and its edges are caused to gape by applying surface diathermy on them. A suture is placed on the lips of the incision (Fig. 13-7). A small knuckle of choroid is then exposed by further deepening the scleral incision, and it is treated with light surface diathermy in order to close choroidal vessels. Then the area is transilluminated as described above to ensure that no patent choroidal vessels remain. The choroidal knuckle is perforated with a fine diathermy needle. As soon as no more subretinal fluid escapes, the suture over the perforation is temporarily tied, the mattress sutures over the silicone implant are pulled up, and any slack in the circling band is eliminated by pulling on the ends of the band. Then the fundus is carefully scrutinized with the ophthalmoscope. If subretinal fluid is still present in the area of the perforation, it is released. If a large pocket of fluid is present elsewhere and none is visible in the area of the perforation, a second perforation may be advisable in order to empty the pocket of fluid. When all the subretinal fluid has

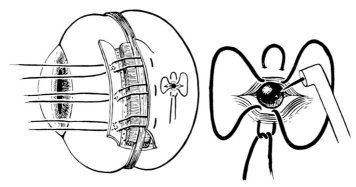

Fig. 13-7. Most frequent method for release of subretinal fluid is through single perforation located on disc side of buckle. (From Schepens, C. L.: Trans. Amer. Acad. Ophthal. Otolaryng. **68:**959, 1964.)

escaped, the suture placed over the perforation is tied permanently, as well as the scleral mattress sutures. It is important not to pull the mattress sutures too tightly.

Before the circling band is pulled up, the ocular pressure must be measured and found to be below 10 mm. of mercury with a Schiøtz tonometer. If it is higher, loosening up of the scleral mattress sutures may be indicated. Each end of the circling band is now pulled in opposite directions. The ocular pressure should be measured again and left no higher than 15 mm. Hg. Sometimes the ocular pressure is much higher than 10 mm. Hg after the mattress sutures are tied, and it may appear inadvisable to loosen them in order to lower the pressure. Under such circumstances the ocular pressure may be lowered with intravenous carbonic anhydrase inhibitors. When indispensable, a careful paracentesis is performed. The circling band should not be pulled up until every effort has been made to lower the pressure under 10 mm. Hg, and pulling the band should not raise the pressure by more than 5 mm. Hg. When the band has been shortened to its final length, the prongs of the clip are closed by flattening them over the ends of the band. To prevent the clip from eroding the ocular coats, a short grooved piece of silicone, or boat (no. 60), is placed beneath it (Fig. 13-6).

Since tissues cannot adhere to silicone, steps must be taken to prevent postoperative exposure of silicone implants. Anteriorly located implants must be covered entirely with the scleral flaps, and Tenon's capsule is carefully resutured over the area of the scleral buckling with buried 5-0 chromicized-gut mattress sutures. When the portion of Tenon's capsule that is around the limbus is very thin, as is frequently observed in old people, the orbital portion of the capsule must be anchored to the sclera or to the edges of the rectus muscles, 6 to 7 mm. from the limbus. Before the wound is closed, it is generously injected with an antibiotic solution containing 5000 units of polymyxin B sulfate per milliliter. (During the course of the operation 6 Gm. of sodium methicillin are given by slow intravenous injection.) A moderately compressive bandage is maintained in place by elastic tape, the unoperated eye is left uncovered, and the patient may be ambulatory the day after operation.

Special techniques used for marked fixed folds and massive preretinal retraction

The first problem is the choice of the method for producing a chorioretinal adhesion. All known methods tend to make preretinal retraction somewhat worse. Because of the frequency of hazy media, photocoagulation is undesirable. Cryoapplications run the risk of being ineffective if the reaction they cause is not continuous. I have the definite impression that the adhesion obtained with cryoapplications is weaker than that produced by diathermy and, consequently, relapses after cryoapplications are more frequent in unfavorable cases. At this time the method of choice appears to be fairly strong diathermy applications (stronger than usual) made with a blunt conical electrode. The applications should be sparse as described above.

The width, length, and height of the scleral buckling must be increased in the area of the retinal breaks. After subretinal fluid is released, the fundus is examined to see if the breaks are closed. If not, a larger silicone implant may be used and the circling band is pulled up until the breaks are closed. If closure of the breaks re-

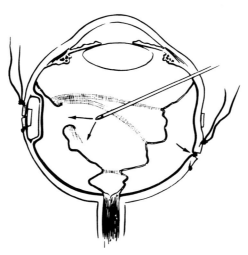

Fig. 13-8. Vitreous injection performed with open choroidal perforation may force back retina, which was maintained detached by vitreous bands.

quires considerable pulling up of the circling band, injection of saline solution into the eye may be indicated.[4] This is done through a small gauge needle (no. 30) after the suture on the perforation site is temporarily tied. A meridional scleral incision is made over the pars plana ciliaris through one half the scleral thickness, and a mattress suture is placed on the lips of the scleral incision. The needle is pushed through the incision, and this step is facilitated by touching the needle with a diathermy electrode. Before the needle is removed from the eye, the suture is temporarily tied over it. If the patient is aphakic and there is no vitreous in the anterior chamber, the injection may be made through a small limbal incision just large enough to permit passage of the needle. When the needle is withdrawn, the ocular pressure is measured, since raising the ocular pressure above 30 mm. Hg with the injection is contraindicated.

Even after much subretinal fluid has been released through a posteriorly located perforation and saline has been injected, the retina may remain detached because it is held in the vitreous cavity by preretinal organization. The perforation site is then reopened and saline solution is reinjected slowly into the vitreous cavity while subretinal fluid continues to escape (Fig. 13-8). This technique may force the retina to settle on the scleral buckling, thereby closing the retinal breaks. Once the retinal breaks are closed, the scleral suture over the choroidal perforation is tied. If indicated, the scleral buckling may then be reduced in size with an additional injection of saline solution.

The injection of air has effects similar to those of saline; however, air makes ophthalmoscopy difficult or temporarily impossible. Therefore, it is tried after saline has failed to help and when the low specific gravity and the elasticity of air may contribute to reattaching the retina.

If these procedures fail, it is better to stop the operation. In rare cases, the fundus appearance improves slowly after operation and the case becomes a success.

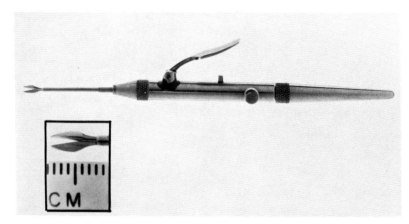

Fig. 13-9. Vitreous scissors. *Insert:* Instrument tip compared to millimeter rule.

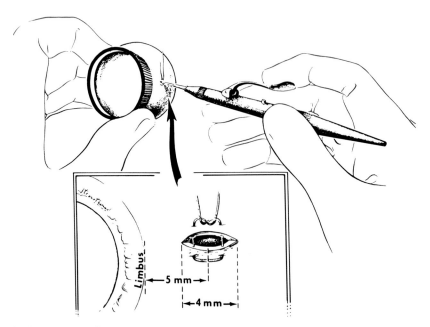

Fig. 13-10. Vitreous scissors penetrate through scleral incision, 4 mm. long, made over pars plana ciliaris. Middle of incision is 5 mm. from limbus, and distance between arms of mattress suture is 1.5 mm. Movements inside globe are controlled through binocular indirect ophthalmoscope. (From Freeman, H. M., and Schepens, C. L.: Trans. Amer. Acad. Ophthal. Otolaryng. **72:**399, 1968.)

Most often, the case remains a failure. In selected cases, vitreous surgery may be attempted weeks or months later.

Surgery inside the vitreous cavity opens up possibilities in cases in which traction on the retina from vitreous bands and membranes causes failure of current methods of retinal detachment surgery. Prerequisite of this surgery is a thorough examination, including binocular indirect ophthalmoscopy with scleral depression, biomicroscopy with a 3-mirror contact lens, and detailed sketching of findings in both retina and vitreous cavity.

The miniature scissors used for cutting vitreous membranes have blades 5 mm. in length and the part that enters the eye has a diameter of 1.6 mm. (Fig. 13-9). A meridional sclerotomy 4 mm. long is made over the pars plana ciliaris. A mattress suture of 4-0 polyester fiber is placed over the sclerotomy, the arms of the suture being 1.5 mm. apart (Fig. 13-10). The exposed choroid is treated with light diathermy to close blood vessels and it is incised with a knife. Then the scissors are introduced through the incision by an assistant. The surgeon wears a headband type of indirect stereoscopic ophthalmoscope and holds a +25D condensing lens in his left hand. As soon as the point of the scissors becomes visible in the pupillary area, the surgeon takes the scissors' handle in his right hand and the assistant pulls up the mattress suture sufficiently to prevent leakage of vitreous. The surgeon moves the tips of the closed blades near the membrane to be cut. The scissors are opened, pushed forward to straddle the membrane, and closed to cut it. If the eye becomes very hypotonic, the cornea may cave in and viewing becomes difficult. Severe hypotony may also result in a reflux of blood from the filtration meshwork into the anterior chamber, which obscures ophthalmoscopy. When marked hypotony occurs, the instrument should be removed from the vitreous cavity and intraocular pressure restored with an injection of physiologic saline through the pars plana ciliaris.

The cases that succeed best are those in which vitreous bands are in completely fluid vitreous, as often happens in high myopes. If bands are continuous with extensive and hard-to-view membranes or if they are embedded in vitreous gel, results are less satisfactory. This underscores the importance of careful preoperative study of the vitreous cavity by slit lamp microscopy.

Thin sclera

Thin sclera may be a localized condition, often limited to the upper temporal quadrant, or it may affect a large area. Thin and weakened sclera resulting from previous surgery is often a complex problem, one that has been discussed in some detail[5] and will not be reviewed here.

Dehiscences of the sclera (Fig. 13-11) appear as radial dark streaks, varying in width from 0.5 to 4 mm. They are usually present anterior to the equator in areas where the sclera is expected to be thick, namely, between the rectus muscles. Equatorial staphyloma (Fig. 13-12) is seen in the same location but involves a larger area, sometimes an entire quadrant. A thin-walled staphyloma may rupture if the intraocular pressure is raised excessively. Scleral dissection is not attempted where the sclera is very thin, and cryoapplications are preferred, over such areas, to weak diathermy applications. Short scleral flaps are dissected on either side of the thin area. They must be of sufficient size to permit the placement of mattress sutures. If

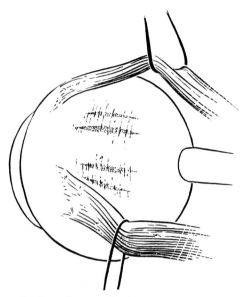

Fig. 13-11. Dehiscences of sclera. Inner scleral layers are absent, so that dark choroid can be seen through outer scleral fibers. As sclera adjacent to dehiscenses may also be thin, it may not be advisable to dissect a flap over such an area. (From Okamura, I. D., et al.: Arch. Ophthal. **75:**615, 1966.)

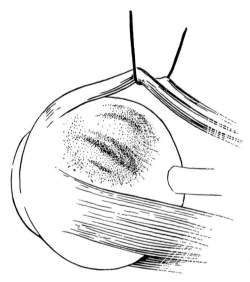

Fig. 13-12. Equatorial staphyloma. Although the actual bulge of a staphyloma may be insignificant, the sclera can be very thin. (From Okamura, I. D., et al.: Arch. Ophthal. **75:**615, 1966.)

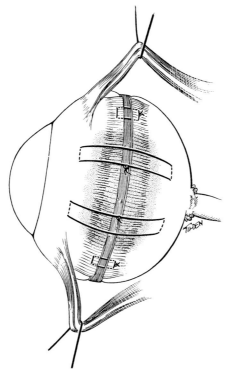

Fig. 13-13. When an implant is located over a large staphyloma, anchoring sutures may have to be placed as indicated, scleral bites being made in tissue of sufficient thickness. If possible, the implant should extend beyond the limits of the staphyloma, where scleral flaps can be cut and sutured as usual.

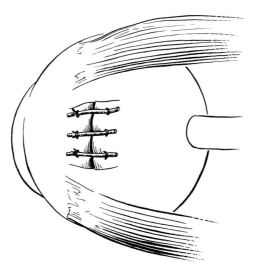

Fig. 13-14. Use of 3-0 plain absorbable gut sutures as reinforcements or bolsters to prevent nonabsorbable polyester mattress sutures from cutting through weak sclera. (From Okamura, I. D., et al.: Arch. Ophthal. **75:**615, 1966.)

the staphyloma is very large, mattress sutures for anchoring the implant are inserted beyond the limits of the staphyloma in normal sclera, without making scleral flaps (Fig. 13-13). When the scleral flaps that can be made are also thin, mattress sutures may cut through. To prevent this complication, a length of 3-0 plain absorbable gut suture is placed under the loop and under the knot of the mattress suture to act as a reinforcement or bolster (Fig. 13-14). When one flap is very weak, the suture may be placed beyond the flap, in undissected sclera, and the scleral bite

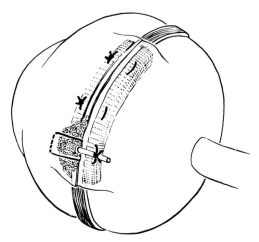

Fig. 13-15. A thin anterior scleral flap did not permit placement of mattress suture in the usual way and a scleral bite was made, parallel to original scleral incision, in healthy sclera. The knot was tied over a reinforcement placed over the healthier scleral flap. (From Okamura, I. D., et al.: Arch. Ophthal. **75:**615, 1966.)

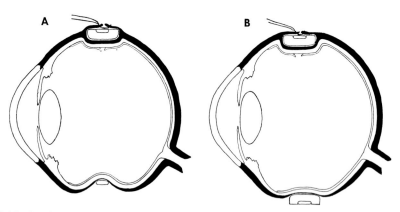

Fig. 13-16. A, If the sclera under the circling element is very thin, excessive indentation by the silicone band may result, but the implant makes only a shallow indentation. B, This situation is corrected by placing a grooved silicone piece (no. 219) under the circling element where it overlies thin sclera. (From Schepens, C. L.: Trans. Amer. Acad. Ophthal. Otolaryng. **68:**959, 1964.)

made parallel to the original scleral incision, as in the case of an extensive staphyloma (Fig. 13-15). A reinforcement is then used under the knot only.

It is essential to use a fairly large implant over a staphylomatous area in order to prevent possible erosion of the ocular wall at a later date. The edges of the implant must be trimmed with particular care. Since the scleral sutures have less holding power in thin sclera than in tissue of normal thickness, a circling element is essential to maintain the buckling effect. If the circling element rests on thin sclera, unsupported by a grooved implant, it tends to indent the globe more deeply in that area than under the implant (Fig. 13-16). This situation gets worse as time goes on, the buckling effect increasing most where it is least desired, that is, where no implant was used. A length of grooved silicone (no. 219) placed under the band will help prevent excessive indentation of the sclera where it is thin. Since this additional implant is not held in place by scleral flaps, it must be secured under one mattress suture in each quadrant. When the sclera underlying either the implant or the circling element is of extreme thinness, it is advisable to suture donor sclera to the globe first. Donor sclera is cut in such a way that it reaches an area where the patient's own sclera is sufficiently thick for suturing. The donor material is secured by four to six sutures, and the implant or circling element is placed over it.

When a buckling effect is not needed and the sclera is thin, either photocoagulation or cryoapplications are used. If the media are clear and the area requiring treatment is at the equator or posterior to it, photocoagulation is the method of choice; in all other cases cryoapplications are preferred.

A question frequently raised concerns the relative merits of using molded silicone rubber rather than silicone sponge[6] as implant material. In silicone sponge of the closed-cell type, most of the little air pockets are closed. However, handling the sponge material during operation often causes some of the cells to rupture and communicate with each other. As a result, when a sponge is removed at a second operation, blood and tissue fluids can nearly always be expressed from it. This point is important because it establishes the existence of dead spaces that can harbor intractable infection.

The alleged advantages of the sponge are that it is softer and easier to suture to the sclera than is molded silicone, which should be buried under scleral flaps. Silicone sponge is most often used without a circling element, and its buckling effect then depends entirely on the use of mattress sutures. The placement of mattress sutures in undissected sclera is always more dangerous than in a scleral flap. Moreover, these sutures are most effective when placed far away from the silicone sponge, but their placement may cause technical difficulties. It is a long established fact that any material sutured to the sclera often fails to produce a permanent buckle. In other words, in most instances, the sutures give way after weeks or months and the silicone sponge forms nothing more than an excrescence on the globe's external surface.

Sometimes the sponge is placed under a circling element and then a permanent ridge is created. However, since there is no groove in which to fit the circling element, it easily slips off the silicone sponge. Because the sponge lacks rigidity, the "wings" of the implanted sponge tend to lift away from the globe as soon as the mattress sutures give way and the buckle remaining is nothing more than a narrow ridge instead of a broad elevation as originally planned (Fig. 13-17).

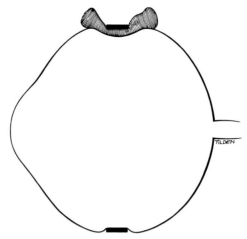

Fig. 13-17. When silicone sponge is placed under a circling band, the sponge tends to form "wings," which lift away from the globe where the sponge is not held down by mattress sutures.

It is impossible with a sponge to shape the buckle so that it fits the case exactly. For instance, a hump cannot easily be obtained over a stubborn meridional fold, and a posterior or anterior extension of the buckle cannot be made easily to cover an extensive break. Finally, with sponge it is difficult, if not impossible, to make a thin anteriorly located implant to cover breaks close to the ora serrata.

Another difficulty with sponge implants relates to reoperations. Because the surface of the sponge is rough, blood and connective tissue stick to it, making recognition of the implant and its removal more difficult than in the case of molded silicone. When placed over very weak or absent sclera, it may stick to the underlying tissue so that its later removal may be accompanied by choroidal hemorrhage or rupture.

In summary, silicone sponge is doubtless easier to implant than molded silicone placed under scleral flaps. However, it is considerably less effective for complex cases, the buckle it creates seldom being permanent. For the same buckling effect it requires a much larger implant and its use is, in my opinion, attended by more dangers.

SPECIFIC PROBLEM CASES
Ehlers-Danlos syndrome[7]

The Ehlers-Danlos syndrome is an inherited disorder of connective tissue that is manifested clinically by hyperelastic, fragile skin and hyperlaxity of the joints. The skin may be stretched some distance from the body, particularly in areas of bony prominence. When released it returns immediately to its former position. Wounds of the skin have a tendency to gape, and poor healing and scarring are common. The fragile skin may split spontaneously over a large hematoma or upon sudden twisting of the wrist. The scars are mobile over the underlying tissues and most marked over areas exposed to trauma, such as forehead, elbows, knees, and tibial surfaces.

Laxity of the joints causes frequent falls, and repeated dislocation of the clavicle, shoulder, radius, hip, or patella may occur. Some patients can extend the thumb and other fingers so that they can touch the wrist. Traction on the fingers may dislocate the joints and on release the fingers snap back into place. Structural abnormalities of the feet, such as clubfoot or flatfeet, are often noted.

The basic connective tissue defect, though most striking in its cutaneous and joint manifestations, also affects other tissues of the body. Most significant, because it suggests a relationship to Marfan's syndrome, is the occurrence of dissecting aortic aneurysm due to cystic median necrosis. The hemorrhagic tendency is generally considered to be caused by abnormalities in the supporting tissues of the blood vessels or the vessel walls. General friability of tissues has often been noted in many organs at operation or autopsy.

Eye abnormalities include keratoconus, blue sclera, posterior staphyloma with high myopia, ectopia of the lens, postoperative dehiscence of cataract wound, and bilateral corneal laceration as a result of minor trauma. Vitreous hemorrhage and retinal detachment also occur in these patients. This connective tissue syndrome appears to be due to abnormal formation of the collagen fibers. The occurrence of vitreous hemorrhage suggests a weakness in the wall of the retinal blood vessels, which bleed when subjected to traction by the vitreous. Retinal breaks seen in patients with Ehlers-Danlos syndrome were accompanied by evidence of strong vitreous traction such as rolled edges, areas of white without pressure, and horseshoe tears with visible adherent vitreous membranes. Premature degeneration and collapse of the vitreous gel were present.

Surgical management

Since there is a definite tendency for vitreous hemorrhage, it is advisable to decrease the intensity of diathermy or to use cryosurgery or photocoagulation. Perforation of the choroid to release subretinal fluid must be done with the utmost care to avoid choroidal bleeding. The exposed knuckle of choroid should be treated with weak surface diathermy, then transilluminated through the cornea, and any patent choroidal blood vessel should be retreated with diathermy. Because of the frequency and prominence of vitreous membranes, a scleral buckling procedure is indicated when possible. The general history of poor wound healing dictates very careful wound closure. Since relatively innocuous areas of retinal disease may rapidly develop retinal breaks, follow-up examinations should be frequent and detailed.

It has been observed that patients without Ehlers-Danlos syndrome but with high myopia may also show an abnormal bleeding tendency from choroidal blood vessels. For this reason it is very important to avoid excessive diathermy and to be extremely careful when perforating the choroid in highly myopic eyes.

Choroidal coloboma[8]

Retinal detachment occurs in about 40% of the patients with choroidal coloboma. The peculiar features of retinal detachment associated with this congenital defect are more easily understood when considering the developmental pathology of choroidal coloboma. During normal development the fetal fissure becomes closed by fusion of the two layers of the optic cup. The inner sensory layer fuses with the

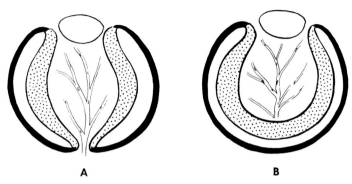

Fig. 13-18. Diagram of section through the fetal fissure. **A,** Before fusion of layers. **B,** After normal fusion. (From Jesberg, D. O., and Schepens, C. L.: Arch. Ophthal. **65:**163, 1961.)

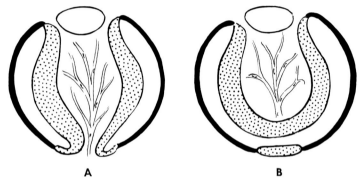

Fig. 13-19. Diagram of section through the fetal fissure illustrating abnormal fusion. **A,** Beginning eversion of sensory layer. **B,** Isolated zone of sensory layer in the outer coat. (From Jesberg, D. O., and Schepens, C. L.: Arch. Ophthal. **65:**163, 1961.)

corresponding inner layer, and the outer pigment epithelium layer fuses with its counterpart on each side of the fissure in a regular fashion (Fig. 13-18). This process begins at the equator and proceeds anteriorly and posteriorly as if a zipper were being closed in each direction.

When the regular process of fusion does not occur at the fissure, a colobomatous defect results. If the inner layer everts and replaces the outer layer at the fusion zone, an island of unpigmented tissue is produced in the pigment epithelial layer (Fig. 13-19). Wherever pigment epithelium is replaced by sensory retinal tissue, the choroid develops poorly and the sclera may also be underdeveloped in this area. The defective layers of the globe tend to fuse and become ectatic. The mature colobomatous defect shows absence of pigmented and vascular tunics. The wall of the globe is usually represented by abnormal retinal tissue and a thin overlying sclera. At the margin of the coloboma there is an abrupt defect of choroid and pigment epithelium, the retina being closely applied over the scleral edge of the coloboma. The retina is not bound or attached to the margins of the defect throughout, however, although there is frequently an incomplete line of hyperpigmentation

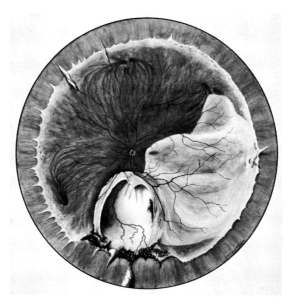

Fig. 13-20. Choroidal coloboma associated with temporal retinal detachment. Anomalies are present in the ora serrata region: abnormal meridional folds at 10, 11, and 3 o'clock; distorted and excessively pigmented ora serrata near 6 o'clock. A small retinal break at 3 o'clock was closed surgically without improving the retinal detachment.

Closer examination of the colobomatous region revealed the following features: The retina was elevated over the scleral edge, on the temporal side, for a short distance into the coloboma. The detached retina was continuous with a very fine membrane that lay over the upper portion of the coloboma and appeared to be detached from the underlying staphylomatous sclera. This membrane was presumed to represent anomalous retina lining the inner aspect of the coloboma. Careful observation by stereoscopic indirect ophthalmoscopy gave the impression that there were breaks (not represented in the figure) in the continuity of the anomalous filmy retina over the temporal edge of the coloboma, near the subretinal hemorrhage. This bleeding did not assume the sharply outlined picture of in situ hemorrhage but was more diffuse as if it had settled in this area from another site. A single line of diathermy was carefully applied over healthy choroid along that portion of the edge of the coloboma that was continuous with the retinal detachment. This was followed by quick and permanent reattachment. (From Jesberg, D. O., and Schepens, C. L.: Arch. Ophthal. **65:**163, 1961.)

suggesting an attachment. Typical fissural defects are below the disc, but they may include the disc or even extend above it. The macula may be eliminated by inclusion in the coloboma.

If marked instances of choroidal coloboma are often associated with microphthalmia, more moderate degrees are frequently found in myopic eyes. The choroidal coloboma itself is generally staphylomatous, a feature easily detected by stereoscopic ophthalmoscopy.

There are two types of retinal detachment associated with choroidal coloboma: In the first type, the coloboma is no more than an incidental finding. Obvious retinal breaks are found, unrelated to the coloboma, and their closure results in reattachment of the retina.

The second type of retinal detachment appears to be definitely related to choroidal coloboma. Retinal detachment, in these cases, is often inferotemporal with demarcation lines, or total. The treatment of visible or suspected retinal breaks does not bring about reattachment of the retina because retinal breaks are present in the colobomatous area. Such breaks easily escape visual detection because of the lack of contrast afforded by the white scleral background and because of the diaphanous nature of the retinal membrane (Fig. 13-20). In addition, a break may occur in the undeveloped retina in an area of the coloboma that is hidden behind the scleral edge of the posterior staphyloma or in the region of the much-distorted inferior ora serrata. The presence of such a break may be signified by a recent hemorrhage in the colobomatous area, and this sign must be given due consideration when present. The edges of the coloboma must be carefully examined by stereoscopic ophthalmoscopy for indications of elevation connected with the retinal detachment. It has been found that diagnosis was helped by the use of slit lamp microscopy as well as binocular indirect ophthalmoscopy.

Breaks in the flimsy membrane that represents the retina in the colobomatous area may be produced by traction exerted on this membrane by abnormal preretinal tissue that may be visible in the area of the coloboma.

Surgical management

Treatment of cases of the second type requires the establishment of a line of chorioretinal adhesion along the edge of the coloboma. The posterior portion of this line is best made by photocoagulation. The anterior portion can be made either with diathermy or with cryoapplications. Accurate minimal applications are essential because all nerve fibers peripheral to an application are sacrificed. When a coloboma involving the disc is encountered, the entire extent of the defect cannot be treated without interfering with the nerve fibers from all quadrants. It might be tried, however, to treat only that portion of the coloboma's edge that appears elevated. It is obvious that adhesive chorioretinitis cannot be produced where choroid and retina are either extremely atrophic or absent. Thus, treatment in the colobomatous area would probably be of no value for closing retinal breaks that might be present over the coloboma.

Since it has been repeatedly noted that colobomatous eyes react poorly to surgical trauma, it is important to operate with great care and to perform the minimal amount of surgery that has a chance of being successful.

REFERENCES

1. Brockhurst, R. J., Schepens, C. L., Okamura, I. D., Regan, C. D. J., and McMeel, J. W.: Scleral buckling procedures. VIII. Preoperative complications, Arch. Ophthal. **74:**792, 1965.
2. Hovland, K. R., El Zeneiny, I. H., and Schepens, C. L.: Clinical evaluation of the small-pupil binocular indirect ophthalmoscope. (In press, Arch. Ophthal.)
3. Schepens, C. L., Okamura, I. D., and Brockhurst, R. J.: The scleral buckling procedures. I. Surgical techniques and management, Arch. Ophthal. **58:**797, 1957.
4. Schepens, C. L.: Scleral buckling with circling element, Trans. Amer. Acad. Ophthal. Otolaryng. **68:**959, 1964.
5. Okamura, I. D., Schepens, C. L., Brockhurst, R. J., Regan, C. D. J., and McMeel, J. W.:

Scleral buckling procedures. IX. Complications during operation, Arch. Ophthal. **75:**615, 1966.

6. Lincoff, M. A.: Modifications to the Custodis procedure for retinal detachment, Arch. Ophthal. **73:**160, 1965.

7. Pemberton, J. W., Freeman, H. M., and Schepens, C. L.: Familial retinal detachment and the Ehlers-Danlos syndrome, Arch. Ophthal. **76:**817, 1966.

8. Jesberg, D. O., and Schepens, C. L.: Retinal detachment associated with coloboma of the choroid, Arch. Ophthal. **65:**163, 1961.

14

Complications of retinal detachment surgery

Edward W. D. Norton

Complications of retinal surgery may be divided into three principal groups: those occurring prior to the surgical procedure and therefore influencing the preoperative management of the patient, those occurring during the surgical procedure, and those occurring in the postoperative period. Unfortunately, these complications can be so numerous that it is not practical to discuss them all in this presentation. Therefore, it is my intent to list the complications in each group and to discuss the management of selected complications.

Preoperative complications

1. General—age, health, etc.
2. Infection
   a. Conjunctivitis
   b. Infected buckle
   c. Dacryocystitis
   d. Lid
3. Opacities of the media
   a. Corneal
   b. Lens
   c. Vitreous
4. Inflammation
   a. Uveitis
      (1) Mild
      (2) Severe
   b. Choroidal detachment
5. Small pupil
   a. Phakic—iridectomy
   b. Aphakic
      (1) Franceschetti procedure
      (2) Photocoagulation

6. Glaucoma
    a. Angle closure
    b. Open angle
    c. Angle recession
    d. Hemorrhagic
7. Vitreous
    a. Hemorrhage
    b. Traction
        (1) Local
        (2) Massive vitreous retraction
8. Previous intraocular surgery
    a. Recent cataract surgery
    b. Thin filtering bleb
9. Subluxated or dislocated lens

OPACITIES OF THE MEDIA

Since the fundamental principles of retinal surgery are to find the retinal breaks, to set up a reaction in the pigment epithelium underlying these breaks, and to bring the retina into contact with this reaction, it is apparent that proper visualization of the entire retina is most desirable. Although this is essential during the preoperative examination, it is particularly true during the operation. Therefore, one must keep in mind that it is usually easier to see the fundus before the operation than during the operation.

Corneal opacifications are rarely of such an extent to present an insurmountable problem. I have never encountered a patient whose corneal clarity was such that a transplant was necessary before retinal surgery could be undertaken. I am certain such cases do occur since I have seen one patient with severe interstitial keratitis, in whom I debated following such a course, but fortunately I was able to resolve his retinal problem by retinal surgery alone.

Lens opacities are much more common, but in general they rarely require cataract surgery prior to the retinal surgery. It is essential for the surgeon skilled in binocular indirect ophthalmoscopy to allocate a great deal of time to the examination of the fundus. With persistence and careful drawing, one can determine the limits of the detachment, locate definite retinal breaks or at least suspicious areas, and outline the appropriate surgical procedure. As a general rule, if the limits of the detachment can be determined, retinal surgery is always the initial procedure.

Vitreous opacities usually represent recent bleeding. Naturally, if the bleeding has been so severe as to give rise to a black reflex, one can only wait until some evaluation of the retina is possible. My usual course for a patient with recent hemorrhage is to hospitalize him, bilaterally patch the eyes, and confine him to bed with his head elevated 60 degrees for a period of 12 to 48 hours. Often at least the upper half of the fundus can be adequately viewed and treated accordingly. If after 48 hours the vitreous shows no evidence of settling or clearing, one has to accept that it may be weeks to months before that fundus can be viewed.

Such patients are made ambulatory, returned to their active environment, and followed regularly. Gross-hand fields are sometimes useful in following the status of the retina. If at any time a retinal detachment is recognized and a compatible break located, surgery is carried out even though the rest of the fundus remains obscured. These patients cannot be seen in routine outpatient visits in the midst of a busy schedule. Sufficient time must be available on each revisit so that persistent and careful ophthalmoscopy can be carried out.

INFLAMMATION

Mild inflammation, with a few cells and flare in the aqueous beam, is relatively common with retinal detachments and presents no problem. Occasionally, however, patients present such severe inflammatory reaction that the anterior chamber is filled with fibrin and cells, the iris is bound down, and the fundus cannot be viewed. These patients usually respond promptly to systemic and topical steroids and cycloplegics. Once the retina is reattached, the anti-inflammatory agents can be discontinued and the eye will remain quiet.

The obvious question is: "Did the inflammatory reaction cause the detachment or did the detachment initiate the inflammatory response?" My clinical impression is that the latter is usually the case.

In some patients, in addition to the severe inflammatory reaction, massive choroidal detachments accompany the detached retina. In the past, my treatment of these patients was, first, to give steroids, systemic and local, then to await the regression of the choroidal detachment. Now I initiate the steroid therapy and operate to close the breaks as soon as feasible. If the choroidal detachments interfere with the process of setting up a reaction in the pigment epithelium underlying the breaks, they are drained and flattened by injecting saline into the vitreous cavity before treatment is applied.

Such cases undoubtedly carry a poorer prognosis for reattachment and visual function, but my present course of early intervention is much more satisfactory.

GLAUCOMA

Glaucomatous eyes commonly develop retinal detachments. This type is almost always open-angle glaucoma and can be either ignored in the preoperative dilation and examination or treated with carbonic anhydrase inhibitors and epinephrine agents.

In the rare patient with angle-closure glaucoma, peripheral iridectomy or, preferably, full iridectomy should be carried out prior to the detachment surgery so that proper dilation and examination can be performed preoperatively and postoperatively. Such an operation probably could be done simultaneously with the detachment surgery, but I have always allowed 48 hours to intervene between the two procedures. A tight closure of the corneal scleral wound at the iridectomy site is imperative.

Although my experience is limited, my preference for the full iridectomy revolves around the occasional tendency for posterior synechia to form following peripheral iridectomy, resulting in difficult viewing.

PREVIOUS INTRAOCULAR SURGERY

Retinal detachments may be recognized after the removal of an opaque lens. Such detachments are usually of longstanding duration and can easily wait 4 to 8 weeks until the cataract incision is sufficiently healed to present no problem to the retinal surgeon. Occasionally, however, the patient develops the retinal detachment in the immediate postcataract extraction period and the surgeon would like to reattach the retina as soon as possible to regain the maximum visual function. In such cases bilateral patches are applied, the retina is studied carefully, and surgery is performed about 4 weeks after cataract surgery. If problems with examination and scleral depression are encountered, such as squeezing, a lid block is often useful. If surgery cannot be delayed until the fourth week, it can be done anytime. The earliest I have done such surgery is on the tenth postoperative day.

In patients with very thin filtering blebs, if the surgeon is careful in exposing the operative field, in applying traction and pressure on the globe, and in draining fluid before tightening the buckling sutures, these procedures can be done without disrupting the integrity of the globe.

Complications during surgery

1. General—anesthetic, etc.
2. Impaired view
   a. Corneal clouding
      (1) Prevention
      (2) Removal of epithelium
   b. Contracted pupil
3. Exposure
   a. Canthotomy
   b. Muscles
      (1) Reoperation
      (2) Radial buckle vs. equatorial buckle
      (3) Superior oblique and inferior oblique
   c. Macula hole
   d. Staphyloma
      (1) Superior temporal
      (2) Reoperation
   e. Infection at reoperation—unrecognized
4. Difficulties with localization
   a. Ideal
   b. Adjustment
5. Treatment—judgment of adequacy
   a. Flat
   b. Highly elevated
6. Placement of sutures
   a. Thin sclera
   b. Relation to hole
   c. Vortex ampulla
7. Fluid drainage
   a. Unplanned
      (1) Suture
      (2) Rupture
      (3) Localization

   b. Planned
      (1) Selection of site
      (2) Technique
      (3) Incarceration and/or vitreous loss
   c. Inadequate drainage—what is adequate?
8. Bleeding
   a. Anterior chamber
   b. Vortex (external)
   c. Drainage site
   d. Intraocular
      (1) Mild
      (2) Massive
   e. Development of choroidal detachments—transilluminate
9. Intraocular pressure—appearance of vessels and blood pressure
   a. After diathermy vs. after cryotherapy
   b. Segmental
   c. Encircling
   d. Air
   e. Keratocentesis
      (1) Phakic
      (2) Aphakic
10. Failure of retina to settle—when to quit?
   a. Meridional folds
   b. "Fish mouth"
   c. Balloon superior temporal
      (1) Leave alone
      (2) Air

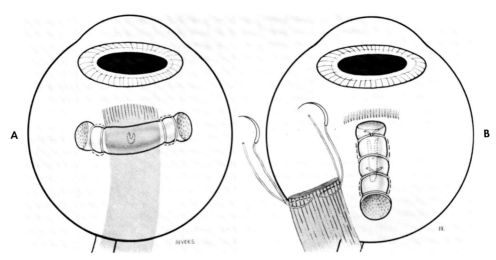

Fig. 14-1

EXPOSURE

Proper exposure facilitates retinal surgery as it does any other surgery, but the routine use of a canthotomy does not seem justified to me. In the great majority of cases it is unnecessary and only contributes to the patient's postoperative discomfort. If indicated, however, there should be no hesitation in its use.

The detachment of muscles is rarely necessary. In fact, the only times that I detach muscles now are in those cases undergoing reoperation following widespread diathermy in which I intend to place an implant under the muscles and in the occasional case in which I intend to place a radial buckle immediately under a muscle (see Fig. 14-1, *B*). There is no problem with equatorially placed implants (Fig. 14-1, *A*), but I have encountered technical difficulties with the radial ones.

Staphylomas are almost always localized and can therefore be treated by placing sutures in thicker sclera on either side, thus supporting the implant over the thinned area.

DIFFICULTIES WITH LOCALIZATION OF THE BREAKS

Ideally, the break should be localized and marked on the sclera so that in the case of small breaks the surgeon knows where the posterior edge is (Fig. 14-2, *A*), and in large breaks where the posterior and anterior limits are. Using this located posterior limit of the break as his guide, the surgeon places the sutures for the implant so that the scleral mark is centered between the scleral bites of the suture (Fig. 14-2, *B*). When the retina settles, the break will lie on the anterior crest of the buckle. In large horseshoe breaks it is essential to locate on the sclera not only the posterior edge but also the anterior edge so that the implant is made wide enough to place the entire break on the buckle, thereby eliminating anterior leaks.

When the retina is highly elevated, finding the exact location of the break is difficult. In such a case, the sclera is always marked as mentioned previously, but

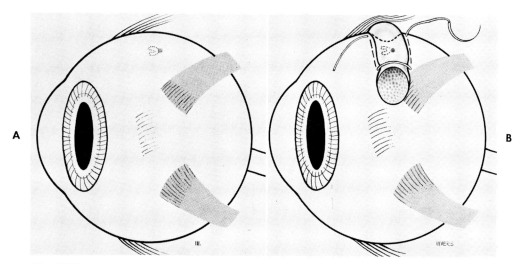

Fig. 14-2

greater leeway is allowed for error by making the scleral suture bites farther apart to accommodate a wider implant.

If fluid is not drained, one can estimate the suitability of the buckle by indenting it with a cotton applicator. If fluid is drained, the relationship is readily apparent. Utilization of cryotherapy and full-thickness scleral implants makes readjustment of the buckle-hole relationship relatively easy, merely by replacement of the sutures.

ADEQUATE TREATMENT WITH CRYOTHERAPY

The judgment of adequate treatment with cryotherapy is still evolving, but use of such treatment is undoubtedly somewhat less than what we are currently using. At the present time, if the retina is flat, the slightest whitening is probably sufficient. When the retina is highly elevated from the choroid, this judgment is more difficult, but the change in choroidal appearance to orange-yellow probably indicates adequate treatment. Certainly the appearance of ice overlying the pigment epithelium and choroid indicates excessive treatment. Although these end points are unrelated to the temperature setting on the dials of the various cryoprobes, I believe that it is an advantage to be able to regulate the maximum temperature drop so that there is less tendency to overfreeze and overtreat.

FLUID DRAINAGE

Most retinal surgeons would agree that fluid drainage is the one aspect of the surgical procedure over which they have the least control, and, although complications are unusual, they can be disastrous. Custodis' demonstration that it was not always necessary to drain fluid certainly was a significant contribution. Today few surgeons will drain fluid if the holes are in contact or almost in contact with the buckle. The problem comes, however, when the subretinal fluid highly elevates the hole from the buckle and the surgeon must decide whether to drain. My indications for drainage of subretinal fluid are variable but they tend to be as follows:
1. Longstanding detachment
2. Posterior break
3. Large break
4. Multiple breaks in different quadrants
5. Inferior break
6. Evidence of vitreous bands and preretinal organization
7. Aphakia

In addition, if the macula has recently detached and I believe it may take some time for the fluid to reabsorb, I will favor drainage.

Once drainage has been initiated, when is it adequate? Once the holes are essentially in contact with the buckle and its treatment, there is no further need to drain fluid. The practice of "drain them dry" can no longer be defended.

Incarceration of the retina, with or without vitreous loss, is a serious complication. Not only does it jeopardize reattachment, incarceration seriously jeopardizes visual prognosis. When it occurs, the area should be surrounded with cryotherapy and the site should be placed on a buckle. If the drainage site was selected in the plane of the planned buckle, extension of this buckle over the incarcerated area is sufficient.

DEVELOPMENT OF CHOROIDAL DETACHMENTS

Occasionally, during the operative procedure, especially if it is prolonged, large choroidal elevations will develop. In general, these are serous and present few problems once they are recognized. If they are not recognized and persistent attempts are made to drain the "subretinal fluid," complications may develop. If these choroidals are hemorrhagic, they have a much more serious prognosis and the postoperative course will be complicated by extension of blood into the vitreous and may result in poor visual function. If the surgeon is doubtful of the nature of the choroidals, he has two guides: intraocular pressure and transillumination. With hemorrhage, the globe becomes firm and there is a dense defect on transillumination.

INTRAOCULAR PRESSURE AT THE END OF SURGERY

Great emphasis has been placed upon the level of the intraocular pressure at the end of surgery. When an encircling element is used, the eye should be normotensive at the end of the procedure. When segmental buckles are used, however, this is less important; if the retinal circulation is apparent at the nerve head, there should not be any vascular difficulties. Similarly, if the intraocular pressure is greatly elevated by air injection into the vitreous cavity, the pressure of the globe will return to safe levels within a few minutes.

Keratocentesis is rarely necessary, but I have done it in phakic eyes with segmental buckles in which the retinal circulation was embarrassed. I would never do a keratocentesis in an aphakic eye because of the danger of incarcerating vitreous in the wound.

WHEN TO TERMINATE THE OPERATION

The decision most dependent upon good judgment is when to terminate the operation. Too much time can be spent, at great risk to the eye, moving or enlarging a buckle in order to eliminate meridional folds or "fish mouth" holes. Most of these, if left alone, will cause no trouble, but they sometimes seem to bother the surgeon more than the retina. The major decision is whether the buckle is posterior enough for the hole to be on the anterior slope when the retina settles. This decision is made by indenting the buckle with a cotton applicator to estimate how it will look postoperatively.

Some detachments, especially those with a large superior break and a high balloon, fail to approach the buckle despite considerable drainage of fluid. I have found, as Rosengren did, that the injection of air into the vitreous in these cases promptly settles the retina against the buckle. The surgeon can often anticipate these cases when making the preoperative drawing if he notices that with scleral depression the balloon disappears and the retina flattens.

Postoperative complications

1. General
2. Infection
   a. Early
      (1) Immediate ℞—antibiotics
      (2) Removal implant

      b. Late—pain
- 3. Uveitis
  - a. Mild
  - b. Severe, with coagulum
  - c. Iris atrophy
  - d. Synechia
- 4. Glaucoma
  - a. Angle closure
  - b. Open angle
  - c. Choroidals and angle closure
- 5. Hemorrhage
  - a. Choroidal
  - b. Retinal
  - c. Vitreous
- 6. Corneal
  - a. Edema
  - b. Anesthesia
  - c. Dellen of Fuchs
- 7. Diplopia
  - a. Symblepharon
  - b. Limitation movement
- 8. Redetachment
- 9. Preretinal and vitreous shrinkage
  - a. Macular pucker
  - b. Massive vitreous retraction
- 10. Exposure of implant
  - a. Early
  - b. Late
    - (1) Fistula formation
    - (2) Extrusion
    - (3) Hemorrhage
- 11. Intrusion of implant
- 12. Refractive changes
- 13. Optic atrophy
- 14. Ptosis
- 15. Enophthalmus

INFECTION

Any surgical procedure carries the risk of infection, and this risk is greatly increased when a foreign body remains. Fortunately, with proper sterilization of relatively nonreactive silicone materials, combined with cryotherapy, the incidence of postoperative infection is less than 1%. For the past several years, we have not used systemic antibiotics either preoperatively or postoperatively. We have irrigated the wound at the time of surgery, however, with a solution of neomycin and bacitracin (neomycin, 500 mg.; bacitracin, 50,000 units in 50 ml. of Ringer's solution). In addition, the silicone implant soaks in this antibiotic solution immediately prior to its use. I have no statistical data to defend or advocate this practice.

Recognition of intraocular infection is sometimes difficult if there is undue reaction to the operative procedure. The presence of a "white puff" in the retina and overlying vitreous, however, should alert the surgeon to the probability of a severe intraocular reaction to a scleral infection. Once this is recognized, intensive systemic and local antibiotics should be initiated and the foreign body removed. It is far better to run the risk of redetachment and subsequent reoperation than to lose the eye to infection—this is not a time for the surgeon to procrastinate.

Late infection of the implant is much more frequent, with pain the characteristic complaint of the patient. Persistent redness of the eye, pain, and localized tenderness almost certainly indicate an infection around the foreign body. These patients can be treated with systemic antibiotics and careful observation if there is no intraocular reaction, but they must be carefully examined daily for evidence of a fistula or developing abscess, and unless there is prompt cessation of the symptoms, the foreign body should be removed. If the foreign body becomes exposed, there is usually good drainage and little risk of immediate intraocular extension. Once the retina is firmly healed, however, probably in 3 weeks, the foreign body should be removed and the problem will promptly be resolved. There is no reason to try to cover an exposed implant with conjunctiva.

POSTOPERATIVE GLAUCOMA

The most common cause for postoperative glaucoma is the appearance of large anterior choroidal detachments displacing the iris root forward against the angle. If the aqueous shows little reaction, as is usual with cryotherapy, the glaucoma can be managed with carbonic anhydrase inhibitors and epinephrine agents. These medications, plus the occasional addition of miotics, have been sufficient to handle this complication. I can visualize a situation associated with severe inflammatory reaction, however, in which it would be advisable to drain the choroidals and reopen the angle.

REDETACHMENT

There are several reasons for unsuccessful retinal surgery. Once an unsatisfactory result is recognized, reoperation in some manner is mandatory. The retinal break may fail to settle on the implant, a misjudgment at the time of surgery. Bilateral patches, with or without bed rest, may be tried for several days, and supplemental photocoagulation may be placed on the choroid through the break, but if fluid begins to reaccumulate, reoperation is inevitable. Of course, the conservative methods will be successful only if the retinal break-buckle relationship is a correct one. If it is not, reoperation should be done immediately.

Occasionally, the break is sealed posteriorly but leaks down the trough anterior to the buckle and balloons the retina inferiorly. If this occurs, judicious use of photocoagulation may seal the break and avoid reoperation (Fig. 14-3).

If in the postoperative period redetachment occurs and a "missed break" is recognized, reoperation is the only course of action. New breaks rarely form unless they are associated with significant changes in the vitreous. In the absence of the develop-

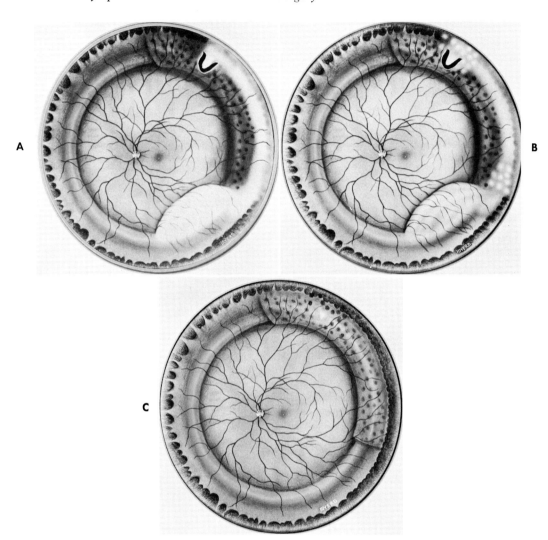

Fig. 14-3. A, Leakage of subretinal fluid anteriorly, producing inferior detachment. **B,** Photocoagulation to break at 1:00 and to ora at 3:30. **C,** Status after observation of fluid and reattachment.

ment of significant vitreous organization and traction, the surgeon should assume the reponsibility for failure. It will usually result from an improperly placed buckle, a buckle not wide enough to cover the break, a missed break, or improper judgment about fluid drainage at the time of surgery.

The nightmare of the retinal surgeon is the patient, "successfully" reattached with good visual function, who on the sixth to seventh postoperative week calls to say that there has been a marked change in the visual function. This almost certainly indicates vitreous traction and preretinal organization. At best, it results in a macular pucker (Fig. 14-4) with loss of acuity; at worst, total retinal detachment,

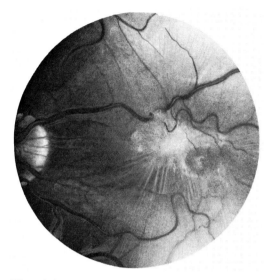

Fig. 14-4

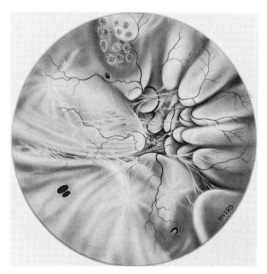

Fig. 14-5

multiple tears, whitening of the retina, and the depressing picture of massive vitreous retraction (M.V.R.) (Fig. 14-5). The reasons for this complication remain unknown. Certainly it occurs without retinal surgery, but its time relationship to retinal surgery, usually about 6 weeks, cannot be fully ignored. I also have the distinct impression that this complication occurs less frequently today, when we have minimal intraocular reaction postoperatively, than it did 15 years ago, when severe intraocular reaction was much more common.

The successful management of severe forms of this complication has yet to be discovered, but a high equatorial encircling buckle will often preserve some useful field of vision. Only the future will determine the value of a direct surgical attack on the vitreous and the preretinal membranes. These procedures, though heroic and occasionally useful, rarely result in useful vision, and maximum effort must be directed toward finding the cause and prevention of this serious complication.

15

Six years' experience with silicone injections into the vitreous cavity

Gerd R. E. Meyer-Schwickerath
O. E. Lund
W. Höpping

The tolerance of silicone oil by the human body has been known to the pharmacologist for more than 20 years. In our country Vonkennel advocated the use of silicone oil for ointments in 1953. There was no reaction in animal experiments when silicone was given intraperitoneally (1953).[17]

For visible and ultraviolet light, silicone is completely transparent. It tolerates several hundred degrees centigrade, which is important for the use of photocoagulation. About 100 years ago, when the first silicone was synthesized, nobody could imagine how widely this substance was going to be used in our day.

The intraocular administration of silicone oil, however, seems to be an unusual step, in spite of the mentioned qualities. Our physiologic knowledge about metabolism of the retina and the lens would lead us to expect severe damage of the retina and lens opacities.

In 1958 Stone was the first one who tried fluid silicone in a rabbit's eye. The silicone was well tolerated. Four years later Cibis, Becker, and Okun reported about the first cases of silicone oil injections into human eyes.

Several articles have been published on this subject: Niesel and Fankhauser (1963), Dufour (1963), Bonnet (1964), Castren (1964), and Moreau (1964, 1965, 1967). In 1964 Höpping presented our material for the first time in relation to photocoagulation. Recently, in 1967, Lund has shown our material at the vitreous symposium of the German Ophthalmological Society.

The indication for this operation was almost the same as stated by Cibis and Okun. We have performed this operation only in those cases in which any other type of operation, including injection of saline into the vitreous, was hopeless. Quite a number of patients who were referred for silicone implant have been treated successfully by other methods. With the exception of *one case* with a very longstanding

235

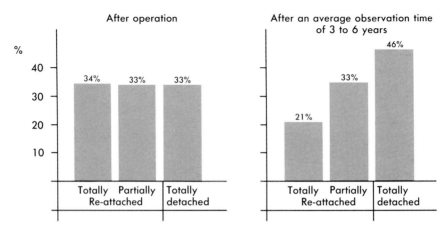

Fig. 15-1. Anatomic results of retinal detachment operations.

detachment, all cases had one or several detachment operations before fluid silicone was used. One fourth of our patients had an aphakic detachment and one fourth a very thick preretinal membrane. The injection technique was the same as that described by Cibis and Okun: Under control of a binocular ophthalmoscope or of the operating microscope with an additional plane contact lens, the silicone was injected into the funnel before the disc. We never emptied the vitreous cavity as Cibis did at the beginning; we emptied only the subretinal space by using electrolysis punctures.

At first we used 2000-centipoise silicone oil; then we found out that the results became better with higher viscosity and we tried the highest viscosity that we could get through an enlarged 2-gauge needle. This was silicone oil of 10,000 cp., which we are still using for this procedure.

The amount of silicone injected varies between 2 and 4 ml. In one large, and high myopic eye, we injected 6.4 ml. without losing a drop of silicone. A second injection of silicone was performed in 5 cases; in 2 cases silicone was injected three times.

RESULTS

As shown in Fig. 15-1, the retina was completely reattached in 35 cases at the time of dismissal from the hospital. In 34 cases there was still some detachment, mainly in the lower half of the fundus. In another 34 cases the reattachment of the retina was impossible. This means that in two thirds of our cases the vision was better than it was before the operation.

If we continue to control our results over a longer period, we find (Fig. 15-1) that only 54% show a completely or partially reattached retina.

We have found out that aphakic detachments, as well as those that have a thick preretinal membrane, have a worse prognosis than the other cases.

As presented in Table 15-1, we also followed the visual acuity of our patients. The visual acuity before the operation was lower than 0.05, with two exceptions. Roughly we can say that in about one third of our cases we were able to prevent

Table 15-1. Functional results

Visual acuity	% of cases
Improved	24
Unchanged	40
Worse	18
Amaurosis	18

blindness of the eye. This means a lot if we consider that almost all of these patients had already lost one eye before the second one was operated on.

COMPLICATIONS

First of all, we have to state that tolerance to the silicone oil is very good. We have never seen inflammatory or allergic reactions against it. Other complications, however, that may occur during the operation, some days later, or even much later, are possible. In 5.5% of the cases, we have seen new tears that occurred during the operation, when the retina was unfolded but stuck together. In one case we probably penetrated the retina with the needle.

The presence of silicone oil in aphakic cases in the anterior chamber was 9%. Oil in this chamber should be avoided, but prevention is not always possible. In one case we could see that a small silicone bubble had passed around the lens in a phakic eye. A rather high percentage of our complications are opacities of the lens. Quite a number of these cases have had lens opacities before the operation, some of them in the type of cataracta complicata. It is certainly not correct to believe that all the lens opacities are due to silicone implant, because we know cataracta complicata may occur in many of those eyes that have undergone several detachment operations. We can see that many of the blind fellow-eyes of our patients without silicone implant also show cataract. In those cases, however, in which silicone is in direct contact with the lens—a rare situation—we may presume that the cataract is due to the silicone.

We have operated on several patients by using implanted silicone because of cataract. We did not find it more complicated than in nonsilicone cases.

In six of our cases a dystrophy of the cornea occurred. Five of them were aphakic eyes with silicone in the anterior chamber, whereas in one case the anterior chamber was absent after a massive hemorrhage. To our surprise, secondary glaucoma was a rare complication and could be controlled mostly by conservative treatment.

To sum up our results, we can find that they are very similar to those of Cibis and Okun. We therefore think that in cases in which the prognosis is hopeless, especially if it is an only eye, the silicone injection can be recommended. Of course, we have to discuss with the patient the possibility of early and late complications.

Nevertheless, we shall look for other better methods giving fewer complications. Quite a number of our patients are extremely grateful. They all honor my friend Paul Cibis, who dared to introduce this type of operation.

REFERENCES

1. Armaly, M. F.: Experimental intraocular uses of the silicone fluids, Invest. Ophthal. **1**:801, 1962.

2. Armaly, M. F.: More ocular uses of silicone forms, Invest. Ophthal. **1**:434, 1962.

3. Armaly, M. F.: Ocular tolerance to silicones, A.M.A. Arch Ophthal. **68**:390, 1962.

4. Armaly, M. F.: The organo-silicones and the eye, Eye Ear Nose Throat Dig., p. 51, 1964.

5. Bonnet, I.: Essais de traitement de certains décollements de rétine par injection de silicone intra-vitréen, Bull. Soc. Ophtal. Franc. **64**:451, 1964.

6. Castren, I. A.: Retinal detachment and intraocular silicone fluid injection, Ann. Med. Exp. Fenn. **42**:1, 1964.

7. Cibis, P. A.: Vitreoretinal pathology and surgery, St. Louis, 1965, The C. V. Mosby Co.

8. Cibis, P. A., Becker, B., Okun, E., and Canaan, S.: The use of liquid silicone in retinal detachment surgery, Arch. Ophthal. **68**:590, 1962.

9. Dufour, R.: L'injection intra-vitréenne de silicone liquide dans le décollement rétinien désespéré, Ophthalmologica **147**:160, 1964.

10. Höpping, W.: Lichtkoagulation nach Glaskörperersatz durch Silikone, Ber. Deutsch. Ophthal. Ges. **65**:336, 1964.

11. Lehmann, H.: Die Verwendung der Silikone in Pharmazie und Medizin, Schweiz. Apoth. Zeitung, p. 459, 1955.

12. Levine, A. M., and Ellis, R. A.: Intraocular liquid silicone implants, Amer. J. Ophthal. **55**:939, 1963.

13. Lund, O. E.: Silicon-Oel als Glaskörperersatz, Ber. Deutsch. Ophthal. Ges. **68**:166, 1967.

14. Moreau, P. G.: Premiers essais d'injections de silicones liquides intra-oculaires dans le décollement de la rétine, Bull. Soc. Ophtal. Franc. **64**:130, 1965.

15. Moreau, P. G.: Les silicones intra-oculaires dans les décollements de rétines désespérés, Ann. Oculist **200**:257, 1967.

16. Niesel, P., and Fankhauser, F.: Zur retrovitrealen Silikoninjektion bei der Behandlung der Netzhautablösung, Ophthalmologica **147**:167, 1964.

17. Polemann, G., and Froitzheim, G.: Tierexperimentelle Untersuchungen zur biologischen Verträglichkeit von Silikonen, Arzneimittelforschung **3**:457, 1953.

18. Stone, W., Jr.: Alloplasty in surgery of the eye, New Eng. J. Med. **258**:486, 1958.

16

Experimental retinal detachment and reattachment*

I. Methods, clinical picture, and histology

Robert Machemer

INTRODUCTION

Nearly 100 years have passed since Chodin[1] in 1875 accidentally found that he could produce a retinal detachment in an animal eye. Many investigators since then have tried to achieve such detachments, and various methods have been described. Especially today, there is great interest in finding a good experimental model for retinal detachment, as publications during recent years show. There is still a great need for a good model, since there are so many unanswered questions, first about pathology—especially of early cases, secondly about the pathophysiology of the eye with a detached retina that cannot be studied on the human eye, and finally it is of the greatest importance to be able to develop new therapeutic methods for those 10% of human detachments that still resist therapy.

Upon perusal of the literature it is interesting to note that nearly all experiments on animals have been performed with rabbits. These animals are inexpensive and their eyes are large, but this is nearly all that can be said in favor of these eyes, because they differ very much from the human eye. I will mention two important differences—not only does the vitreous have a much more gel-like consistency than the human eye, but the blood supply of the retina is also very different. The result was that, although detachments were achieved, these detachments never formed the impetus for further intensive investigation.

*This investigation was supported in part by U. S. Public Health Service research grant NB-06841 from the National Institute of Neurological Diseases and Blindness, Bethesda, Md., in part by Research to Prevent Blindness, Inc., 598 Madison Avenue, New York, N. Y., in part by the Florida Lions' Eye Bank, Inc., Miami, Florida, and in part by Deutscher Akademischer Austauschdienst, Bonn, Germany.

Attempts to reattach detached retinas experimentally were very seldom reported. We know of only one successful attempt. It was made in 1911 by Birch-Hirschfeld,[2] who reattached long-lasting detachments in two rabbit eyes by means of electrolysis.

In the following paper we want to present an experimental retinal detachment that we consider a useful model for large-scale investigation. This model contributes to our knowledge of human detachment because:

1. It presents a clinical picture that is very similar to the human one.
2. It offers an investigation not only of simple cases of detachment but also of complicated ones such as giant tears, dialysis, and massive vitreous retraction.
3. It permits histologic study of the early stages of retinal detachment, of which so little is known.
4. It permits reattachment of the retina and, thus, similar studies of early stages that are nearly unknown.

The animal that was selected for the experiments was the owl monkey *(Aotus trivirgatus)*. This small monkey is not very expensive and has rather large eyes. The anatomy of the eye is very similar to that of the human eye, the only difference being the lack of a fovea.

CLINICAL PICTURE
Materials and methods

Our methods of producing a retinal detachment followed the original idea of Alajmo and Auricchio[3] and of Foulds,[4] who injected 150 to 600 units of hyaluronidase into the vitreous, with the expectation that this enzyme, together with mechanical destruction, would destroy the vitreous and then, following the production of a retinal hole, a permanent retinal detachment would be easily achieved. In the following description of our technique the main changes are the use of a monkey instead of a rabbit, the drastic reduction of hyaluronidase to 1 unit, and a different technical approach.

The owl monkey was generally anesthetized and then placed into a box from which the head projected. Under the operating microscope a 26-gauge needle on a tuberculin syringe filled with one unit of hyaluronidase diluted in 0.1 ml. of saline was inserted through the pars plana usually on the nasal side. Then a contact lens was placed on the eye. The hyaluronidase was carefully injected into the vitreous. Under continuous observation of the fundus, vitreous was aspirated and reinjected into the vitreous cavity several times. During aspiration the needle was carefully guided, in a circular pattern, along the surface of the retina in the area where the retinal hole was to be produced. Finally, the needle was put as closely as possible to the retina on the temporal side. It is of paramount importance that the needle be absolutely vertical to the retinal surface. Then 0.2 ml. of aspirated vitreous was injected, with pressure against the temporal retina. This action immediately resulted in a small retinal hole and a surrounding detachment (Fig. 16-1). The needle was then withdrawn and the animal returned to its cage.

During the first week the media of the eye were very cloudy, so that it was often impossible to see the details. This cleared up within 1 week. The original area of retinal detachment became enlarged between the third and fourteenth day and usually total detachment resulted.

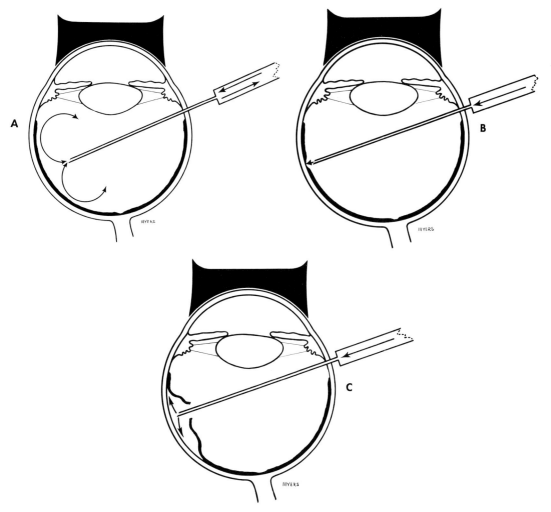

Fig. 16-1. Schematic drawing of the manipulations in the vitreous. **A,** After insertion of the needle through the pars plana, the needle is guided in a circular motion in proximity to the retina. Hyaluronidase is injected and the vitreous aspirated and reinjected. **B,** Then the needle is placed very close to the retinal surface and vitreous is injected with pressure. **C,** This results in a retinal hole with surrounding detachment. (From Machemer, R., and Norton, E. W. D.: Amer. J. Ophthal. **66:**388, 1968.)

Nine eyes were treated in exactly the same way, with the only exception that instead of hyaluronidase only saline was used.

The reattachment operations were performed 1, 2, 4, 8, and 12 weeks after the production of the detachment. Each group consisted of two or three eyes. Those eyes that had a small retinal hole were selected. The operations were performed under general anesthesia, together with a retrobulbar injection of Xylocaine. For easy access to the temporal sclera a part of the temporal orbit was opened by removing some of the zygomatic bone. Then the Custodis[5] procedure was performed.

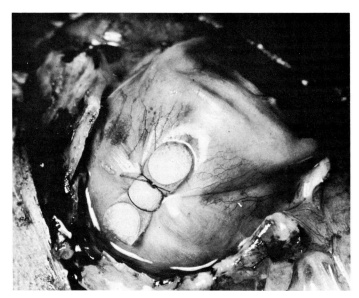

Fig. 16-2. The orbit has been opened on the temporal side for easier access to the temporal sclera. After localization of the retinal hole a Silastic sponge is sutured on the full-thickness sclera. Subretinal fluid is removed by diathermy puncture. (From Machemer, R.: Amer. J. Ophthal. **66:**1075, 1968.)

After localization of the retinal hole, the sclera in the immediate vicinity of the hole was diathermized as little as possible. A Silastic sponge was sutured on the sclera and all subretinal fluid was carefully released (Fig. 16-2). Sometimes it was necessary to refill the vitreous cavity with saline, which was injected through the pars plana. Then the wounds were closed and penicillin applied locally and systemically. To prevent proptosis, the lids were closed for 2 days with two sutures.

Results and comment

Out of 63 eyes successfully operated on in the above-described manner, 50 eyes developed progressive retinal detachment, i.e., 79% of the eyes operated on. Out of 52 eyes that were observed over a period of at least 14 days, 44 eyes were totally or nearly totally detached after 14 days. The detachments, once they had become progressive, did not show any tendency toward spontaneous reattachment, even in eyes observed as long as 20 weeks.

Four different types of retinal detachments developed:

1. In the first group the original small detachments enlarged (Fig. 16-3) and usually progressed to total detachment. The retinal hole remained its original small size. The retina was hazy from the beginning. Usually, large folds developed, radiating from the center, but sometimes the detachment remained flat. The retinal surface itself did show some wrinkles, but generally it was rather smooth, whereas the posterior side of the retina showed a shagreenlike pattern in high, detached areas which, as will be demonstrated later, was due to wrinkles of the outer layers of the retina (Fig. 16-4).

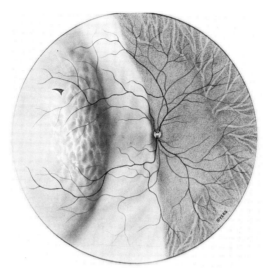

Fig. 16-3. Fundus painting of a 3-day-old detachment. The retinal hole is the original size. (From Machemer, R., and Norton, E. W. D.: Amer. J. Ophthal. **66:**388, 1968.)

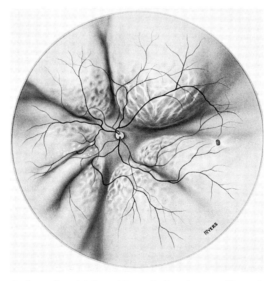

Fig. 16-4. Fundus painting of a 14-day-old total detachment. Note the radiating folds and the shagreen-like pattern of the higher detached bullae. (From Machemer, R., and Norton, E. W. D.: Amer. J. Ophthal. **66:**388, 1968.)

2. The second type had large retinal holes. Usually the original hole had already been large, but these holes had a tendency to enlarge spontaneously to the periphery. They always had edges that were rolled inward, something that happened immediately after the production of a larger hole. Beneath these holes a pigment epithelium defect could be seen. This defect corresponded to

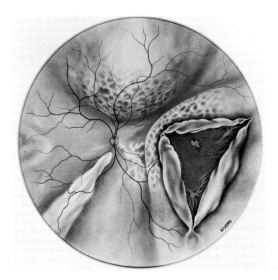

Fig. 16-5. Fundus painting of a 6-week-old total detachment. The original hole has enlarged into a giant tear. Note the inwardly rolled retina at the edges and the tendency of the hole to tear toward the periphery. (From Machemer, R., and Norton, E. W. D.: Amer. J. Ophthal. **66:**388, 1968.)

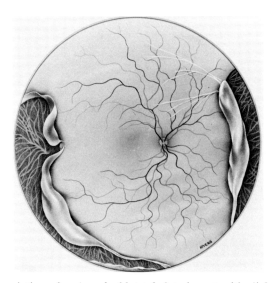

Fig. 16-6. Fundus painting of a 4-week-old total detachment with dialysis. The hole on the temporal side (9 o'clock) enlarged to the periphery and caused the dialysis. The dialysis on the nasal side was possibly caused by vitreous strands pulling at the retina. (From Machemer, R., and Norton, E. W. D.: Amer. J. Ophthal. **66:**388, 1968.)

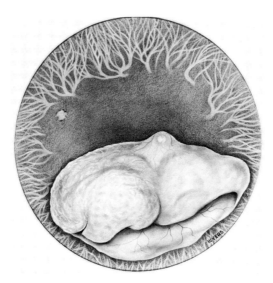

Fig. 16-7. Fundus painting of a 4-week-old total detachment with 360-degree dialysis. The retina floats easily in the vitreous. The back of the retina is corrugated. (From Machemer, R., and Norton, E. W. D.: Amer. J. Ophthal. **66:**388, 1968.)

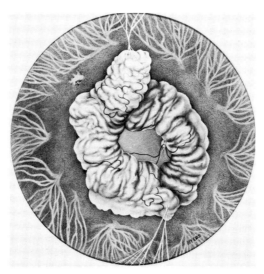

Fig. 16-8. Fundus painting of a 14-day-old total detachment and 360-degree dialysis with the appearance of massive vitreous retraction. Note the compactly folded peripheral retina. (From Machemer, R., and Norton, E. W. D.: Amer. J. Ophthal. **66:**388, 1968.)

the original hole and was caused by the jetstream that produced the retinal hole (Fig. 16-5).

3. In the third type a dialysis developed, probably by peripheral enlargement of the original retinal hole (Fig. 16-6). These dialyses tended to enlarge very rapidly, and soon there was a 360-degree dialysis. The superior part of the retina tended to fall down, thus hiding the disc, but the entire funnel, following gravity, moved around in the eye. In these eyes it was possible to observe directly what had caused the shagreenlike pattern. There were irregularly distributed valleys and elevations of the outer retina (Fig. 16-7).

4. Finally, in four cases with 360-degree dialysis we were able to observe the development of what simulated massive vitreous retraction, which started in a localized manner, with some puckering on the retinal surface. The full picture of a massive vitreous retraction developed within 14 days after production of the detachment, whereas the posterior retina was flatly detached and smooth, the anterior retina consisted of densely packed thick folds, and the retina did not move because it was immobilized by vitreous strands (Fig. 16-8).

Those nine eyes that were treated with saline alone instead of hyaluronidase did not develop a retinal detachment.

Twenty-five eyes with retinal detachment were operated on with the Custodis method to reattach their retinas; 19 of these eyes were treated successfully. After the operation the media remained clear. Residues of subretinal fluid were absorbed after 2 days. The retina was flatly attached. Sometimes small folds were visible. The buckle was usually rather prominent. The coagulated areas turned into partly pigmented scars within 14 days (Fig. 16-9).

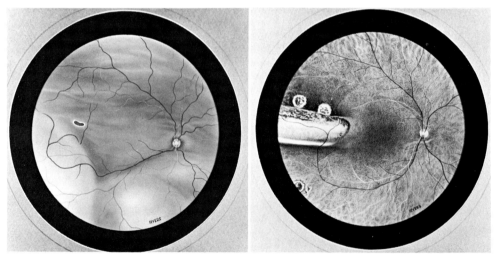

Fig. 16-9. Fundus painting of the pre- and postoperative situation of the first monkey eye in which a Custodis procedure was performed to reattach the retina. (From Machemer, R., and Norton, E. W. D.: Amer. J. Ophthal. 66:388, 1968.)

HISTOLOGY

It is astonishing how little is known about early serial histologic findings in the detached and reattached retina and in the pigment epithelium. This dearth is probably due to the fact that relatively few eyes with early retinal detachments are seen by the pathologist, so that it has never been possible to observe a sequence of histologic changes. The second reason is that human eyes are usually fixed in formalin, a fixative that does not preserve the structure of the retina and pigment epithelium very well. Finally, in the past the interest was focused on localized retinal lesions, such as degenerations and retinal holes.

Materials and methods

A sequence of detachments of different age was studied (1 hour; 1 and 3 days; 1, 2, 3, 4, 8, 12, and 20 weeks; each group consisting of two or three eyes). Retinas previously detached for a period of 1, 2, 4, 8, and 12 weeks were examined after they had been reattached for 4 weeks (each group consisting of two eyes). Four normal eyes served as controls. Two eyes were treated with hyaluronidase alone, and four eyes were treated with hyaluronidase plus vitreous destruction but without hole production.

The enucleated eyes were fixed in Kolmer's fixative, embedded in paraffin, and finally stained with hematoxylin-eosin and PAS.

Results and comment

The normal retina of an owl monkey is very similar to that of a human eye (Fig. 16-10). Mere intravitreal injection of hyaluronidase or vitreous destruction, together with hyaluronidase, does not present any changes in the retina. This point has to be emphasized as proof that the changes in eyes with retinal detachment are due to the detachment itself.

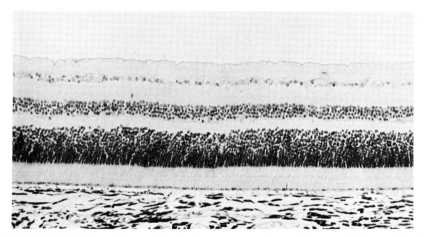

Fig. 16-10. The histology of normal retina in an owl monkey looks very similar to that of the human. Kolmer fixation preserves the structure of the retina very well. (PAS, ×190.) (From Machemer, R.: Amer. J. Ophthal. **66:**396, 1968.)

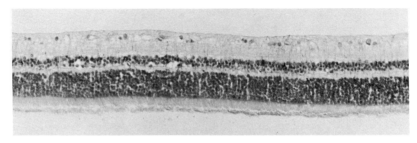

Fig. 16-11. Retina of a 1-day-old detachment. The inner parts of the retina, including the inner nuclear layer, show a diffuse loosening of their structure caused by edema. (PAS, ×190.) (From Machemer, R.: Amer. J. Ophthal. **66:**396, 1968.)

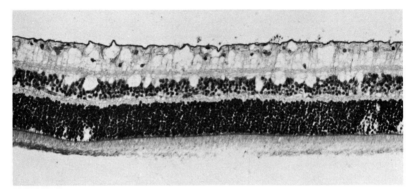

Fig. 16-12. In a 3-day-old detachment, cystoid spaces develop mainly in the ganglion-cell layer and in the inner nuclear layer. (PAS, ×190.) (From Machemer, R.: Amer. J. Ophthal. **66:**396, 1968.)

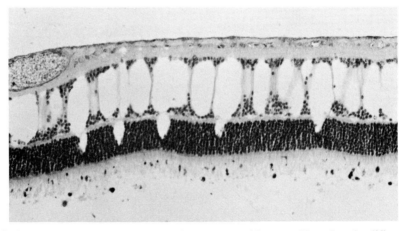

Fig. 16-13. Fourteen-day-old detachment with large cystoid spaces. Note that the diffuse edema has vanished in the inner retinal layers, that the spaces are separated only by thin walls of nerve fibers, and that the cystoid spaces have enlarged into the outer nuclear layer. (PAS, ×190.) (From Machemer, R.: Amer. J. Ophthal. **66:**396, 1968.)

Retinal detachment

Retina. Immediately after production of the detachment, the retina looks normal in the detached part, with the exception of changes in the immediate vicinity of the retinal hole with which we do not deal today. The most prominent change, beginning with the first day of detachment, is an edema. On the first day it is a diffuse loosening of the retinal structure in the inner retinal layers (Fig. 16-11). But as early as 3 days after the production of the detachment, cystoid spaces have developed. In the beginning they are found in the ganglion-cell layer and more numerously in the inner nuclear layer (Fig. 16-12). Later only the inner nuclear layer is affected and at the same time the diffuse edema has disappeared in this area. The spaces enlarge more and more so that 14 days after the detachment they break through the outer plexiform layer into the outer nuclear layer (Fig. 16-13). They are often so large that the walls between them become acellular and consist only of a thin layer of nerve fibers. The nuclei are found on the inner and outer sides of the spaces. Finally, these spaces can enlarge so much that many septa break down and huge empty spaces are formed. The cysts reach from the ganglion-cell layer to the outer nuclear layer. Only a few cells of the inner nuclear layer and the outer nuclear layer are left (Fig. 16-14).

It is important to mention that these changes are not apparent throughout the whole detached retina. The older a detachment is, the more different changes of edema can be found, so that nearly normal-looking retina, diffuse edema, and small and huge cystoid spaces occur all in one retina. It is not quite clear why some areas develop these intensive changes and others remain fairly normal, but one of the reasons seems to be the distance of the retina from the pigment epithelium.

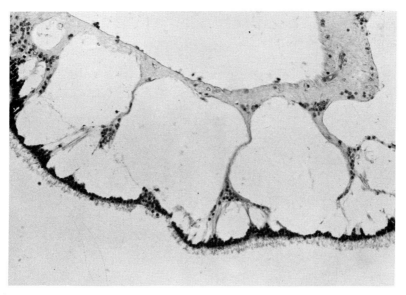

Fig. 16-14. Huge cystoid spaces with loss of cells in the inner and outer nuclear layer are formed in a 14-week-old detachment. (PAS, ×190.) (From Machemer, R.: Amer. J. Ophthal. 66:396, 1968.)

An interesting finding is that the edema never causes the inner side of the retina to bulge but only the outer side. Thus the back of the retina has a wavy appearance, and we think this appearance corresponds to the clinical observation of the shagreen-like pattern in a detached retina (Fig. 16-15).

Of special interest are the changes that occur in the photoreceptor layer of the retina. In a normal retina the inner and outer segments are arranged parallel and single rods and cones can easily be distinguished (Fig. 16-16). Beginning with the first day after the detachment, there is a progressing irregularity in the layer of the outer segments. It is no longer possible to distinguish single outer segments (Fig.

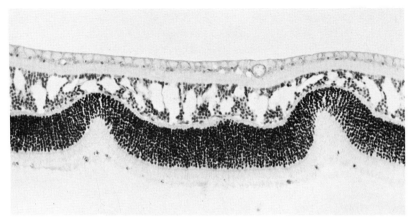

Fig. 16-15. Edema as well as cystoid spaces may outwardly bulge the posterior side of the retina. This structure causes the shagreen-like appearance of the retina as shown in Figs. 16-3 to 16-5 and 16-7. (PAS, ×190.) (From Machemer, R.: Amer. J. Ophthal. **66:**396, 1968.)

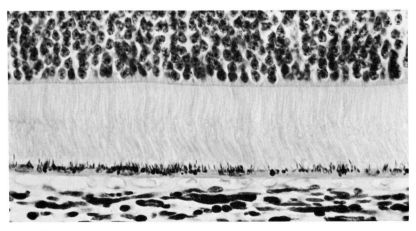

Fig. 16-16. The photoreceptors of the normal retina consist mainly of parallel-arranged rods that can be easily distinguished. (PAS, ×750.) (From Machemer, R.: Amer. J. Ophthal. **66:** 396, 1968.)

16-17). The older the detachment becomes and the heavier the cystic changes are, the more destruction will take place in the layers of the outer segments. The inner segments look quite normal for a long time, but finally, with heavy cystoid space formation in the retina, they become thicker and shorter (Fig. 16-18). Macrophages are found in the outer segment layer as early as 3 days after the beginning of the detachment, and they become much more numerous later on.

The changes in the outer segments depend very much on how high the detachment is. For example, in one 14-day-old high detachment the outer segments were very irregular and full of macrophages; in another eye of the same age with very flat detachment the retina showed many intact outer segments that were still parallelly arranged (Fig. 16-19).

Three observations concerning the above-described changes seem to be of special interest: The first is that a part of the photoreceptor cell, the outer segment, degenerates, but the cell, as indicated by its otherwise well-preserved structure, is still alive. This partial degeneration is probably due to the lack of normal nourishment of the photoreceptor cells by the pigment epithelium. The next finding is that edema of the retina occurs in an area that is well supplied by blood vessels. Capillaries penetrate toward the outside of the inner nuclear layer. Not only the outer parts of the retina

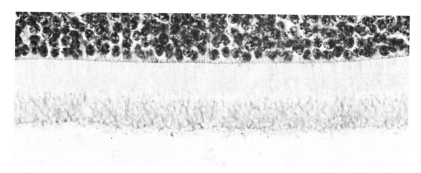

Fig. 16-17. One day after detachment of the retina the outer segments become irregular and cannot be separated from each other. (PAS, ×750.)

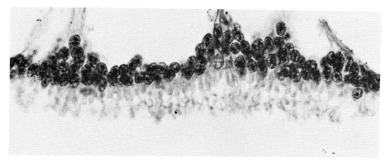

Fig. 16-18. In a 14-week-old detachment with large cystoid space formation the inner segments are fewer, shorter, and thicker. The outer segments are almost totally degenerated. (PAS, ×750.) See also Fig. 16-14. (From Machemer, R.: Amer. J. Ophthal. 66:396, 1968.)

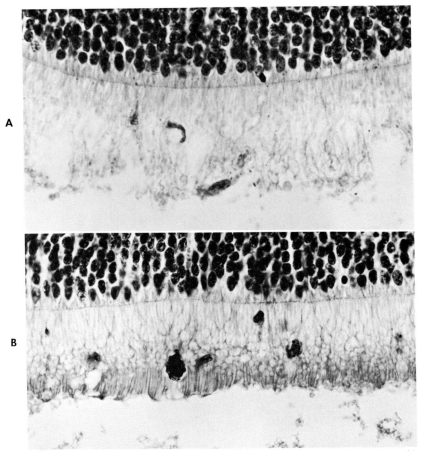

Fig. 16-19. Fourteen-day-old detachments. Compare the degeneration of the photoreceptors in an area of high detachment, **A,** with the fairly well-preserved photoreceptors in a very flat detachment, **B.** Note the macrophages. (PAS, ×750.) (From Machemer, R.: Amer. J. Ophthal. **66:**396, 1968.)

seem dependent on the metabolic activity of the pigment epithelium but also the inner parts. Finally, it is important that the degeneration of the outer segments and the edema of the retina are always fewer when the retina is flatly detached. This seems to indicate that the detached retina still receives some nutrition from the pigment epithelium that not only can delay the development of an edema in the inner part of the retina but also can maintain the structure of the outer segments of the retina.

Pigment epithelium. The pigment epithelium in an eye with a retinal detachment looks different from that which is usually seen in eyes with an artificial detachment due to the histologic process. The latter shows flat pigment cells, the base of which has a rather clear cytoplasm and a partly visible nucleus. The inner part of the cell is pigmented with vertically oriented pigment granules (Fig. 16-20). In the de-

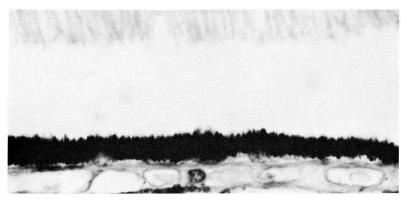

Fig. 16-20. Artificial retinal detachment caused by the fixation process. The pigment epithelium seems to consist of two parts: the base clear, with partly visible nuclei, and the top full of pigment granules. (PAS, ×1900.) (From Machemer, R.: Amer. J. Ophthal. **66**:396, 1968.)

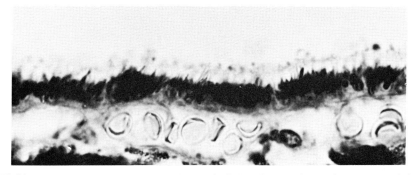

Fig. 16-21. Pigment epithelium 1 hour after retinal detachment. A translucent part of the cell overlying the pigmented part becomes visible. It represents the cytoplasmic processes of the pigment epithelial cell. (PAS, ×1900.) (From Machemer, R.: Amer. J. Ophthal. **66**:396, 1968.)

tached retina immediately after the detachment a third part overlying the pigmented part of the cell is visible. It stains faintly but has a vertical structure and has about one third the thickness of the cell (Fig. 16-21). This translucent part becomes more prominent in the older detachments.

After 3 days of detachment the pigment epithelium cell surface becomes protuberant, and the pigment granules are no longer mainly vertically oriented but often very irregular. The protuberant cells can have the shape of a button (Fig. 16-22), but with the increase of the detachment period and with thickening of the translucent layer, the pigment epithelial cell finally tends to flatten out again.

We think that the translucent layer, which is so well visible after Kolmer fixation of the eye, represents cytoplasmic processes of the pigment cell that, in an attached retina, interdigitate with the outer segments. In an artificial detachment caused by the fixation they are probably pulled off the pigment cell and are therefore never seen.

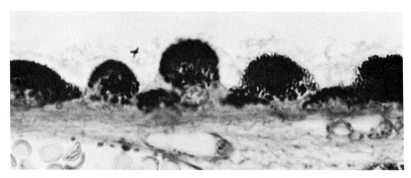

Fig. 16-22. Fourteen-day-old detachment. Pigment epithelial cells tend to protrude. (PAS, ×1900.)

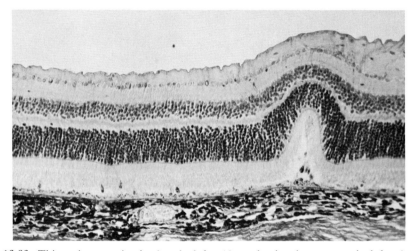

Fig. 16-23. This retina, previously detached for 12 weeks, has been reattached for 4 weeks. In the flatly attached part the retina looks normal. The fold reminds one of the previous detachment. (PAS, ×190.)

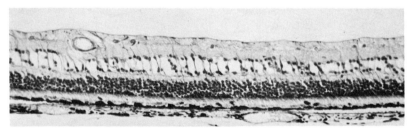

Fig. 16-24. After 2 weeks of detachment and 4 weeks of reattachment this retina still has a few areas with small cystoid spaces in the inner nuclear layer. (PAS, ×190.)

It is important to emphasize that over a period of at least 20 weeks no signs of degeneration of the pigment epithelium could be found; on the contrary, we had the impression that the pigment epithelium was still highly functional. This corroborates very well the above-described observation that a flatly detached retina undergoes less intensive changes.

Reattachment

The findings in the reattached retina are much more monotonous. It is usually flatly attached, sometimes with a little fold (Fig. 16-23). Older detachments occasionally reattach somewhat wavily. The edema and the cysts that were so prominent in the detached retina have disappeared, irrespective of the detachment period. Only occasionally a little diffuse edema or small cysts remain (Fig. 16-24). In old detachments there is an infrequent loss and displacement of cells in a few places. The most important finding is that the photoreceptor layer looks nearly normal. Inner

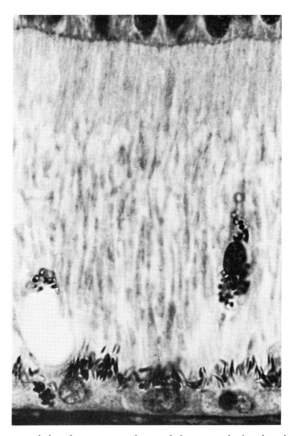

Fig. 16-25. High power of the photoreceptor layer of the reattached retina shown in Fig. 16-23. The inner and outer segments are again arranged in a parallel pattern, are of normal length, and are in good contact with the pigment epithelium. Macrophages remind one of the previous detachment. (PAS, ×1900.) (From Machemer, R.: Amer. J. Ophthal. 66:1075, 1968.)

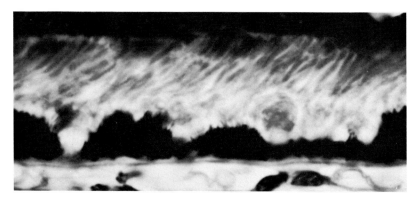

Fig. 16-26. Only in a few areas are the outer segments of the reattached retina clumped. This retina was detached for 2 weeks and reattached for 4 weeks. (PAS, ×1900.)

and outer segments are parallelly arranged, and they are in good contact with the pigment epithelium (Fig. 16-25). The only three reminders of a previous detachment are as follows: a few areas where clumping in the outer segment layer can be seen (Fig. 16-26), macrophages that are still visible in the outer segment layer, and pigment epithelium cells that are sometimes still protuberant although most of the cells are flattened out. The pigment granules are vertically arranged as in the normal eye, and they project into the outer segment layer.

What has happened in the reattached retina? The edema of the inner layers, irrespective of the detachment period, has been absorbed very quickly, mostly without leaving behind any microscopically visible destruction. It is most striking that after only 4 weeks of reattachment the outer segments of the photoreceptor layer look nearly normal. This appearance cannot be due only to a rearrangement of outer segments that are still intact. These findings suggest very strongly that there must have taken place a regeneration of outer segments.

SUMMARY

It is possible to produce a permanent and progressive retinal detachment in the owl monkey very similar in its clinical picture to that of the human retinal detachment: total detachment with small holes, development of giant tears and dialyses, and, finally, pictures that simulate M.V.R. It is possible to reattach these retinas by conventional surgical techniques. The most prominent features in histologic sections of detached retina are diffuse edema and cystoid space formation in the inner retinal layers, together with degeneration of the outer segments of the photoreceptor layer. The changes seem to depend on the age and height of the detachment. The pigment epithelium has an inner translucent portion, demonstrates no signs of degeneration, and shows metabolic activity. The edema in the reattached retina vanishes very quickly, and the outer segments seem to regenerate.

• • •

I wish to acknowledge the patient craftsmanship of Mr. John McGuinness Meyer who did the fundus paintings and the assistance of Mrs. Marcelia Halley during the operative procedures and in the preparation of histologic slides.

REFERENCES

1. Chodin, A.: Einige Versuche über den Glaskörpervorfall, Zbl. Med. Wiss. (Berlin) **5:**704, 1875.
2. Birch-Hirschfeld, A., and Inouye, T.: Experimentelle und histologische Untersuchungen über Netzhautabhebung, Graefe Arch. Ophthal. **70:**486, 1909.
3. Alajmo, A., and Auricchio, G.: Sul distacco di retina sperimentale, Rass. Ital. Oftal. **22:** 192, 1953.
4. Foulds, W. S.: Experimental retinal detachment, Trans. Ophthal. Soc. U. K. **83:**153, 1963.
5. Custodis, E.: Beobachtungen bei der diathermischen Behandlung der Netzhautablösung und ein Hinweis zur Therapie der Amotio retinae, Ber. Deutsch. Ophthal. Ges. **57:**227, 1952.

17

Experimental retinal detachment and reattachment*

II. Electron microscopy

Arnold J. Kroll
Robert Machemer

INTRODUCTION

It has been shown in the preceding paper that experimental retinal detachment in the owl monkey produced characteristic histologic changes and that surgical re-attachment of the retina reversed them.† In the present paper, we shall describe the electron microscopic characteristics of the retina and pigment epithelium in these eyes.

MATERIALS AND METHODS

In a series of owl monkeys (*Aotus trivirgatus*), retinas were experimentally de-tached as previously described.† Eyes were enucleated, without regard to conditions of light or dark adaptation, at intervals ranging from 1 hour to 14 weeks. In addition, a series of retinas of varying ages of detachment was surgically reattached and all of these eyes were enucleated 4 weeks postoperatively.

Control eyes were subjected to intravitreal hyaluronidase injection alone or in-jection plus vitreous aspiration and reinjection. Areas of attached retina in eyes with partial detachment also served as controls.

After enucleation, each globe was opened near the ora serrata. A portion of mid-peripheral retina and pigment epithelium remote from the retinal breaks was excised with a sharp razor blade. The specimens were then fixed in 2% phosphate-buffered osmium tetroxide, dehydrated in a graded series of ethanol, embedded in Epon 812

*This investigation was supported by research grants NB-05918 and NB-06841 from the National Institute of Neurological Diseases and Blindness, U. S. Public Health Service; by Fight for Sight, Inc., Grant-in-Aid Special Fellowship no. F-211; and by funds from Research to Prevent Blindness, Inc., and the Florida Lions Eye Bank, Inc.
†See Chapter 16.

and sectioned and stained for both phase-contrast and electron microscopy, as described elsewhere.[1]

OBSERVATIONS

The detailed observations are recorded as legends that accompany the figures. In essence, experimental retinal detachment produced the following changes:

1. The horizontally layered saccules in the photoreceptor outer segments underwent marked degeneration. This degeneration included loss of horizontal orientation, fragmentation, and eventual atrophy.
2. Macrophages phagocytized fragments of outer segments.
3. The pigment epithelial lamellar inclusion bodies[2-4] degenerated and disappeared.
4. The apical surface of the pigment epithelial cells became convexly protuberant, and the apical processes increased in number and became thickened.
5. Melanin granules withdrew from the apical processes.
6. Cystoid extracellular spaces of varying sizes appeared in the middle and inner retina. These spaces consisted of enlargement of extracellular spaces. They were bordered by the cytoplasmic membranes of contiguous retinal cells.

Surgical reattachment of the retina resulted in reformation of the normal horizontally layered photoreceptor outer segment saccules. Inclusion bodies reappeared in the pigment epithelium, and melanin granules returned to the apical processes. The latter resumed their normal length, shape, and morphologic relationship to the photoreceptor outer segments. The cystoid retinal spaces disappeared.

Text continued on p. 274.

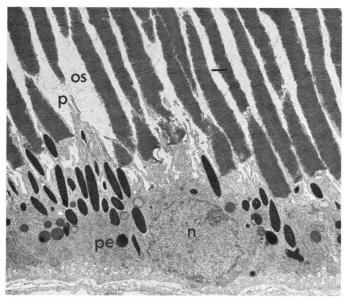

Fig. 17-1. Control eye. Low-power survey of region of photoreceptor outer segments *(os)* and pigment epithelium *(pe)*. Note the close morphologic relationship of the outer segments to the apical processes *(p)* of the pigment epithelial cells. *n,* Nucleus of pigment epithelial cell. (Mark is equivalent to 1 μ. ×6000.)

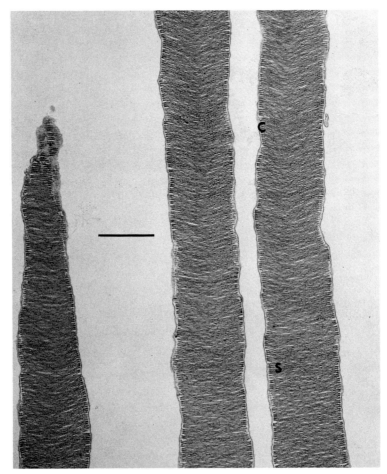

Fig. 17-2. Control eye. The photoreceptor outer segment in radial section at higher magnification consists of stacks of flattened membranous saccules *(s)* enclosed by the cytoplasmic membrane *(c)*. (Mark is equivalent to 1 μ. ×20,000.)

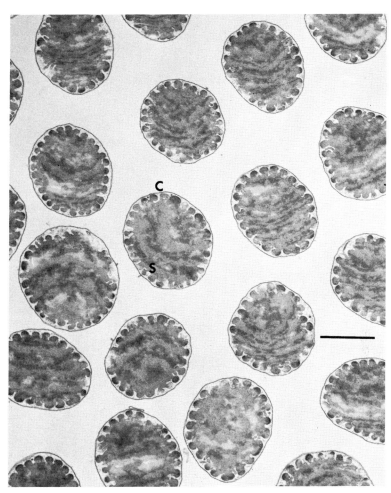

Fig. 17-3. Control eye. The photoreceptor outer segment in flat section consists of a circular structure with scalloped edges *(s)* enclosed by the cytoplasmic membrane *(c)*. Comparing this with Fig. 17-2 permits the three-dimensional construction of the outer segment as similar to a stack of coins enclosed in a closely fitting thin bag. (Mark is equivalent to 1 μ. ×20,000.)

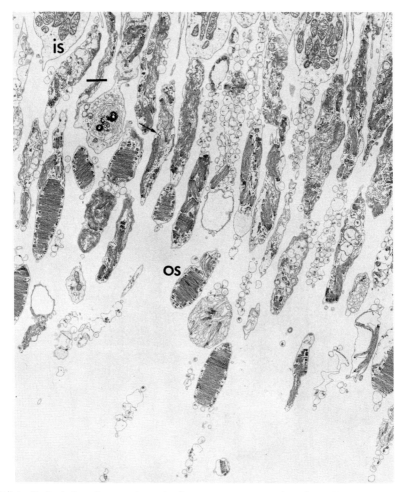

Fig. 17-4. Retinal detachment, 1 week. Low-power survey of region of outer segments (cf. Fig. 17-1). Some outer segments *(os)* retain a relatively normal configuration. Others *(arrow)* contain saccules that are fragmented, loosely bound, vertically arranged, and irregular. In still others the cytoplasmic membrane has ruptured and the discs have become swollen and globular. The inner segments *(is)* are morphologically normal. (Mark is equivalent to 1 μ. ×7000.)

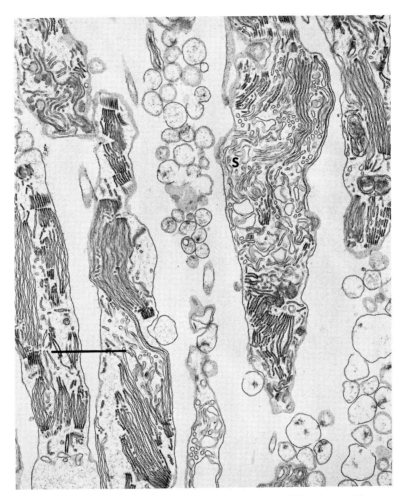

Fig. 17-5. High-power micrograph of one region of Fig. 17-4. The abnormally arranged and fragmented saccules *(s)* of the outer segments still retain a layered appearance in some cells. In other cells the cytoplasmic membrane has ruptured. (Mark is equivalent to 1 μ. ×26,000.)

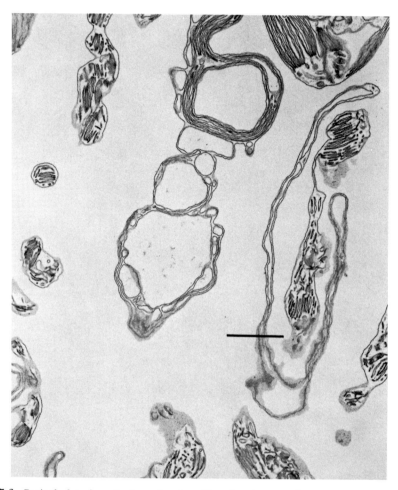

Fig. 17-6. Retinal detachment, 4 weeks. In older detachments the outer segments become attenuated, become cystic, or assume bizarre forms. (Mark is equivalent to 1 μ. ×20,000.)

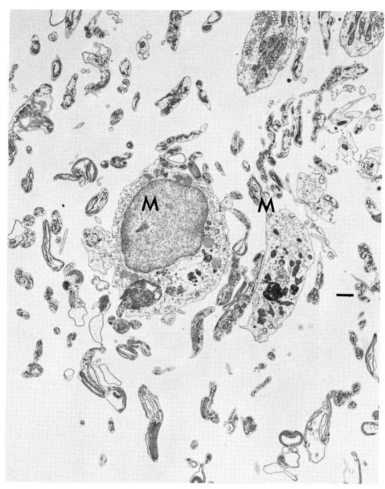

Fig. 17-7. Retinal detachment, 4 weeks. Low-power survey of region of outer segments show-ing the presence of macrophages *(M)* in this layer. The latter appear within a few days after retinal detachment. (Mark is equivalent to 1 μ. ×6000.)

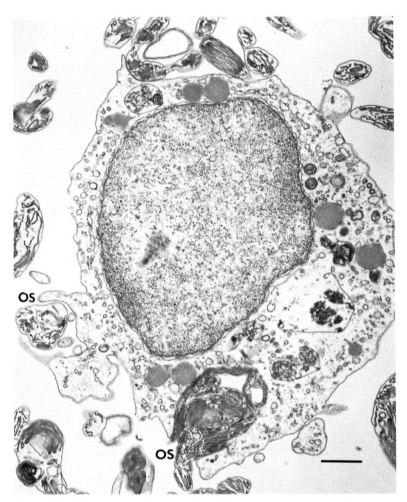

Fig. 17-8. High-power micrograph of a macrophage seen in Fig. 17-7. The cell is in the process of phagocytizing two portions of outer segment material *(os)*. (Mark is equivalent to 1 μ. ×15,000.)

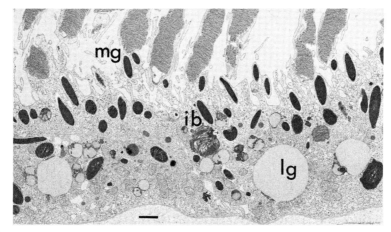

Fig. 17-9. Control eye. Low-power survey of pigment epithelium. The cells contain several kinds of cytoplasmic inclusions: (1) inclusion bodies (*ib*), which consist of stacked flattened saccules, (2) melanin granules (*mg*), which are dense homogeneous elliptical bodies enclosed by a single membrane, and (3) lipofuscin granules (*lg*), which are spherical and less dense. (Mark is equivalent to 1 μ. ×6000.)

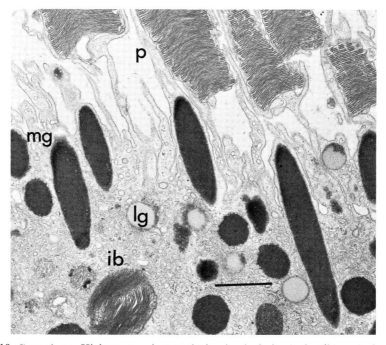

Fig. 17-10. Control eye. High-power micrograph showing inclusion body *(ib)*, melanin granules *(mg)*, and lipofuscin granules *(lg)* in the pigment epithelium. The apical processes of the pigment epithelial cells *(p)* are long, thin, and in close contact with the photoreceptor outer segments. The dense elliptical melanin granules tend to lie in the apical processes. Note the structural similarity between the outer segments and the inclusion body.[3-5] The latter may be a portion of a photoreceptor outer segment engulfed by a pigment epithelial cell.[2-4] (Mark is equivalent to 1 μ. ×20,000.)

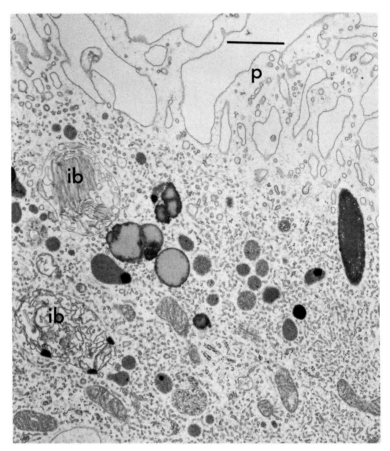

Fig. 17-11. Pigment epithelium in eye with detached retina, 1 day. Two degenerate inclusion bodies *(ib)* are present. The apical processes *(p)* are thickened and no longer contain melanin granules. In older detachments, the inclusion bodies have completely disappeared. (Mark is equivalent to 1 μ. ×20,000.)

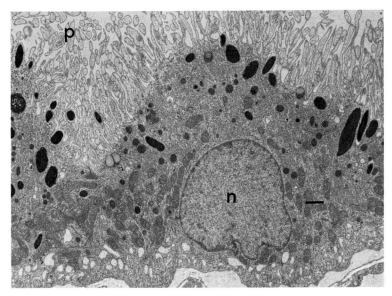

Fig. 17-12. Pigment epithelium in eye with detached retina, 8 weeks. Low-power survey (cf. Fig. 17-9). The pigment epithelium is taller. Inclusion bodies are absent, but melanin and lipofuscin granules are present. The melanin granules have withdrawn from the apical processes *(p)*, leaving a melanin-free apical zone. The apical processes are thickened and increased in number. The pigment epithelial cell apices are convexly protuberant. *n*, nucleus. (Mark is equivalent to 1 μ. ×6000.)

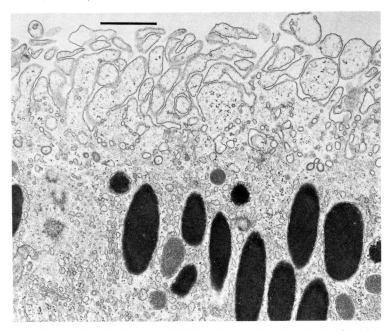

Fig. 17-13. Apical region of pigment epithelium in eye with detached retina, 2 weeks (cf. Fig. 17-10). There is a melanin-free zone of pigment epithelial apical processes. (Mark is equivalent to 1 μ. ×20,000.)

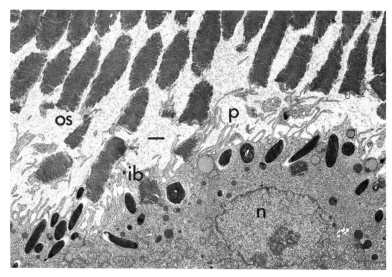

Fig. 17-14. Surgically reattached retina, 4 weeks postoperative. Low-power survey of pigment epithelium (cf. Figs. 17-4 and 17-12). The retina had been detached for 2 weeks prior to surgery. The photoreceptor outer segments *(os)* have returned to their normal configuration and are once again in close relation to the pigment epithelial apical processes *(p)*. Inclusion bodies *(ib)* have reappeared in the pigment epithelium. The apices of the latter remain convexly protuberant. *n*, nucleus. (Mark is equivalent to 1 μ. ×6000.)

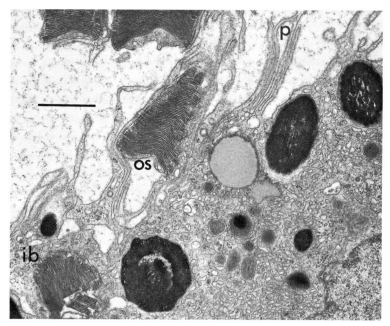

Fig. 17-15. High-power micrograph of a portion of Fig. 17-14 (cf. Figs. 17-5 and 17-13). Note the presence of an inclusion body *(ib)*, the normal lamellated structure of the photoreceptor outer segments *(os)*, and the close association of the outer segments with the apical processes *(p)* of the pigment epithelium. (Mark is equivalent to 1 μ. ×20,000.)

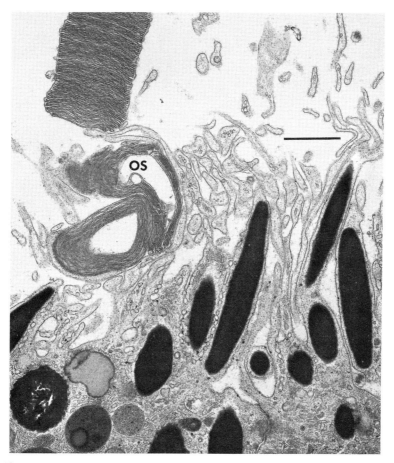

Fig. 17-16. Surgically reattached retina, 4 weeks postoperative (cf. Fig. 17-13). The retina had been detached for 4 weeks prior to surgery. In this micrograph of pigment epithelium, note the return of the dense melanin granules into the apical processes and the close association of the processes to some still abnormal outer segment material *(os)*. (Mark is equivalent to 1 μ. ×20,000.)

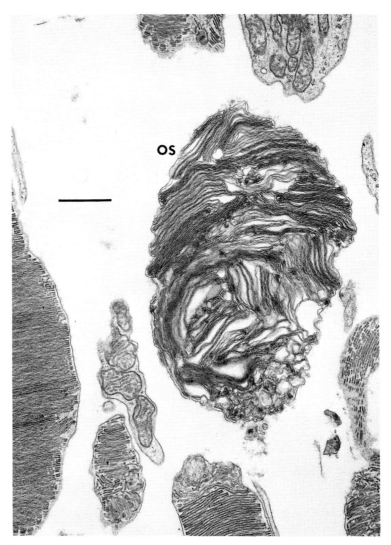

Fig. 17-17. Surgically reattached retina, same eye as in Fig. 17-16. Not all the outer segments have yet returned to their normal configuration. The outer segment *(os)* in the center of the micrograph remains disorganized. It closely resembles an inclusion body of the pigment epithelium. (Mark is equivalent to 1 μ. ×20,000.)

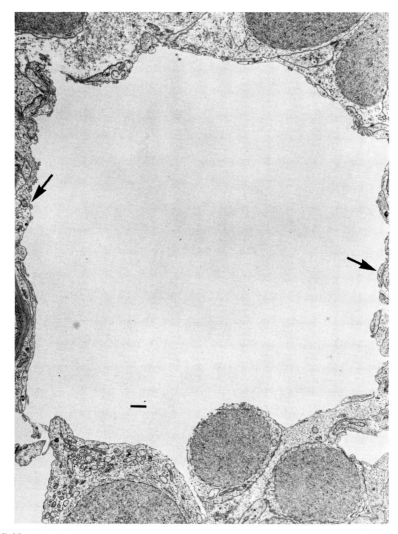

Fig. 17-18. Retinal detachment, 4 weeks. Low-power micrograph of a cystoid space in the bipolar cell layer. Note that the borders of the space *(arrows)* have no lining structure. The space is an enlargement of the extracellular space. Surgical reattachment of the retina results in the disappearance of these cystoid spaces. (Mark is equivalent to 1 μ. ×5000.)

COMMENT

It has been known by light microscopists for many years that degeneration of photoreceptor cells follows detachment of the retina.[5] In the present study, electron microscopy has shown that the portion of the photoreceptor primarily affected is the outer segment. (In the relatively short periods of detachment studied, some, but not many, photoreceptor cell bodies degenerated.) The visual pigments are found in the outer segments.[6] The recovery of the fine structure of outer segments with reattachment of the retina suggests that proximity to the pigment epithelium and choroid is essential for the maintenance of outer segment morphology.

Electron microscopy in the present study has also shown that the lamellar inclusion bodies of the pigment epithelium degenerate and disappear after retinal detachment and that they reappear after reattachment of the retina. Inclusion bodies are spherical membrane-bound cytoplasmic inclusions of the pigment epithelium that

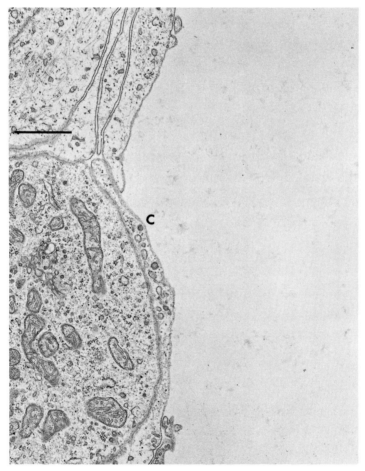

Fig. 17-19. Detached retina, 8 weeks. The border of a cystoid space may be smooth. It consists of the cytoplasmic membrane *(c)* of the adjacent retinal cells. (Mark is equivalent to 1 μ. ×20,000.)

measure approximately 1.5μ in diameter and consist of stacked flattened saccules, not dissimilar to those of photoreceptor outer segments. They may be broken or detached portions of photoreceptor outer segments engulfed by the pigment epithelial cells.[2-4]

It is impressive that retinal detachment produces disintegration primarily of only two structures, the outer segments of the photoreceptors and the inclusion bodies of the pigment epithelium, and that on reattachment of the retina these structures return together to their normal morphology. There is only one other experimental

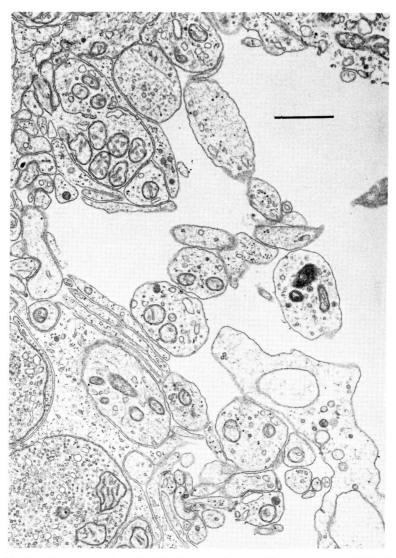

Fig. 17-20. Detached retina, 4 weeks. The border of a cystoid space may be highly irregular. It nevertheless consists of the cytoplasmic membrane of adjacent retinal cells. (Mark is equivalent to 1 μ. ×20,000.)

condition known to cause outer segment degeneration and disappearance of inclusion bodies—vitamin A deficiency—and these changes can be reversed by administration of vitamin A.[7] What could retinal detachment and vitamin A deficiency have in common?

It is well established that the close morphologic relationship between the photoreceptors and the pigment epithelium is an important one.[6] The processes of light and dark adaptation involve exchanges of vitamin A between the outer segments of photoreceptors and the pigment epithelium. That is, in light adaptation the amount of retinine (vitamin A aldehyde) in the retina falls, and the amount of vitamin A in the pigment epithelium rises. In dark adaptation the amount of retinine in the retina rises and the amount of vitamin A in the pigment epithelium falls.[8]

It is conceivable that the separation of the photoreceptor and pigment epithelial layers by subretinal fluid in retinal detachment interferes enough with the exchange of vitamin A, and possibly other materials between them, that a situation mimicking a localized deficiency of the vitamin is present. This interference is supported, perhaps, by the observation that the photoreceptors in areas of flat detachment are much better preserved than in areas of high bullous detachment.*

In any event, the present work suggests that the pigment epithelial inclusion body does indeed originate from the photoreceptor outer segment. Recently, it has been reported that prolonged exposure of albino rats to light caused a temporary marked increase in the number of inclusion bodies in the pigment epithelium, associated with degenerative changes in the photoreceptor outer segments.[9]

It is not likely that ischemia resulting from the separation of the photoreceptors from their blood supply in the choroid could account for the observed changes. It is difficult to postulate that ischemia would selectively damage the outer segments only and not the photoreceptor cells proper. In addition, ischemia could not account for the changes observed in the pigment epithelium. Finally, retinal ischemia is known to produce mitochondrial and cytoplasmic swelling,[10] neither of which was seen in the present study. The reasons for the other changes noted in the pigment epithelium after retinal detachment and the recovery after reattachment are not clear.

The appearance of cystoid spaces in the retina after retinal detachment also occurs in the human disease.[11, 12] In the present work, the cause of the retinal hydration with detachment and dehydration with reattachment is unknown. It is possible that one function of the pigment epithelium and choroid is to keep the retina in a normal state of dehydration. The presence of a retinal break and subretinal fluid apparently interferes with this function. Closure of the retinal break and resorption of subretinal fluid only then may permit dehydration of the retina to take place. Apparently, the blood supply to the retina is not the determining factor in cystoid space formation. The spaces form in the inner and middle retina, where the blood supply from the central retinal artery is intact, and not in the outer retina.

SUMMARY

Electron microscopy of a series of experimentally detached retinas in the owl monkey (*Aotus trivirgatus*) revealed fine-structure changes in the retina and pig-

---

*See Chapter 16.

ment epithelium. The photoreceptor outer segments degenerated, lamellar inclusion bodies disappeared from the pigment epithelium, melanin granules withdrew from the pigment epithelial apical processes, and cystoid extracellular spaces appeared in the middle and inner retinal layers. Control eyes did not show these changes, and surgical reattachment of the retinas reversed them.

• • •

The authors acknowledge the capable technical assistance of Mr. Barry Davis and Mrs. Marcilia Halley.

REFERENCES

1. Kroll, A. J.: Fine structural classification of orbital rhabdomyosarcoma, Invest. Ophthal. **6:**531, 1967.
2. Dowling, J. E., and Gibbons, I. R.: The fine structure of the pigment epithelium in the albino rat, J. Cell Biol. **14:**459, 1962.
3. Bairati, A. J., and Orzalesi, N.: The ultrastructure of the pigment epithelium and the photoreceptor-pigment epithelium junction in the human retina, J. Ultrastruct. Res. **9:** 484, 1963.
4. Cohen, A. I.: Vertebrate retinal cells and their organization, Biol. Rev. **38:**427, 1963.
5. Birch-Hirschfeld, A., and Inouye, T.: Experimentelle und histologische Untersuchungen über Netzhautabhebung, Graefe Arch. Ophthal. **70:**486, 1909.
6. Wald, G.: Photochemical aspects of visual excitation, Exp. Cell Res. **5:**Suppl.:389, 1958.
7. Dowling, J. E., and Gibbons, I. R.: The effect of vitamin A deficiency on the fine structure of the retina. In Smelser, G., editor: The structure of the eye, New York, 1961, Academic Press.
8. Dowling, J. E.: Chemistry of visual adaptation in the rat, Nature (London) **188:**114, 1960.
9. Kuwabara, T., and Gorn, R. A.: Retinal damage by visible light—an electron microscopic study, Arch. Ophthal. **79:**69, 1968.
10. Kroll, A. J.: Experimental central retinal artery occlusion, Arch. Ophthal. **79:**453, 1968.
11. Hogan, M., and Zimmerman, L. E.: Ophthalmic pathology, an atlas and textbook, Philadelphia, 1962, W. B. Saunders Co.
12. Keith, C. G.: Retinal cysts and retinoschisis, Brit. J. Ophthal. **50:**617, 1966.

18

Therapy of retinal detachment complicated by massive preretinal fibroplasia*

(Long-term follow-up of patients treated with intravitreal liquid silicone†)

Edward Okun and Neva P. Arribas

INTRODUCTION

Until Paul Cibis introduced the concept of intravitreal surgery utilizing liquid silicone to loosen up preretinal membranes, retinal detachments complicated by massive preretinal fibroplasia were considered hopeless. Today, many of these cases are cured, and as our techniques and material improve, we can look forward to the day when all retinal detachments are amenable to some type of treatment.

INDICATIONS

Intravitreal surgery for reattachment of the retina should be undertaken only after it becomes apparent that a surgical cure cannot be accomplished by an ab externo approach. Simple vitreous supplementation with balanced salt solution should first be tried to see whether the fixed folds can be pushed back into a more normal position (Fig. 18-1). If this supplementation does not change the appearance of the central retina, the indication is that the preretinal membrane is too resistant to be overcome by the push and will, therefore, have to be separated from the retina. For this purpose, liquid silicone has proved to be the most adequate material by virtue of its relatively high surface tension and perfect transparency.

*This investigation was supported in part by research grant NB-01789, from the National Institute of Neurological Diseases and Blindness, National Institutes of Health, Bethesda, Maryland.

†This material, now called Dow Corning no. 360 Medical Fluid, is not yet available for general use. It can presently be used only with the consent of the Food and Drug Administration, U. S. Public Health Service.

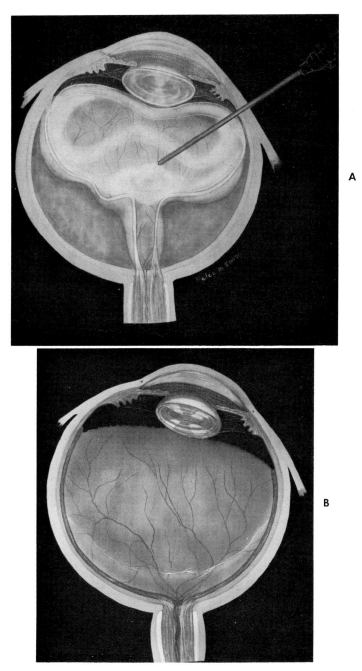

Fig. 18-1. A, Intravitreal saline used to expand shrunken vitreous space. **B,** In some instances the preretinal membrane will be fractured and stretched enough by this push to allow closure of retinal breaks and permit cure of early massive preretinal fibroplasia.

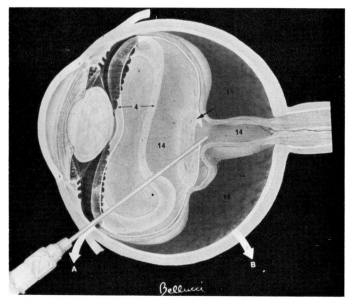

Fig. 18-2. Needle properly positioned for initial injection of liquid silicone *(A)*. Subretinal fluid has been released in part *(B)*.

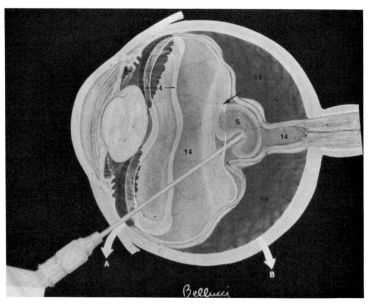

Fig. 18-3. Beginning of injection. View of the disc can now be obtained through the silicone bubble.

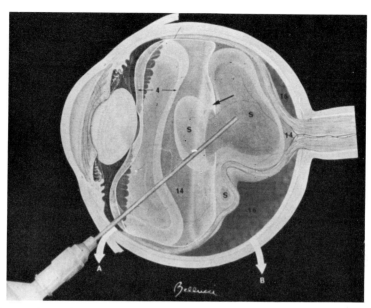

Fig. 18-4. Superior retina flattened. Membrane being pushed anteriorly. (From Cibis, P. A.: Vitreoretinal pathology and surgery in retinal detachment, St. Louis, 1965, The C. V. Mosby Co.)

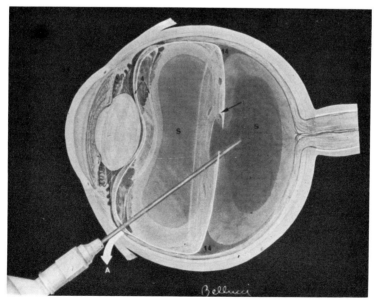

Fig. 18-5. Appearance at end of procedure. 1 to 2 ml. of liquid silicone used. All liquid silicone deposited in posterior vitreous space. (From Cibis, P. A.: Vitreoretinal pathology and surgery in retinal detachment, St. Louis, 1965, The C. V. Mosby Co.)

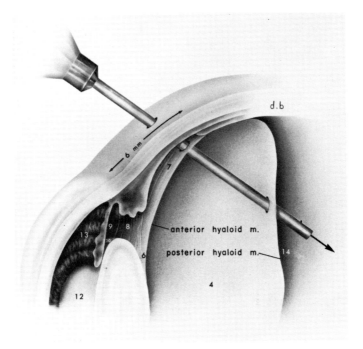

Fig. 18-6. Site of intravitreal injection through the pars plana approximately 6 mm. posterior to the limbus.

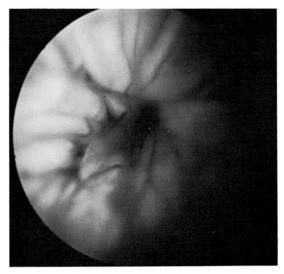

Fig. 18-7. Preoperative photograph of patient successfully treated by intravitreal liquid silicone procedure. Note dark cavity in the depths of which the disc is situated.

Under direct visual control, the liquid silicone can be deposited between this membrane and the retina, thus moving the membrane forward into a transvitreal plane and allowing the retina to settle back into its normal position once again (Figs. 18-2 to 18-5).

TECHNIQUE

The technique used is essentially that which was described by Paul Cibis in his monograph on vitreoretinal surgery.[1] The site for injection of the liquid silicone is first prepared approximately 5 to 6 mm. posterior to the limbus over the pars plana. A 4-0 silk traction suture is placed 3 mm. from the limbus, and the site for injection is marked off on the sclera approximately 2 mm. posterior to this suture (Fig. 18-6). A site for release of subretinal fluid is then selected and subretinal fluid is drained in part. The patient is then turned on his side and a Graefe knife is used to create a 2 to 3 mm. radial sclerochoroidal opening 5 to 6 mm. from the limbus. Under indirect ophthalmoscopic control, the tip of the knife is directed into the center of the vitreous, and when it is seen clearly, it is withdrawn. A 20-gauge blunt needle is then introduced through this incision and carried deep into the eye directly over the optic nerve head (or into the cavity in the depths of which the disc is situated) (Figs. 18-7 and 18-8). Liquid silicone (Dow Corning no. 360 Fluid) of 2000-centistoke viscosity is then pumped into the eye while the needle is moved slowly over the optic nerve in an attempt to help with the dissection of a translucent membrane from the surface of the retina. Free silicone will escape and rise as a small bubble if the membrane is not penetrated. Once the membrane is penetrated, the bubble remains central and, through it, a good view of the disc and posterior retina

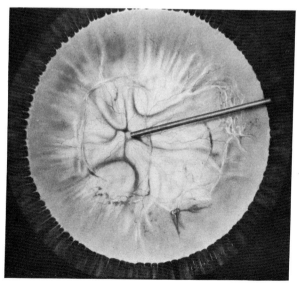

Fig. 18-8. Fundus painting indicating correct placement of needle before injection of liquid silicone is begun.

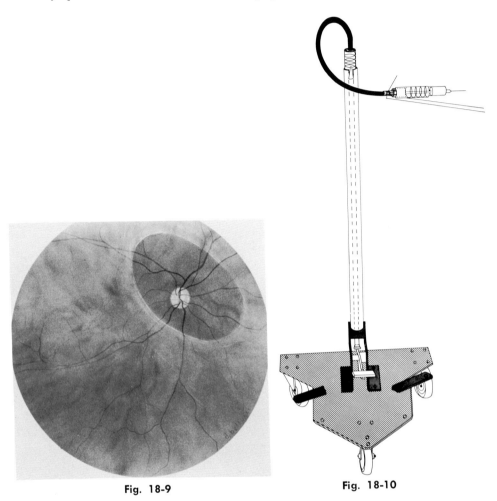

Fig. 18-9   Fig. 18-10

Fig. 18-9. Appearance of fundus after preretinal membrane has been moved to a transvitreal postequatorial plane.
Fig. 18-10. Drawing and diagram of foot-operated pump for delivery of liquid silicone.

is obtained. As the membrane is lifted off from the retina, small retinal hemorrhages usually appear on the surface of the retina. When the silicone is well positioned, one must use only 1 to 1.5 ml. The operation is terminated when the membrane reaches a transvitreal postequatorial plane (Fig. 18-9). Usually only minor scleral surgery is done at the time of the liquid silicone injection, since failure at this stage of the operation would make any ab externo surgery superfluous.

The actual injection of the liquid silicone has been greatly facilitated by the development of a foot-operated pump[2] (Figs. 18-10 to 18-14). This pump is so designed that the rate of injection is controlled solely by the force applied to the foot pedal, thus allowing the hand to perform the delicate task of teasing and dissecting the vitreous membranes. It is essential that every step of this procedure be visually

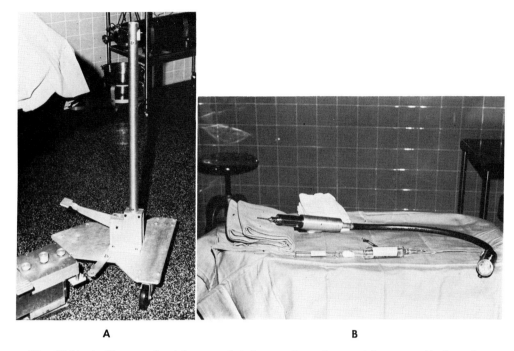

Fig. 18-11. A, Photograph of foot stand, before sterile syringe and hose assembly have been connected. **B,** Sterile syringe and hose assembly.

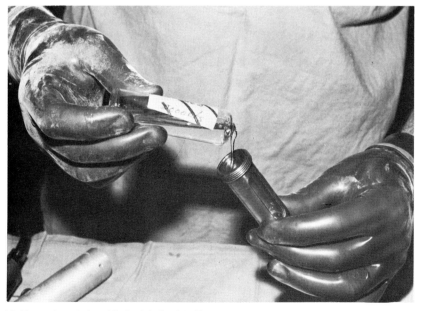

Fig. 18-12. Syringe being filled with liquid silicone.

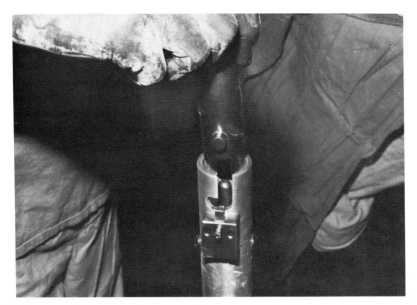

Fig. 18-13. Hose being connected to foot stand.

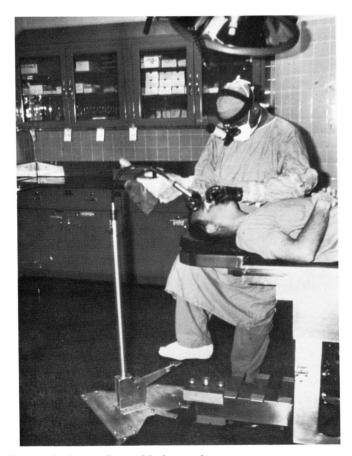

Fig. 18-14. Photograph of pump in use. Mock procedure.

monitored by means of an instrument that affords excellent stereopsis. For this purpose, we have used the binocular indirect ophthalmoscope worn on the head, thus freeing both hands for maneuvers. One hand holds the lens loop and the other directs the blunt-tipped needle that admits the liquid silicone and, at the same time, is used to tease membranes from the surface of the retina.

RESULTS

At the time of this writing, intravitreal surgery utilizing liquid silicone has been used in 311 patients (Fig. 18-15). An anatomic improvement has been accomplished initially in 186 patients (60%). Fifty-one of these patients (16%) showed no visual improvement despite anatomic reapposition of the retina. Fifty-four patients (17%) showed early improvement in visual function, but vision deteriorated subsequently, secondary to either recurrent retinal detachment or other complications. Sixty-seven

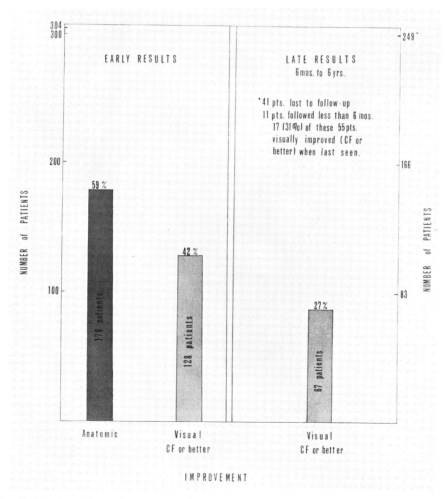

Fig. 18-15. Chart illustrating results of intravitreal surgery utilizing liquid silicone.

Table 18-1. Long-term follow-up of visual function in eyes that were treated with intravitreal liquid silicone

Year of surgery	Number of eyes treated	Number followed	Visual improvement c.f. min.	Percentage	Inadequate follow-up
1967	18	18	12	66	0
1966	17	15	5	33	2
1965	41	34	6	18	7
1964	43	31	8	26	12
1963	90	77	25	32	13
1962	80	73	19	26	7
1961	22	19	4	21	3
Total	311	267	79	28	44

of 249 patients (27%), who were followed for 6 months to 5 years, had maintained visual acuity of finger counting or better (walking vision). Thirty-five patients had maintained usable vision for more than 4 years (Table 18-1). Of 44 patients who had been lost to follow-up and 11 who had been followed less than 6 months, 31% were visually improved when last seen. Nine were deceased, three from myocardial infarction, one from a kidney condition, and two from far-advanced carcinoma. The cause of death was unknown in the other three. In all six cases in which the cause of death was known, the disease process that led to death anteceded the liquid silicone operation.

COMPLICATIONS

Complications of intravitreal surgery can be divided into those occurring during the surgical procedure and those occurring late. At the time of surgery the injection can be poorly placed, with most of the silicone going anterior to the membrane. This misplacement usually results in persistent retinal detachment (Fig. 18-16). Too vigorous an injection or excessive tug against the vitreous membranes can result in iatrogenic retinal breaks. Other retinal breaks can be produced either by too posterior an entry incision or by direct trauma from the delivery needle. Liquid silicone may gain access to the subretinal space either through one of these iatrogenic breaks or through one that had not been closed, leading to failure. Vitreous hemorrhages can occur at the injection site if a large ciliary vessel is inadvertently injured. A poorly directed injection needle can cause lens injury either at the time of injection or during its removal. Overfilling with liquid silicone can push the membrane too far anteriorly and lead to an extrusion of the vitreous base and subsequent disinsertion of the retina. Liquid silicone in the posterior chamber can cause a pupillary-block glaucoma.

Late complications included (1) Recurrent retinal detachment (Fig. 18-17), usually inferior, observed frequently in patients treated with liquid silicone (Dow Corning no. 360 Fluid), viscosity 2000 cs. with specific gravity 0.972. (2) Cataract formation occurred in 51% of the phakic patients. The usual cataract seen is that of a combination of nuclear sclerosis and posterior subcapsular opacification. These

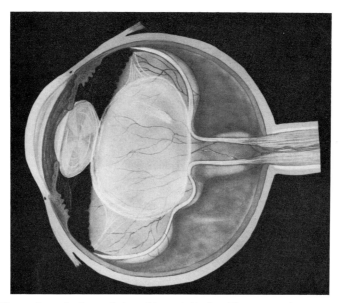

Fig. 18-16. Illustration of effect of deposition of liquid silicone anterior to preretinal membrane. Note persistence of retinal detachment and failure to move membrane.

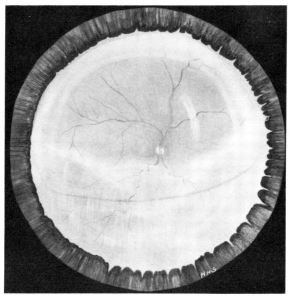

Fig. 18-17. Recurrent inferior retinal detachment in some cases associated with fibrous proliferation from inferior edge of silicone to inferior retina.

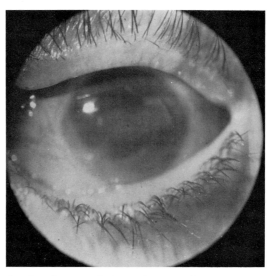

Fig. 18-18. Photograph of early corneal dystrophy secondary to presence of silicone in the anterior chamber. (From Cibis, P. A.: Vitreoretinal pathology and surgery in retinal detachment, St. Louis, 1965, The C. V. Mosby Co.)

Table 18-2. Late complications—intravitreal liquid silicone

Cataracts	Corneal dystrophy	Glaucoma	Enucle-ations	Recurrent retinal detachments
78/156 phakic (50%) 10/78 cataract ext. 5 extracapsular 1—glaucoma 5 intracapsular 2—corneal dystrophy 1—glaucoma	(Only in aphakia) 27/165 (16%)—2, in otherwise successful cases	32 (all but 3 aphakic)	10	45 (recurrence needing revision and refill)

took 6 months to 3 years to develop enough opacity to alter the patient's visual acuity. (3) Corneal dystrophy occurred in 17% of the aphakic patients. It started as a horizontal band-shaped area of edema just above the horizontal and gradually spread to involve the entire cornea (Fig. 18-18). Many of these patients also developed secondary glaucoma. (4) Secondary glaucoma occurred in 31 of the 311 patients. All but two of the patients were aphakic. The superior angle in these eyes always showed peripheral anterior synechiae, and, in addition, many contained fine, foamy-appearing globules of liquid silicone (Fig. 18-19).

MANAGEMENT OF COMPLICATIONS

Many of the operative complications can be avoided by careful selection of sites for injection, attention to landmarks, and working very slowly under visual control.

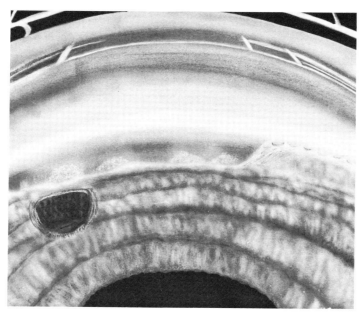

Fig. 18-19. Appearance of tiny silicone globules (foam) in the superior anterior chamber angle.

If retinal breaks occur during surgery, they can sometimes be closed by photo-coagulation therapy, with or without plombage, provided the retina can be flattened. Retinal hemorrhages can sometimes be stopped by light coagulation. Should liquid silicone get into the anterior chamber, it should be aspirated and replaced by air. Formed vitreous, which is extruded through the injection sclerotomy, should be excised.

The late occurrence of an inferior retinal detachment is not treated unless visual function is altered. If visual function begins to deteriorate, this fluid should be drained and an inferior imbrication performed to take up the volume. Of 44 such operations, there have been good results in 20.

When cataract formation becomes so dense that visual function is lost, a cataract extraction is performed. An extracapsular procedure is recommended since this is most effective in preventing liquid silicone from entering the anterior chamber. In children and young adults, a needle aspiration is recommended. Corneal dystrophy has occurred in two patients who have had intracapsular cataract extractions but in none of those who have had extracapsular procedures. However, the best visual acuity was achieved following an intracapsular cataract extraction 3 years after liquid silicone surgery (20/100).

The best therapy for corneal dystrophy is to avoid it. If liquid silicone enters the anterior chamber, as a late complication, an attempt should be made to force it back into the vitreous by the combination of dehydration of the vitreous with osmotic agents and massaging the eye while the patient maintains a prone position. If this procedure does not work, an attempt should be made to remove it by aspiration combined with air replacement. Bed rest is maintained in supine position until all

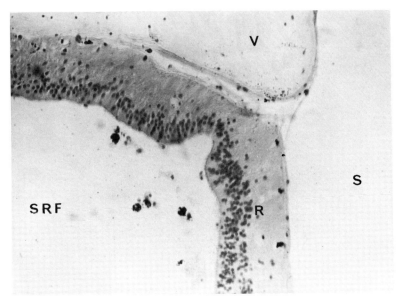

Fig. 18-20. Histopathologic appearance of ocular tissues in contact with liquid silicone. Note lack of cellular reaction. *V*, Vitreous; *S*, liquid silicone; *R*, retina; *SRF*, subretinal fluid.

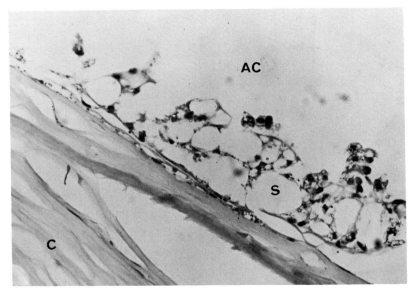

Fig. 18-21. Histopathologic appearance of corneal dystrophy secondary to deposition of fine silicone globules on endothelium. Note macrophages surrounding these globules. *AC*, Anterior chamber; *S*, silicone globules; *C*, cornea.

air is absorbed. If corneal edema persists, one must attempt to remove as much of the intravitreal silicone as possible and replace it with air, for the corneal dystrophy, if not checked, will result in complete loss of visual function.

Late glaucoma must be watched for, since it comes on quite insidiously and can destroy what little vision is left within several months. Several otherwise successful cases lost all useful vision because of undetected glaucoma. Once discovered, it usually responds to medical management. Only one patient has come to glaucoma surgery; his tension was brought under control with cyclodialysis.

Ten eyes that had liquid silicone injection were enucleated. Careful, histologic study of these eyes revealed minimal, if any, reaction to the silicone (Fig. 18-20). In two eyes, the liquid silicone broke up into foamy globules and some cellular activity could be seen surrounding these globules (Fig. 18-21).

COMMENTS

The most significant finding that comes from this critical review of surgery with liquid silicone is that some patients continue to do quite well and are still walking about on their own, 4 or 5 years after their surgery. A critical study of these patients reveals that (1) the silicone has remained posterior to the transvitreal membrane, (2) the retina has flattened without residual fixed folds, and (3) the silicone has remained in one large globule. In general, the earlier that one intervenes in the process of preretinal fibroplasia, the better and more durable are the functional results. In the present series no eyes were treated with liquid silicone if we felt there was a chance of cure by any other procedure. Poor functional results are built into such a series. There was a high incidence of complications and the visual results were frequently less than we had been accustomed to seeing after perfect anatomic reattachment of the retina. But these were eyes that were considered hopeless from the start, and the return of any vision would make such a procedure worthwhile for a one-eyed individual. The two-eyed patients in the present study found it very annoying and exasperating when late complications requiring active therapy occurred in the eye that they were not using. For this reason, we have limited our intravitreal surgery to essentially one-eyed patients.

We are hopeful that new materials and techniques will be forthcoming that will produce results less plagued by complications than is liquid silicone; but until this comes about, liquid silicone will continue to be used in the treatment of those hopeless cases of retinal detachment complicated by massive preretinal retraction.

REFERENCES

1. Cibis, P. A.: Vitreoretinal pathology and surgery in retinal detachment, St. Louis, 1965, The C. V. Mosby Co.
2. Okun, E., Boniuk, I., and Lambert, G.: A foot-operated pump for delivery of viscous fluids into the eye. (In preparation.)

19

Prevention of detachment and proliferation in diabetic retinopathy

Gerd R. E. Meyer-Schwickerath

The first case of diabetic retinopathy was treated with photocoagulation in 1955. In my booklet in 1959 I recorded four cases with a late proliferative stage that were treated without effect, but in a case presenting microaneurysms and exudates, partial disappearance of the latter was achieved by coagulation of the microaneurysms. Since then, with skeptical interest, we have continued to treat cases of diabetic retinopathy with photocoagulation. We knew how difficult it was to judge the therapeutic effect in a disease in which the natural course is so different from one case to another and in which spontaneous regression may occur.

In the meantime the literature and experience on this subject was gathered by François and Weekers in their monograph, "La photocoagulation en ophtalmologie." Pischel and Colyear (1960), along with Clark (1961), have not seen any good results. Others, as Moura Brasil and Rezende (1961), Lopez de Andrade and De Sá (1962), as well as Wetzig and Worlton (1963), have advocated this treatment. I do not want to give you a detailed report of the literature on this subject, but I would like to continue to report how our experience developed in this field.

The first thing we realized during this period of "skeptical interest" was the fact that complications of this treatment in cases of diabetic retinopathy without proliferation into the vitreous were almost absent. Secondly, a most striking observation was that even in cases with several hundred coagulations the objective reduction of the visual field was rather small and subjective scotomas were almost absent. This observation is also true for cases in which photocoagulations were performed in the vicinity of the disc and the macula. Of course, the coagulations have to be performed with a small (1.5 mm.) diaphragm and with the lowest intensity that gives a visible effect.

Between 1963 and 1964 my co-worker Klaus Schott worked up the whole ma-

294

Table 19-1. Comparison in 1963 of 58 patients treated with photocoagulation

6 months to 5 years	50 treated eyes	16 untreated eyes
Better	6	2
Unchanged	33	8
Worse	11	6

Table 19-2. Restricted comparison of patients treated with photocoagulation

2 to 5 years	14 treated eyes	10 untreated eyes
Better	4	1
Unchanged	8	3
Worse	2	6

terial on diabetic retinopathy, which was presented at the German Ophthalmological Society in 1964. Fifty-eight patients had been treated, 33 of them we were able to follow up sufficiently. In 50 eyes of these 33 patients, photocoagulation was performed (Table 19-1). After a follow-up of 6 months to 5 years in the 50 treated eyes there were six cases of improvement, 33 were unchanged, and 11 had become worse. At the same time, of 16 untreated fellow-eyes, two eyes became better spontaneously, eight remained unchanged, and six became worse.

If we take only those cases that have an observation time between 2 and 5 years (Table 19-2), we have treated 14 eyes, of which four became better, eight remained unchanged, and two became worse. In the same period 10 untreated fellow-eyes showed improvement in one case, three remained unchanged, and six became worse.

Much more convincing than this small statistic was a checkup of our old and new fundus photographs. This is a good example of the great value of fundus photography for the evaluation of long-time observations and for the detection of very slow-acting changes. Case by case, we simultaneously projected fundus photographs having intervals of several years. This, of course, was only possible in those cases in which vitreous and lens were sufficiently clear to get good photographs.

We noticed that the yellowish deposits in most of the eyes that were treated sufficiently had considerably regressed. We considered this a reason for improvement in some of our first cases. We also noticed that retinal edema, which at the beginning of the treatment was hiding the choroidal pattern, subsided more and more. This subsidence did not occur within a few months, but even after years, the process of improvement was still detectable. At the same time the enlargement of the retinal veins, which is always a very early symptom of diabetic retinopathy, disappeared more and more. This interesting observation can be drawn from most of our cases.

At this time we asked ourselves whether the coagulation of microaneurysms and new-formed vessels in the level of the retina was at all the reason for the improvement of these cases. This question so far has remained unsolved because we did not dare to destroy normal structures of the retina in cases of diabetic retinopathy. Since we have studied diabetic retinopathy with fluorescein angiography, we know that many of the aneurysms are self-occluded.

In 1965 my co-worker Hans Yoerg Schneider did a second checkup of our diabetic retinopathy cases treated with photocoagulation. Out of 85 treated cases, 49 could be followed up sufficiently. This checkup showed, on the other hand, that statistical analysis as we had done it before was very difficult with our material.

The main reason for the difficulty was as follows: In the beginning we had treated mainly cases in which the fellow-eye was worse and we treated only one eye of the same patient. When we had more experience and when we knew that the frequency of complication was low, we treated more and more early cases and more and more both eyes in the same patient. For this reason it is difficult to compare our old results with the new ones and to compare the treated eyes with the untreated eyes.

Two points, however, were evident: The first is that, within an observation time between 6 months and 67 months, out of 73 eyes treated with photocoagulation *only one case developed proliferative diabetic retinopathy and none of these 73 eyes developed retinal detachment.* Second, out of 25 not photocoagulated fellow-eyes, six cases developed retinal detachment besides proliferating diabetic retinopathy. The starting position for both of these groups of course was not the same. Quite a number of these 25 eyes were not treated because they already had a proliferating diabetic retinopathy.

From this checkup we can conclude that after treating an early stage of diabetic retinopathy with photocoagulation it is rare that a proliferating stage may develop and that the occurrence of a retinal detachment is rare too.

From several publications, as from Beetham (1963), from Caird and Garret (1963), as well as from Fischer (1966), we know about the natural course of diabetic retinopathy without specific treatment, which is certainly worse than that of our treated cases.

Before I show you some of our photographic observations, I would like to draw your attention to some observations that throw some light on the question of how photocoagulation may act in this disease.

Amalric and Mylius have published cases in which a unilateral high myopic eye developed no diabetic retinopathy whereas the emmetropic fellow-eye showed an advanced stage of diabetic retinopathy. The same holds true for some cases of unilateral chorioretinitis and for optical atrophy. I think it might be possible that the beneficial effect of photocoagulation in diabetic retinopathy may be due to the destruction of normal retinal tissue and thereby reduction of the metabolic activity of the retina.

So far this is a hypothesis. Further long-time observations and photographic controls will help us to find out the optimal time and the optimal amount of treatment that is necessary. Our observation should encourage also those who have treated later and proliferative stages of diabetic retinopathy, as Wetzig and Amalric have done.

We are aware of course that this treatment is destructive and not specific. But I think so long as we do not have any better treatment we should continue to gain experience with photocoagulation in diabetic retinopathy.

CASE REPORTS

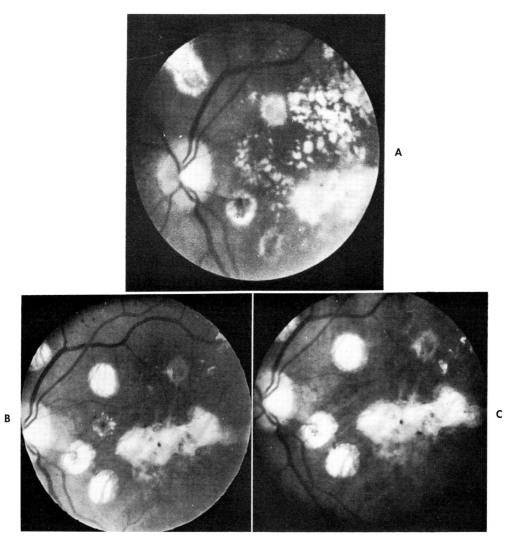

Fig. 19-1. Sixty-three-year-old woman. The left eye was treated three times in 1959 and 1960. A shows the condition after the first treatment. B shows the same area 4 years later. No further coagulations have been performed. C presents the same area 8 years later. There is still a remarkable improvement between the fourth and eighth year. Visual acuity in this eye increased from 1/20 to 5/35. The untreated better eye became worse from 5/20 to 1/20.

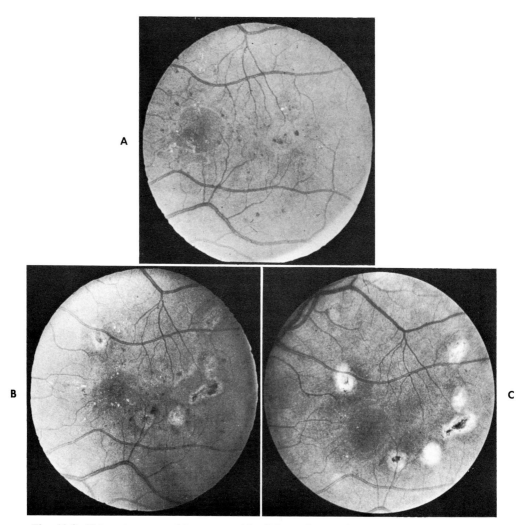

Fig. 19-2. Thirty-three-year-old woman with diabetes known for 16 years. Both eyes were treated once with photocoagulation in December 1963. **A** shows the left eye before photocoagulation. A considerable edema is hiding the choroidal pattern. **B** shows improvement 8 months later. **C** shows a still considerable decrease of retinal edema and aneurysms. The choroidal pattern is much more visible than in **A**. Note how few coagulations have been necessary to improve the macular area.

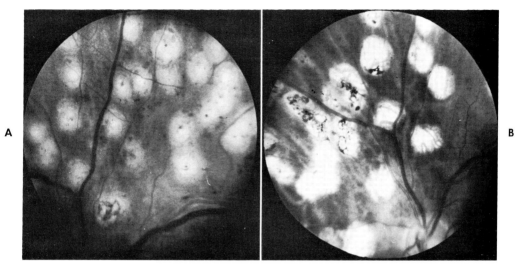

Fig. 19-3. Twenty-five-year-old man with diabetes known for 15 years. Severe diabetic retinopathy of the juvenile type with numerous aneurysms and new-formed vessels in the level of the retina. **A,** Two days after photocoagulation. **B,** Seven months after photocoagulation. The fellow-eye is still under treatment.

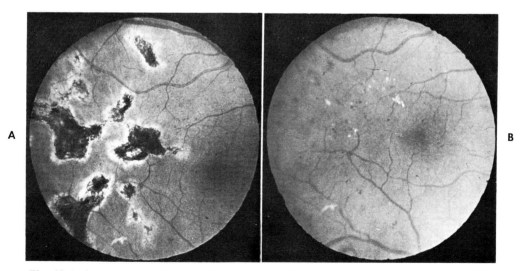

Fig. 19-4. **A,** Forty-year-old man with diabetes for 12 years. First photocoagulation in 1964. **B,** Eight months later, decrease of edema and yellowish deposits.

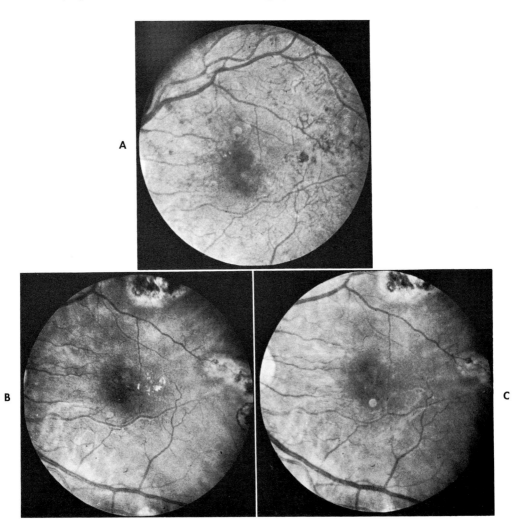

Fig. 19-5. Twenty-five-year-old woman with diabetes known for 7 years. Severe diabetic retinopathy of the rubeosis retinae type. Severe edema, numerous new-formed vessels and engorged veins and capillaries as seen in Fig. 19-4, *B*, before photocoagulation. **A**, One and one-half years after treatment, with considerable decrease of new-formed vessels. **C**, Continuous improvement of the retinal condition 1 year later. Note how new-formed vessels disappear, even if they are not coagulated. Note also the decrease of the tortuosities and enlargement of the blood vessels.

REFERENCES

Amalric, P.: Nouvelles considérations concernant l'évolution et le traitement de la rétinopathie diabétique, Ophthalmologica **154:**151, 1967.

Beethan, W. P.: Visual prognosis of proliferating diabetic retinopathy, Brit. J. Ophthal. **47:** 611, 1963.

Caird, F. I., and Garret, I. C.: Prognosis for vision in diabetic retinopathy, Diabetes **12:**389, 1963.

Clark, G.: Evaluation of photocoagulation, Amer. J. Ophthal. **51**:714, 1961.

Fischer, F.: Einst und jetzt: die historische Entwicklung der Retinopathia diabetica, Munchen Med. Wschr. **96**:1287, 1954.

Fischer, F.: Die diabetische Retinopathie im Lebensflusse (Biorheotische Nosologie von Max Bürger), Ber. Deutsch. Ophthal. Ges. **60**:190, 1956.

Fischer, F.: Eine besondere Verlaufsform der Retinopathia diabetica, Graefe. Arch. Ophthal. **167**:607, 1964.

François, J., and Weekers, R.: La photocoagulation en ophtalmologie, Bull. Soc. Belg. Ophtal. **139**:1, 1965.

Lopes de Andrade, A., and De Sá, S.: Alguns resultatos clínicos da fotocoagulação, Arq. Portug. Oftal. **14**:63, 1962.

Meyer-Schwickerath, G.: Neue Indikationen der Lichtkoagulation, Ber. Deutsch. Ophthal. Ges. **60**:197, 1956.

Meyer-Schwickerath, G.: Lichtkoagulation, Buech. Augenarzt. **33**:1, 1959. (English translation by S. M. Drance, 1966.)

Moura Brazil, N., and De Rezende, J.: Le rôle de la photocoagulation en ophtalmologie, Bull. Soc. Franc. Ophtal. **74**:699, 1961.

Pischel, D. K., and Colyear, B. H.: Clinical results of lightcoagulation therapy, Amer. J. Ophthal. **50**:590, 1960.

Schneider, H. Y.: Behandlung der Retinopathia diabetica durch Lichtkoagulation, Inaugural dissertation, Essen, Germany, 1967.

Schott, K.: Weitere Erfahrungen mit der Lichtkoagulation bei Retinopathia diabetica, Ber. Deutsch. Ophthal. Ges. **66**:349, 1964.

Wetzig, P., and Jepson, C. N.: Further observations on the treatment of diabetic retinopathy by light-coagulation, Amer. J. Ophthal. **62**(3):459, 1966.

Wetzig, P. C., and Worlton, J. T.: Treatment of diabetic retinopathy by light-coagulation. A preliminary study, Brit. J. Ophthal. **47**:539, 1963.

20

Traumatic retinal detachment: clinical and experimental study*

Charles L. Schepens

T his presentation is a review of a continuing investigation carried out by a group of physicists and clinicians in the Department of Retina Research of the Retina Foundation. Traumatic changes in the peripheral fundus caused by ocular contusion were studied in particular detail.[1-3] Other types of trauma, such as perforating injuries and indirect trauma in which a patient developed a retinal detachment after injury to another part of the body, were not considered in this paper. The main reason for eliminating cases of indirect trauma was that they did not differ statistically from spontaneous retinal detachment.[4] They had the same age and sex incidence and the same type of retinal detachment.

Our presentation is divided into two parts, clinical and experimental.

CLINICAL OBSERVATIONS ON RETINAL DETACHMENT BY CONTUSION

It has long been known that contusion of the globe may cause pathognomonic intraocular changes such as recession of the filtration angle,[5, 6] hyphema, iridodialysis, subluxation of the lens, retinal tears in the region of the ora serrata often leading to avulsion of the vitreous base,[7] irregular equatorial retinal breaks following hemorrhage in this area, choroidal tears, and macular retinal breaks.[2]

In a recent study,[2] the characteristics of retinal detachment following contusion of the globe were studied in a group of 160 patients, selected as follows: (1) unilateral retinal detachment preceded by ocular contusion, (2) objective signs of contusion in the affected eye, (3) absence in both eyes of visible spontaneous vitreoretinal degeneration of a type known to cause retinal breaks. Many of the findings in this study were later confirmed by Dumas.[8]

*From the Retina Foundation, Department of Retina Research. This work was supported by U. S. Public Health Service research grant NB-03489.

At least one of the following signs of ocular contusion was required in order to make the reported injury acceptable for the purpose of this study: vitreous hemorrhage, hyphema, traumatic chorioretinal atrophy and pigmentation, traumatic cataract or lens subluxation, lid laceration or ecchymosis, corneal abrasion or scarring, iridodialysis, cyclodialysis, and angle recession.

A statistically significant prevalence of males (86.7%) was found, in contrast to the more nearly equal sex distribution noted in 1390 patients with nontraumatic retinal detachment.[4] The median age of patients with retinal detachment due to contusion was 35 to 40 years younger than a population of 2016 patients[9] with unilateral retinal detachment of any type.

In 138 of 160 patients with retinal detachment due to contusion, the refractive error was known. The incidence of myopia was 21%, which was significantly lower than the incidence of 34.6% found in 1784 patients with unilateral nontraumatic retinal detachment.[4] There were no patients with myopia over 8.00 D. in the group showing retinal detachment as a result of contusion, whereas this degree of myopia was frequently associated with unilateral nontraumatic retinal detachment.

The time interval between ocular contusion and clinical appearance of retinal detachment was variable. Twelve percent of the detachments occurred immediately, 50% within 8 months, and 80% within 2 years. Even the group with long latent periods contained many eyes with classic signs of retinal detachment due to ocular contusion, including five with avulsion of the vitreous base. A long latent interval, therefore, is perfectly consistent with a retinal detachment caused by an ocular contusion.

When cases due to contusion were compared to nontraumatic cases, significant differences were noted in the type and location of retinal breaks. As Table 20-1 shows, ocular contusion causes a marked increase of retinal breaks at the ora serrata and at the posterior pole, retinal breaks near the equator being relatively rare.

Retinal breaks produced by traction at the borders of the vitreous base were the most frequent. Breaks smaller than one ora bay, representing small retinal dialyses, were uncommon at the posterior border of the vitreous base (Fig. 20-1, *A*). Complete retinal dialyses larger than one ora bay (Fig. 20-1, *B*) were more common than linear breaks in the ciliary epithelium at the anterior border of the vitreous base (Fig. 20-1, *C*). Simultaneous dialysis and linear break at the anterior border

Table 20-1. Comparison between contusion cases and nontraumatic cases

Location of retinal breaks	*Detachment by contusion*		*Nontraumatic detachment*	
	Number	*Percent*	*Number*	*Percent*
Near ora serrata	85	59.4	320	21.5
Near equator	12	8.4	896	60.2
Near posterior hole	13	9.1	20	1.3
Other	33	23.1	253	17.0
Totals	143*	100.0	1489	100.0

*Of 160 eyes, 17 could not be fitted in any of the above categories.

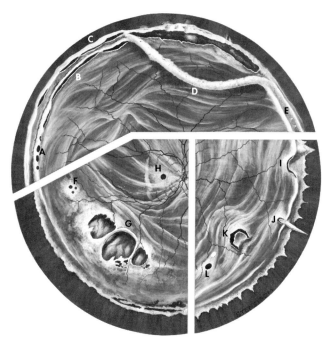

Fig. 20-1. Top, Retinal breaks at borders of vitreous base. *A,* Small breaks at posterior border of vitreous base. *B,* Retinal dialysis at posterior border of vitreous base. *C,* Linear break at anterior border of vitreous base. *D,* Avulsion of vitreous base, which lies free in vitreous cavity. *E,* Tenting-up of retina and epithelium of pars plana ciliaris forming ridges at posterior and anterior borders of vitreous base. **Bottom left,** Retinal breaks unrelated to vitreoretinal attachment. *F,* Round holes in atrophic retina. *G,* Irregular retinal holes in equatorial zone associated with chorioretinal degeneration and with vitreous and retinal hemorrhage. *H,* Atrophic macular hole with nearby pigmentary changes and choroidal rupture. **Bottom right,** Retinal tears associated with abnormal vitreoretinal attachments. *I,* Horseshoe-shaped tear at posterior end of meridional fold. *J,* Horseshoe-shaped tear at posterior end of meridional fold. *K,* Horseshoe-shaped tear in equatorial zone. *L,* Tear with operculum in overlying vitreous. (From Cox, M. S., et al.: Arch. Ophthal. **76:**678, 1966.)

of the vitreous base, resulting in avulsion of the vitreous base, was found in about 25% of the patients (Fig. 20-1, *D*).

Traumatic retinal dialysis had a significant preference for the upper nasal quadrant. It was frequently accompanied by chorioretinal atrophy in the area of the ora serrata, pigmentation, and a small vitreous hemorrhage. Shreds of nonpigmented and pigmented epithelium of the pars plana ciliaris often remained attached to the avulsed vitreous base and could be seen in the vitreous cavity. Less severe traction on the vitreous base caused tenting-up of the peripheral retina and epithelium of the pars plana ciliaris, forming a ridge at the posterior and anterior borders of the vitreous base (Fig. 20-1, *E*).

Equatorial holes were frequent and often associated with vitreous and retinal hemorrhage, retinal edema, and severe underlying choroidal degeneration. Such holes were significantly more common in the inferotemporal quadrant, which is the most frequent site of impact. They were characteristically irregular and were pathognomonic of traumatic cases (Fig. 20-1, *F* and *G*).

Breaks at the macula or near the posterior pole, overlying atrophic choroid, were found in 9.1% of the patients (Fig. 20-1, *H*).

A number of retinal tears developed at the site of abnormal vitreoretinal attachments. These tears were similar to those seen in nontraumatic retinal detachments, except that they were significantly more frequent nasally (Fig. 20-1, *I* to *L*).

The preceding observations establish as fact the clinical impression that the most frequent type of retinal break produced by contusion is located on either side of the vitreous base and most often in the upper nasal quadrant. Retinal detachment caused by breaks near the ora serrata is often flat and progresses insidiously, particularly when located nasally. It may not be noted by the patient until the macula is involved. Signs of long-standing retinal detachment are therefore common in these eyes, such as demarcation lines, subretinal fibrin deposits, and intraretinal cysts. Contusion may cause multiple tears, located in all quadrants, along the vitreous base. In rare cases, the vitreous base is totally avulsed with a 360-degree tear.

From a diagnostic standpoint the most difficult problems arise when a flat retinal detachment is accompanied by tenting-up of a portion of the vitreous base, with slit-like breaks in the ciliary epithelium, along the anterior border of the vitreous base. Breaks of this type are difficult to see and may be hidden by the tented-up vitreous base. However, tenting-up of the vitreous base is in itself pathognomonic of ocular contusion. Morphologically it is quite different from the spontaneous detachment of the ora serrata that is occasionally seen in nontraumatic cases of retinal detachment. In the latter case, the ora line is distorted, being pulled backward in the middle of the ora bays. In traumatic cases, the ora line is not distorted. Two other signs indicative of the traumatic origin of a tented-up vitreous base are: scattered retinal and choroidal hemorrhages in the area of tenting-up and depigmented spots, often surrounded by hyperpigmentation, located in the pars plana ciliaris.

The reasons why contusion of the globe tends to cause damage to the area of the vitreous base were obscure. Consequently an experimental study was performed in an attempt to clarify the pathogenesis of these changes.

EXPERIMENTAL OBSERVATIONS

The experimental observations consisted first of a study of the intraocular damage done by contusion to enucleated pig eyes. It was established that damage to the vitreous base could be reduplicated experimentally in the pig eye, and another investigation was carried out to analyze the deformations of the ocular coat of pig and human eyes under high-speed impact.

Damage to pig eyes by contusion

The eyes were removed from freshly slaughtered pigs, mounted, traumatized, and placed in formalin fixative before 1 hour had elapsed. They were examined with the aid of an operating microscope a few days later when fixation was complete. The eyes were opened equatorially, which permitted study of the ora serrata and pars plana ciliaris over 360 degrees.

In the area of the anterior retina, the anatomy of the pig eye resembles that of the immature human eye. The ora serrata is relatively smooth with occasional serrations as in the human infant. The pars plana ciliaris of the pig eye is wide on the temporal side, whereas on the nasal side the ora serrata is close to the ciliary processes. The vitreous has its firmest attachment to the nonpigmented epithelium of the pars plana ciliaris. Temporally this attachment is wide and lies entirely within the pars plana ciliaris. Nasally the area of adherence is narrow and coincides with the ora serrata for some distance (Fig. 20-2). As in the human, the vitreous also adheres to the posterior lens capsule.

A standard ocular injury was produced by a specially modified air rifle that fired a BB (weight, 0.345 gm.) at an average muzzle velocity of 66.44 meters per second

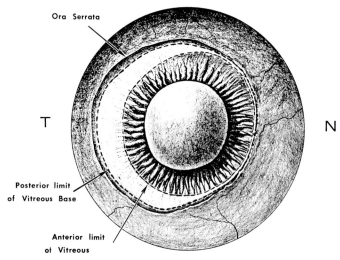

Fig. 20-2. Diagram of fundus periphery of pig eye, seen from the back. (*T*) Temporal; (*N*) nasal. The vitreous base is much wider temporally than nasally. On the temporal side it is entirely located in the pars plana ciliaris, whereas on the nasal side its posterior border coincides with the ora serrata. (From Cox, M. S., et al.: Arch. Ophthal. **76:**678, 1966.)

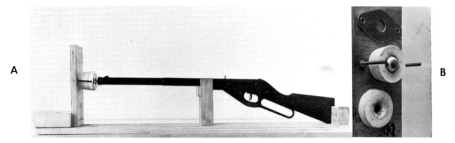

Fig. 20-3. Air rifle mounted in front of enucleated pig eye. **A,** General view; **B,** detail of bracket with gelatin mold containing pig eye—*(below)* front half of mold and *(above)* metal plate designed to hold front half of mold. (From Cox, M. S., et al.: Arch. Ophthal. **76:**678, 1966.)

(Fig. 20-3, *A*). This muzzle velocity was selected to ensure ocular contusion without rupture of the globe.[5]

An examination of 48 pig eyes traumatized in situ was carried out so that various materials used for mounting the enucleated eyes could be evaluated. The findings with eyes so traumatized were most closely reproduced by mounting the enucleated eyes in a 10% gelatin mold.

A window in the anterior section of the mold provided direct access to the cornea for causing a contusion (Fig. 20-3). The position of the eye in the mold could be

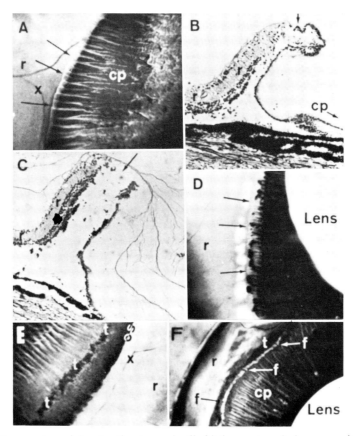

Fig. 20-4. Damage to peripheral retina by projectile hitting center of pig cornea. **A**, Traumatic tenting of ora serrata *(arrows)* on nasal side; *(r)* retina, *(x)* retinal vessel, *(cp)* ciliary processes. **B**, Photomicrograph of traumatic tenting of ora serrata *(vertical arrow)*; *(r)* retina, *(cp)* ciliary processes (×126). **C**, Photomicrograph of retinal tear *(arrow)* in crest of tented area; *(r)* retina (×126). **D**, Traumatic tenting *(arrows)* of the ora serrata; pieces of pigment epithelium adherent to detached nonpigmented epithelium; *(r)* retina. **E**, Extensive tear *(t)* in nonpigmented ciliary epithelium temporally, along posterior edge of vitreous base. *(OS)* ora serrata; *(x)* marginal retinal blood vessel; *(r)* retina. **F**, Nasal festoon of nonpigmented epithelium *(f)* adherent to vitreous base; on the posterior edge of the festoon is a tear *(t)* in the ciliary epithelium; *(r)* retina; *(cp)* ciliary processes. (From Weidenthal, D. T., and Schepens, C. L.: Amer. J. Ophthal. **62:**465, 1966.)

adjusted so that it was struck either near the center of the cornea or near the temporal limbus.

There were three main areas of visible intraocular damage when the BB projectile struck the pig eye near the center of the cornea: lens capsule, nasal ora serrata, and temporal pars plana ciliaris.

Lens damage was usually found near the equator and consisted of rupture of its capsule. Damage to the nasal ora serrata took the form of tenting of the retina and of the nonpigmented epithelium of the pars plana ciliaris (Fig. 20-4, *A* and *B*). Retinal dialysis was frequently present at the peak of the tented area (Fig. 20-4, *C*). Some specimens showed pieces of pigment epithelium adherent to the tented nonpigmented epithelium. Grossly, multiple pale patches were visible where the pigment epithelium had been pulled off the pars plana ciliaris (Fig. 20-4, *D*). Damage to the temporal portion of the pars plana ciliaris consisted of linear tears in the ciliary epithelium that ran parallel to the ora serrata, along the posterior border of the vitreous base (Fig. 20-4, *E*). A festoon made by the ciliary epithelium attached to the vitreous gel was occasionally seen suspended in the vitreous cavity (Fig. 20-4, *F*).

A statistically significant protective effect was exerted on the crystalline lens by mounting the eyes in a stone mold that was either closed or contained a posterior aperture 20 mm. in diameter. A lesser protection was afforded by a stone mold covering the posterior half of the globe to the equator (Fig. 20-5).

When the BB projectile struck the temporal limbus, the incidence of temporal retinal dialysis was high. Such dialysis was never observed in eyes struck near the center of the cornea. Temporal dialysis was frequently associated with tears in the temporal portion of the pars plana ciliaris, a few millimeters anterior to the ora serrata. When hit near the limbus, the eye was not protected by a closed stone mold. Dialysis on the temporal side probably resulted from the violent indentation of the

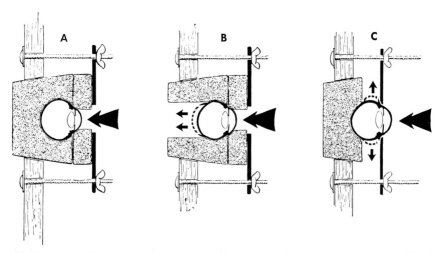

Fig. 20-5. Cross section of protective stone molds with enucleated pig eye in place. **A,** Closed stone mold; **B,** stone mold with posterior aperture, which permits eye to expand posteriorly; **C,** stone mold with equatorial aperture, which permits eye to expand equatorially. (From Weidenthal, D. T., and Schepens, C. L.: Amer. J. Ophthal. **62:**465, 1966.)

ocular coats in that area. This hypothesis explains why a closed stone mold gave the eye no protection. The frequency of clinical retinal dialysis in the lower temporal quadrant due to trauma is explained by the configuration of the human orbit, which renders this area most vulnerable.[10]

These experiments simulate many of the clinical fundus changes ascribed to ocular contusion in humans. Tears of the nasal pars plana ciliaris and avulsion of the vitreous base could be reproduced. Patchy absence of pigment epithelium in the pars plana ciliaris and irregular pigment spots located on the outer aspect of the vitreous base were, in an equally frequent manner, observed clinically in human eyes and experimentally in pig eyes.

Deformation of pig and human globes by high-speed impact

A study was performed of the deformations of pig and human eyes by high-speed impact in the hope of uncovering the mechanism of damage to the region of the vitreous base.

Materials and methods

Two human eyes and 75 pig eyes were each placed in a container made with flat glass plates. Each eye was suspended in its container by threads, and liquid 10% gelatin was poured into the container, leaving the anterior part of the eye exposed. The liquid gelatin was then allowed to coagulate.

Projectiles. The ocular injury was produced by an air rifle as described previously (Fig. 20-6). A magnesium projectile of greater length but of identical speed and weight as the steel BB (Fig. 20-7) was used to measure the corneal indentation during impact because this indentation was deeper than 4.5 mm., which was the diameter of the steel BB. With either projectile, the same amount of kinetic energy was delivered to the eye (K.E. $= \frac{1}{2}mv^2 = 0.68$ joule). The mold containing the eye was rigidly mounted at a distance of 2 to 3 cm. from the muzzle of the gun to ensure alignment of the center of the cornea with the missile path. In this series of experiments the eye was not hit at the limbus.

Photographic recordings. Photographic recordings consisted of high-speed single-

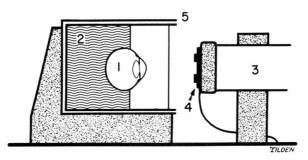

Fig. 20-6. Enucleated pig eye *(1)* mounted in 10% gelatin *(2)*, in a glass container *(5)*. Muzzle of the air rifle *(3)*, with its electrical contact assembly *(4)*. (From Weidenthal, D. T., and Schepens, C. L.: Amer. J. Ophthal. 62:465, 1966.)

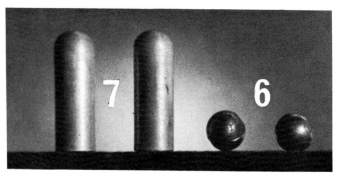

Fig. 20-7. Steel *(6)* and magnesium *(7)* projectiles of same weight. (From Weidenthal, D. T., and Schepens, C. L.: Amer. J. Ophthal. **62:**465, 1966.)

flash photography and cinematography. In single flash high-speed photographs, the object was illuminated during a very short time so that all motion seemed to have "stopped" on the photograph. The experiment took place in complete darkness. The camera focused on the eye was opened for 1 second, during which the gun was fired. When the bullet left the gun, it closed momentarily a pair of electrical contacts (see *4* in Fig. 20-6), and this caused a short but powerful flash of light. The exposure time was thus equal to the length of the light pulse (3 microseconds), and the intensity of the flash was about 7 million candlepower. The light flash was intentionally produced between 0.1 and 10 milliseconds after closing the electrical contacts, depending on the phase of motion to be photographed. The delay was measured for each exposure with a cathode-ray oscilloscope. The use of direct-development film with high sensitivity made the procedure very versatile. The same eye was used for five repeated impacts and photographs. Pictures of the undistorted eye were taken before and after a series of impacts.

With high-speed cinematography the object to be photographed was continuously illuminated, and the film was exposed during very short times by a fast shutter. The camera was driven by a motor at speeds between 5000 and 9000 frames per second. When the film reached the desired speed, the gun was fired by a pair of solenoids actuated by an event synchronizer inside the camera. The high-speed negative films used were 100 feet long. Their relatively low sensitivity required powerful illumination by three 625-watt projectors. This method was more informative than the single flash procedure since the complete event was recorded in one film strip. The picture quality, however, was inferior because of the lower sensitivity of the film and the longer exposure time (50 to 70 microseconds instead of 3 microseconds).

Most experiments recorded deformations of the sagittal plane and a few recorded changes in the equatorial plane of the eyes. The two human eyes available for this work were studied with the high-speed movie technique.

Thirty eyes traumatized by single impact were placed in formalin fixative immediately after trauma. They were examined with the aid of a dissecting microscope a few days after fixation in order to determine what gross damage could be observed to the zonule and lens capsule and in the area of the vitreous base.

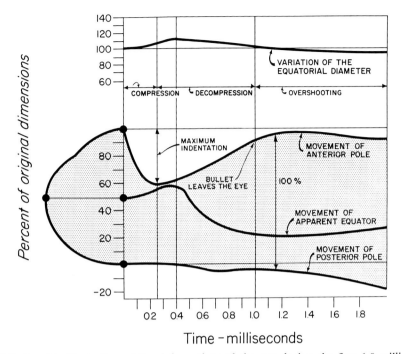

Fig. 20-8. Graphic illustration of the deformations of the eye during the first 1.8 millisecond after impact. *Ordinate:* dimensions of the eye expressed as percentages of their original value. *Abscissa:* time after impact in milliseconds. The graph is divided into two parts. In the lower part, an anteroposterior cross section of one half the eye before impact is represented on the left of the ordinate *(shaded area)*. The posterior pole is on the zero point of the ordinate, the equator is on the 50% point, and the anterior pole is on the 100% point.

The thick black curve starting from the 100% point indicates the movement of the globe's anterior pole, which shows maximum indentation .25 msec. after impact. The movement of the equator of the globe is indicated by the thick black curve that starts at the 50% point. The movement of the globe's posterior pole is indicated by the thick black curve that starts at the zero point.

The upper portion of the graph contains two elements: the thick black curve shows the variations in the length of the equatorial diameter, and below the curve, the sequence of events during the first 1.8 msec. is divided into its three main components (see text). (From Delori, F., et al.: Invest. Ophthal. 8:290, 1969.)

Results

In the eyes examined under the microscope after formalin fixation, the damage was qualitatively the same as that observed by Weidenthal and Schepens,[1] but the percentage of damaged eyes was smaller. Lower ocular pressure before the experiment and somewhat lower missile speed may account for this difference.

The study of globe deformation under the impact of a BB is presented under two headings: interpretation of photographic recordings and graphic reconstruction of the phenomena observed.

Interpretation of photographic recordings. The anteroposterior and equatorial diameters of the eyes were measured during deformation and expressed as a per-

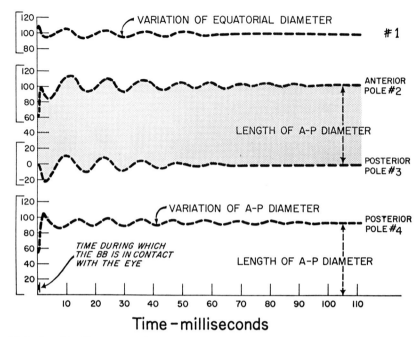

Time – milliseconds

Fig. 20-9. Graphic illustration of changes in the dimensions and positions of various parts of the eye during the second phase after impact, from 1.8 to 100 msec. Details of events during the first phase (0 to 1.8 msec.) are recorded in Fig. 20-10. *Abscissa:* time from impact in milliseconds. *Ordinate:* percentage of original equatorial or anteroposterior diameter, original diameters being equal to 100%. Starting position of posterior pole is at zero on the ordinate and that of anterior pole is at 100. Curve 1 shows variations of equatorial diameter; curve 2 shows displacement of anterior pole; curve 3 shows displacement of posterior pole; the distance between curves 2 and 3 measures the A-P diameter of the globe; curve 4 represents variations of globe's A-P diameter. (From Delori, F., et al.: Invest. Ophthal. 8:290, 1969.)

centage of their original values. Results are presented in a graph (Fig. 20-8) as a function of time after impact. Measurements of equatorial diameters were made in pictures of the posterior pole and showed no significant differences between the relative deformations of the apparent horizontal and vertical diameters.

Movement of the posterior pole was measured with reference to a fixed point in the mold and was expressed as a percentage of the original anteroposterior diameter. Measurement of the distance between the apparent equator and the posterior pole was also expressed as a percentage of the original anteroposterior diameter. After the first 1.8 millisecond, the eye displayed long oscillations in gelatin, which were measured with a frame-by-frame analysis of two high-speed films (Fig. 20-9). Measurements of the anteroposterior and equatorial diameters of two human eyes showed similar results. The complete phenomena that followed impact of the cornea could be divided into four periods: compression, decompression, overshooting, and long-time oscillations.

Compression (between 0 and 0.25 millisecond). The cornea does not present a marked resistance to the impacting bullet. Even the blast of the gun causes a small

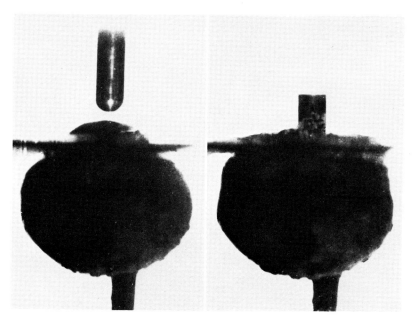

Fig. 20-10. Single flash photographs illustrating the long magnesium missile .1 msec. before and .25 msec. after impact, when the cornea is indented 8.5 mm. The fuzzy area between cornea and sclera is due to irregular refraction at the level of the air-gelatin interface. (From Delori, F., et al.: Invest. Ophthal. 8:290, 1969.)

deformation before impact. A rapid expansion of the anterior sclera compensates for the volume decrease caused by the corneal indentation. The BB stops after about 0.25 millisecond (Fig. 20-8) due to the transient gradient of pressure developed by inertia of the tissues and liquids accelerated by the bullet and by tension in the cornea. At this moment, the globe's anteroposterior diameter is reduced to 59% of its original length, which corresponds to a corneal indentation of 8.5 mm. (Fig. 20-10). It is probable that during this period the posterior surface of the cornea comes in contact with the anterior lens capsule.

Decompression (between 0.25 and 1.00 millisecond). The eye acts as a tension spring and pushes the bullet out (Fig. 20-8). The equatorial diameters continue their expansion until 0.40 millisecond, when they reach their greatest values, 111% of their original length. Simultaneously the vitreous body starts to move posteriorly until the eye assumes a pear shape about 1.0 millisecond. At the same time, the bullet leaves the eye with a speed 5.4 times less than the impacting speed.

Analysis of recordings for this period shows a deformation wave traveling posteriorly in the sclera. It originates most probably at the limbus and is generated by the sudden radial outward movement of the aqueous, produced by the indentation.

Overshooting (between 1.0 and 2.5 milliseconds). The anteroposterior diameter overshoots up to 112% of its original length, whereas the equatorial diameter decreases, giving the globe an ellipsoid shape (Fig. 20-8).

Oscillations (from 2.5 to 100 milliseconds). Curve 3 in Fig. 20-9 represents the

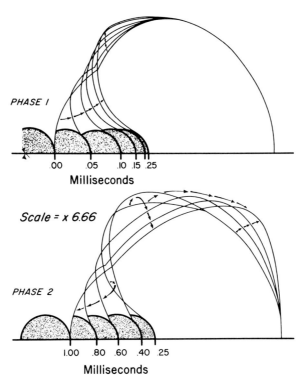

Fig. 20-11. Graphic reconstruction of the changes in shape of the eye based upon a constant volume assumption. The shaded area represents the impacting BB. Phase 1 shows changes in shape during the first .25 msec. (compression phase). Phase 2 shows changes during decompression (from .25 to 1.00 msec.). Arrows indicate the direction in which the ocular coats are moving. Note that the greatest stretching of the anterior portion of the sclera occurs during phase 2 at .40 msec. (From Delori, F., et al.: Invest. Ophthal. 8:290, 1969.)

oscillations of the posterior pole, which may be considered as the oscillations of the whole globe. Their frequency was estimated at 85 cycles per second. In addition to these oscillations, the fluids inside the eye oscillate also, expanding periodically in the anteroposterior and equatorial directions, as represented in curves 1 and 4 (Fig. 20-9). In these curves, the maximum anteroposterior elongation corresponds to the minimum equatorial diameters. The frequency of intraocular fluid oscillations is approximately 90 cycles per second. The oscillations of the whole globe in gelatin stop after 50 milliseconds (curves 1 and 3), whereas the corneal and anteroposterior diameter oscillations are fully attenuated by 100 milliseconds (curves 2 and 4).

Graphic reconstruction. These experimental data and further analysis of shape changes in the eye after impact made it possible to reconstruct graphically the phenomena resulting from the impact. Average measurements in 10 nontraumatized pig eyes after fixation were used as original values (100%) in this reconstruction. The volume of the globe was assumed to remain constant during its deformation. This assumption rested on the fact that during the event (about 100 milliseconds) no fluid could leave the eye by forced diffusion through its walls. The constant vol-

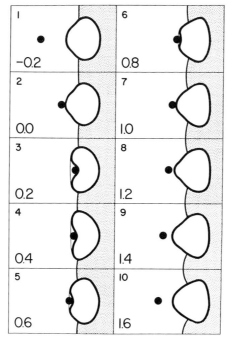

Fig. 20-12. Simulated film strip of the changes in shape of the eye based upon a constant volume assumption. Zero time is when the BB touches the cornea. For each picture, time is noted in the lower left corner in milliseconds. (From Delori, F., et al.: Invest. Ophthal. **8:**290, 1969.)

ume assumption was used to determine shapes that were not visible on the recordings. Fig. 20-11 shows the results obtained during compression (phase 1) and decompression (phase 2). All volumes were computed within 2% of the original volume of 6.88 cc., by graphic integration. Fig. 20-12 is a simulated film strip that was constructed by combining measured and computed changes in shape. With the help of this reconstruction, it was possible to compute the relative length of the 12 o'clock meridian of the eye and the relative surface of the globe. Computation showed elongations up to 5% for the cornea and up to 3% for the equatorial sclera.

By comparing the speed of impact of the BB and the speed at which it left the eye 1 millisecond after impact, it was computed that 95.8% of the impacting energy was used by the system and dissipated in free oscillations, heat absorption due to friction, and damage to the structures of the eye. It was experimentally demonstrated that the amount of energy absorbed by the eye, in such a case, varies with the acceleration of the projectile. Since movement of the anterior pole of the eye was identical to that of the bullet during impact, it was possible to estimate that a force of 28 kg. was applied to the eye by the bullet.* Similar computations were performed to investigate the acceleration of different points of the eye. Both tangential

---

*The force $F = mj$, where m is the mass of the bullet and j its acceleration.

and normal accelerations of the sclera were found to be greatest in the area of the vitreous base. The meridional distension of the sclera was also maximal in this zone. This distension would cause shearing forces between the ocular coats if their moduli of elasticity were different.

Discussion

It was initially thought that damage at the vitreous base occurred when the lens was pushed anteriorly, at the end of the decompression period and during the over-shooting (between 0.70 and 2.50 milliseconds after impact). This damage was ascribed to the forced mass movement caused by wall deformation. The same theory, called the return-shock theory,[11] was used to explain rupture of the zonule as a result of blunt trauma. Our experiments, however, do not support this view. When the lens was pushed anteriorly, the anterior part of the eye was relatively contracted because the intraocular fluid had accumulated in the posterior segment. At that moment the vitreous base was not tugging on the choroid and retina. In fact, distance measurements computed from the recorded shape of the eye, at that stage, even show that the vitreous base was probably in a relaxed state during the phase of overshooting.

Because of the viscosity and inertia of the intraocular fluids, it is possible that negative pressures could be responsible for some of the damage. A theory of formation and sudden collapse of cavities has been proposed to explain brain damage that results from an impact on the skull.[12] However, this theory assumes the existence of a shockwave and no shockwave was observed in the experiments described. Measurements have indicated that if a shockwave were present it would occur within microseconds after impact and it could not be the cause of the marked deformations of the ocular coats that were maximum around 0.4 millisecond after impact. The cause of the damage should be looked for between 0 and 0.60 millisecond after impact, because it is during this period that the most rapid and extensive deformations of the anterior portion of the sclera are observed. Another element of evidence is that damage at the vitreous base strongly indicates severe traction on this structure fol-

Table 20-2. Variations of distance: posterior pole of lens to vitreous base

Time in milliseconds	Percentage of distance before impact
.00	100
.05	105
.10	111
.15	118
.25	125
.40	128
.60	107
.80	94
1.00	87
1.20	89
1.40	94
1.60	94
1.80	94

lowing impact. The vitreous body is firmly attached to the peripheral retina and epithelium of the pars plana ciliaris, in the region of the ora serrata, and to the posterior lens capsule. Between 0 and 0.40 millisecond after impact the lens is pushed backward, at the same time as the envelope of the globe overlying the vitreous base is pushed outward. It is at 0.40 millisecond that the scleral perimeter is largest in this part of the globe (Fig. 20-11). This must cause a considerable increase of the distance between the vitreous base and the posterior pole of the lens. The variation of this distance during the total event was computed, and it turns out that at 0.40 millisecond it is the greatest with 128% of its initial value (Table 20-2 and Fig. 20-13). At that time the intraocular pressure in the area of the vitreous base is markedly increased and exerts a force that is smaller than the traction on the base and in an opposite direction. Since the zonule and lens capsule are quite distensible, the effect of traction on these structures is less than that of traction on the vitreous base, which is poorly distensible. The greatest shearing forces in the retina are located along the posterior border of the vitreous base, which explains why damage occurred frequently in this region. In that particular phase of the impact, shearing forces are especially effective in causing damage because the ocular coats, including the retina, are markedly distended.

From a clinical standpoint it is important to realize that the damage due to contusion of the globe by a high-speed projectile occurs within less than 1 millisecond of impact. Fundus examination performed immediately after contusion should reveal the full extent of damage to the vitreous base. However retinal detachment does not necessarily occur immediately after retinal breaks are produced by this mechanism. Clinical observation shows that there is often a delay of weeks, months, or years before retinal detachment appears. In case of contusion injury the delay tends to be more prolonged than in idiopathic cases because the vitreous gel and the retina are relatively normal and because the location of the retinal breaks is in the extreme fundus periphery and on the nasal side.

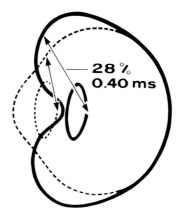

Fig. 20-13. Shape of globe at maximum deformation (.40 msec. after impact) is drawn over shape of eye at rest. At this stage, the distance between vitreous base and posterior pole of the lens is increased by 28%. (From Delori, F., et al.: Invest. Ophthal. **8:**290, 1969.)

REFERENCES

1. Weidenthal, D. T., and Schepens, C. L.: Peripheral fundus changes associated with ocular contusion, Amer. J. Ophthal. **62:**465, 1966.
2. Cox, M. S., Schepens, C. L., and Freeman, H. M.: Retinal detachment due to ocular contusion, Arch. Ophthal. **76:**678, 1966.
3. Delori, F., Pomerantzeff, O., and Cox, M. S.: Deformation of the globe under high speed impact—its relation to contusion injuries, Invest. Ophthal. **8:**290, 1969.
4. Schepens, C. L., and Marden, D.: Data on the natural history of retinal detachment: further characterization of certain unilateral nontraumatic cases, Amer. J. Ophthal. **61:** 213, 1966.
5. Weidenthal, D. T.: Experimental ocular contusion, Arch. Ophthal. **71:**77, 1964.
6. Wolff, S. M., and Zimmermann, L. E.: Chronic secondary glaucoma associated with retro-displacement of iris root and deepening of the anterior chamber angle secondary to contusion, Amer. J. Ophthal. **54:**547, 1962.
7. Schepens, C. L.: Symposium: retinal detachment; diagnostic and prognostic factors as found in preoperative examination, Trans. Amer. Acad. Ophthal. Otolaryng. **56:**398, 1952.
8. Dumas, J. J.: Retinal detachment following contusion of the eye, Int. Ophthal. Clin. **7:** 19, 1967.
9. Schepens, C. L., and Marden, D.: Data on the natural history of retinal detachment. I. Age and sex relationships, Arch. Ophthal. **66:**631, 1961.
10. Neubauer, H.: Die Netzhautablösung nach umschriebener Augapfelprellung mit kurzer Manifestationszeit, Klin. Mbl. Augenheilk. **141:**122, 1962.
11. Frenkel, H.: Etude sur le syndrome traumatique du segment antérieur de l'oeil, Ann Oculist. **155:**78, 1918.
12. Ward, J. W., Montgomery, L. H., and Clark, S. L.: A mechanism of concussion; theory, Science **107:**349, 1948.

21

*Therapy of diabetic retinal detachment**

Edward Okun and Wayne E. Fung

R INTRODUCTION

etinal detachment secondary to proliferative retinopathy is one of the leading causes of blindness in the diabetic eye. Since this detachment is secondary to traction forces that originate from fibrous proliferations within the vitreous cavity, it is not surprising that this stage of the disease does not benefit very much from either pituitary ablative therapy or photocoagulation. The purpose of this paper is to present the ophthalmoscopic findings and histopathology of diabetic retinal detachment, the rationale for surgical treatment, and the results of scleral buckling procedures performed on 50 patients.

PATHOGENESIS AND OPHTHALMOSCOPIC APPEARANCE

Once preretinal fibrovascular proliferations have formed, the accompanying neovascularization may become completely sclerosed with time or, more rapidly, following pituitary ablation or photocoagulation. However, following vitreous detachment or localized vitreous shrinkage, these avascular membranes are pulled into the vitreous, creating a certain amount of pull on the surrounding retina.[1-4] This traction can produce retinal detachment with or without retinal tears or retinoschisis. This same mechanism can lead to vitreous hemorrhages secondary to torn retinal blood vessels. Retinal detachment without retinal breaks first occurs in the area of greatest intravitreal traction, usually sparing the macula. It may remain localized for months or years, or it may gradually spread to involve most of the posterior retina and, finally, the macula. When retinal tears are produced, the detachment spreads more rapidly. These tears are characteristically very small and posterior in location, frequently somewhat obscured by overlying intravitreal proliferations.

In the typical diabetic retinal detachment these proliferations can be seen elevating the retina maximally, approximately halfway between the disc and equator

*This investigation was supported in part by research grant NB-01789, from the National Institute of Neurological Diseases and Blindness, National Institutes of Health, Bethesda, Maryland.

(Fig. 21-1). The retina usually remains flat between the equator and the ora. Long-standing detachments eventually become complete, with the formation of additional membranes that adhere the central retina together in a tight ring (Fig. 21-2).

Histopathologic study of autopsy eyes with diabetic retinal detachment revealed in certain fortuitous sections that the same vitreous strands that are attached to the intravitreal proliferations also insert into the vitreous base just anterior to the

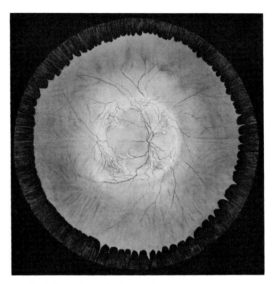

Fig. 21-1. Drawing of typical diabetic retinal detachment.

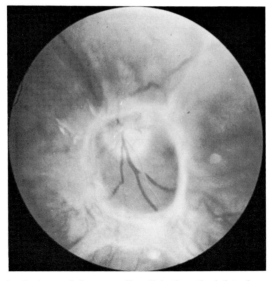

Fig. 21-2. Photograph of advanced, long-standing diabetic retinal detachment.

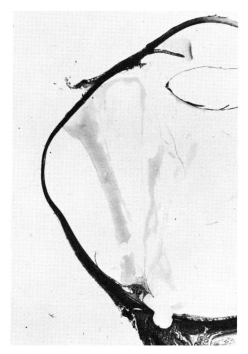

Fig. 21-3. Histopathologic section of eye with proliferative diabetic retinopathy. Note vitreous adhesion to proliferative tissue and insertion at vitreous base.

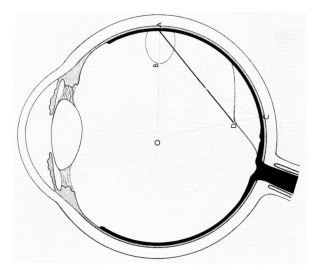

Fig. 21-4. Drawing to illustrate how indentation of the sclera in the region of the vitreous base releases the traction on the detached retina.

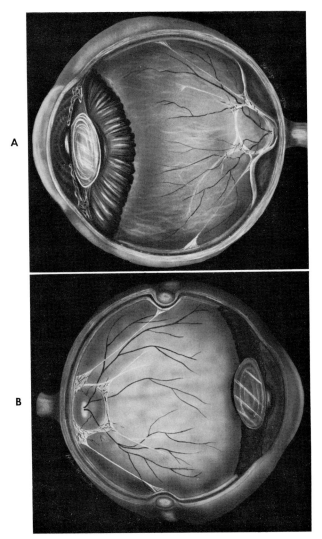

Fig. 21-5. **A,** Schematic drawing of eye with retinal detachment secondary to proliferative diabetic retinopathy. **B,** Same eye after scleral buckling procedure designed to relieve the vitreous traction in the area of proliferation.

equator (Fig. 21-3). Theoretically, indentation of the sclera in the region of the anterior insertion of these vitreous fibrils should release some of the traction being transmitted through the proliferations to the retina (Figs. 21-4 and 21-5, *A* and *B*). In addition, shortening of the sclera in the area of most marked traction should bring the choroid closer to the retina.

INDICATIONS FOR THERAPY

Patients were operated on for diabetic retinal detachment without breaks only after the detachment reached the macula. If retinal breaks were present, they were

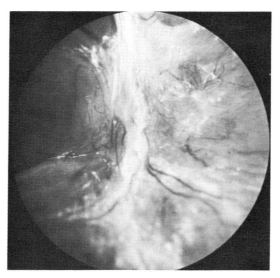

Fig. 21-6. Photograph of eye with grade IV proliferative retinopathy, in which proliferative membrane obscures the fundus, a contraindication to surgery.

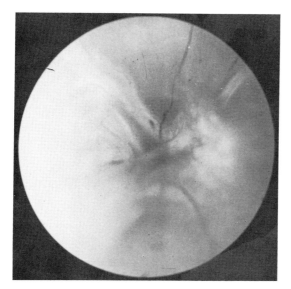

Fig. 21-7. Photograph of eye with longstanding retinal detachment with extremely dense pre-retinal membranes holding bullae together, a contraindication to surgery.

operated on as soon as it became apparent that the detachment was spreading. Patients with localized detachments were followed at intervals of 3 months and told to come in immediately if they lost central vision. The only contraindications to therapy of diabetic retinal detachment were (1) a preretinal membrane that obscured most of the retina, including the macular area (Fig. 21-6), (2) eyes with too much blood and fibrin in the vitreous to allow adequate viewing for an operative procedure, and (3) long-standing retinal detachment with very dense preretinal membranes (Fig. 21-7).

OPERATIVE PROCEDURE

The type of operative procedure performed on any specific case depended upon the location of the traction bands responsible for the detachment of the macular

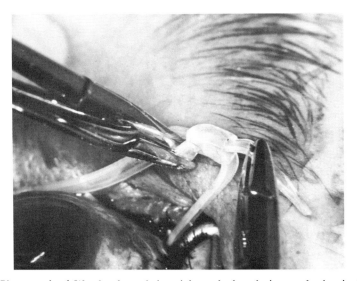

Fig. 21-8. Photograph of Watzke sleeve being tightened after drainage of subretinal fluid.

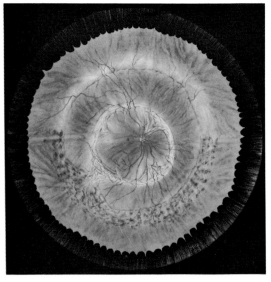

Fig. 21-9. Appearance of fundus at end of scleral buckling procedure. Note persistent slight retinal elevation at site of most marked vitreous traction.

area. If traction appeared to be originating from several points around the equator, an encircling procedure was employed. The majority of cases fell into this category. The presence of retinal breaks determined the location of additional buckling effect. In several cases the traction forces appeared to originate in one narrow segment, necessitating only a localized buckle.

Adequate drainage of subretinal fluid was felt to be an essential part of the procedure. Before fluid was drained, the encircling silicone band was placed in position and the ends united with a short tubular Silastic sleeve[5] (Fig. 21-8). The site for the sclerotomy was then selected at a point where there was adequate subretinal fluid to avoid retinal perforation or incarceration. This usually resulted in a very posterior sclerotomy. The incision was not quite down to choroid, sparing the last few scleral fibers. The lips of the sclerotomy were separated by a preplaced suture, the underlying choroid inspected for large vessels, and the perforation made with a sharp, cold needle. As fluid was drained, the intraocular tension was maintained, first, by a cotton stick applicator pressed against the sclera and, next, by shortening the encircling band. Intravitreal balanced salt, or air, was used to help take up some of the volume lost by drainage in the very advanced cases. In this way, marked hypotony was avoided.

Frequently at the end of the operative procedure a portion of the retina remained elevated, secondary to vitreous traction (Fig. 21-9). Overly enthusiastic attempts to flatten these areas were not made so long as the macular area and most of the posterior pole had been reattached. In general, these eyes required higher buckles than those with routine rhegmatogenous retinal detachment.

RESULTS

Table 21-1 shows the types of procedures and the results of each. The longest follow-up is 8 years and the shortest, 3 months. The average is 30 months. Thirty-

Table 21-1. Surgical procedures used in the treatment of diabetic retinal detachments

Type of buckling	Number of eyes	Number of eyes with useful vision (%)	Average length of follow-up	Number of eyes with 20/400 or better
Encircling with resection	34	22 (65%)	32 mos.	16
Encircling without resection but with plombage	7	5 (71%)	18 mos.	1
Episcleral encircling	4	2 (50%)	13 mos.	1
Resection alone	5	4 (80%)	46 mos.	2
Totals	50	33 (66%)	30 mos.	20 (40%)

Table 21-2. Results as related to the preoperative presence or absence of retinal holes

Preoperative condition	Number of eyes	Number of eyes with useful vision
Detachments without breaks	29	19 (66%)
Detachments with breaks	19	12 (63%)

three of the 50 eyes (66%) maintained useful vision (finger counting or better), and the remainder ended with hand movements or worse. Retinal breaks were present in 19 of the eyes and, of these, 63% have useful vision. No retinal breaks were found in 29 eyes and 19 of these (66%) have useful vision (Table 21-2).

DISCUSSION

Patients with proliferative retinopathy can maintain localized retinal detachments for long periods of time without severe visual impairment. However, once the detachment becomes more generalized and the macula becomes involved, it is unusual for the eye to keep useful vision for as long as 1 year. In the present series of patients on whom surgery has been performed in an attempt to reattach the central retina, useful vision has been maintained in two thirds of these patients for an average of 30 months. There is no question that this procedure has benefited these patients.

The next question of great importance is that of prophylaxis of the diabetic detachment. The best prophylaxis would be that which prevents the proliferations. In the early cases of proliferative retinopathy, photocoagulation has been shown to slow down the progression of the disease process by eliminating the neovascularization before it has had a chance to either bleed into the vitreous or give rise to firm membranes.[6-10] Pituitary ablative therapy also decreases the frequency of vitreous hemorrhage and appears to slow down the progression of the retinopathy by its ability to bring about sclerosis of the newly formed vessels.[11-14] However, once proliferations extend into the vitreous and fibrous membranes become prominent, retinal detachment may ensue.*

Photocoagulation becomes somewhat dangerous in the face of dense intravitreal membranes, and in some of our cases retinal detachment may have been hastened by the therapy. In some patients the chorioretinal adhesion produced by the photocoagulation scar continued to hold, despite increasing vitreous traction. Seven of the patients in this series had received photocoagulation prior to the detachment. The average time between photocoagulation and retinal detachment was 11 months. Five patients with diabetic retinal detachment received uniocular prophylactic photocoagulation to the fellow-eye. None of these eyes suffered retinal detachment.

Whether prophylactic scleral buckling is indicated in eyes with grade IV proliferative changes and marked traction has not yet been decided. Several of the patients who have had successful scleral buckling procedures for their retinal detachments have also shown a marked regression in hemorrhagic activity. Relieving the traction on the retina in eyes with impending retinal detachment might also reduce the incidence of traction-induced hemorrhage, thus benefiting the vasculopathy as well as reducing the chances for future retinal detachment.

CONCLUSION

Retinal detachment secondary to proliferative diabetic retinopathy is one of the leading causes of diabetic blindness. The classical teaching for this condition has

---

*Three of the patients in this series had undergone stalk section of the pituitary prior to the development of retinal detachment.

been the avoidance of surgery unless a retinal break could be found. In this series, the detachments in which breaks were not found did as well as those in which retinal breaks were found. Approximately two thirds of each group retained useful vision following the appropriately designed scleral buckling procedure. Such a procedure should be performed as soon as possible after the macula detaches. Consideration is being given to prophylactic scleral buckling procedures in eyes with advanced proliferative changes.

REFERENCES

1. Larsen, H. W.: Atlas of diabetic retinopathy. A photographic study, Acta Ophthal. **55:** Suppl.:1, 1959.
2. Davis, M. D.: Vitreous contraction in proliferative diabetic retinopathy, Arch. Ophthal. **74:**741, 1965.
3. Tolentino, T., Lee, P. F., and Schepens, C. L.: Biomicroscopic study of vitreous cavity in diabetic retinopathy, Arch. Ophthal. **75:**238, 1966.
4. Gartner, S.: Ocular pathology of diabetes, Amer. J. Ophthal. **33:**727, 1950.
5. Watzke, R. C.: An encircling element connection, Amer. J. Ophthal. **56:**989, 1963.
6. Okun, E., and Cibis, P. A.: The role of photocoagulation in the therapy of proliferative diabetic retinopathy, Arch. Ophthal. **75:**337, 1966.
7. Okun, E.: The effectiveness of photocoagulation in the therapy of proliferative diabetic retinopathy, (PDR): (a controlled study in fifty patients), Trans. Amer. Acad. Ophthal. Otolaryng. **72**(2):246, Mar.-Apr. 1968.
8. Meyer-Schwickerath, G.: Treatment of Eales' disease and diabetic retinopathy with photocoagulation, Western J. Surg. Obstet. Gynec. **72:**76, 1964.
9. Thornfeldt, P. P.: Treatment of retinitis proliferans by photocoagulation, Northwest Med. Dec. 1965.
10. Wetzig, P. C., and Jepson, C. N.: Treatment of diabetic retinopathy by light coagulation, Amer. J. Ophthal. **52:**459, 1966.
11. Contreras, J. S., Field, R. A., Hall, W. A., and Sweet, W. H.: Ophthalmological observations in hypophyseal stalk section, Arch. Ophthal. **67:**428, 1962.
12. Field, R. A.: Role of hormonal suppression in managing diabetic retinopathy, Trans. Amer. Acad. Ophthal. Otolaryng. **72**(2):241, Mar.-Apr. 1968.
13. Speakman, J. S., et al.: Pituitary ablation for diabetic retinopathy, Canad. Med. Ass. J. **94:**627, 1966.
14. Pearson, O. H., et al.: Hypophysectomy for the treatment of diabetic retinopathy, J. Amer. Med. Ass. **188:**116, 1964.

22

General summary of the symposium

Bradley R. Straatsma

This symposium has featured such extensive and elaborate discussions by experienced and knowledgeable scientists that to recapitulate their material would be both redundant and presumptuous. Rather than attempt that, I would like to review this meeting in terms of *systems analysis*—the emerging skeleton of science that endeavors to draw together seemingly disparate aspects and to view every subject, no matter how complex, as a single unit or entity. In this way, observations that may have appeared at scattered points in the program can be drawn together, and emphasis can be given to supporting opinions and common conclusions.

It is appropriate to start this review with the beginning of the clinical appraisal of the retina—the examination—and to point out that during this meeting several aspects of this procedure received particular attention. First, regarding ophthalmoscopy, there was a description of a recently developed binocular indirect ophthalmoscope that permits stereoscopic examination of the ocular fundus through a pupil as small as 1.5 mm. in diameter. This small-pupil ophthalmoscope, presented by Dr. Schepens, is not yet commercially available, but when it becomes obtainable, members of the profession will try it with enthusiasm and eagerness.

Second, we heard a detailed description by Dr. Cockerham of the technique for biomicroscopy of the posterior ocular segment. Supplementing ophthalmoscopy, biomicroscopy is of particular value in study of the vitreous, study of the retina, and study of fundus areas where scleral depression cannot be employed (for example, on the crest of a scleral buckle).

Finally, transillumination was considered by Dr. Norton. He described transillumination by use of a retrobulbar light, which is viewed through the pupil with a condensing lens and an unilluminated binocular indirect ophthalmoscope. This method of transillumination is particularly useful when there are opacities in the media and there is a differential diagnosis between a solid tumor mass and a rhegmatogenous retinal detachment.

Retinal characteristics seen with ophthalmoscopy, biomicroscopy, transillumination, and other forms of examination must, for appropriate interpretation and analysis, be related to the structures of the retina. During the early portion of this symposium, Dr. Foos, Dr. Spencer, and I reviewed topography of the retina, discussed the major regional variations in retinal anatomy, and emphasized the importance of the relatiosnhip between the retina and the vitreous base.

Thereafter, we presented a classification, a systematic description, and a statistical review of the principal variations and the degenerations that occur in the peripheral retina. This material demonstrated that retinal breaks and lesions predisposing to retinal breaks are far more common than retinal detachments. In regard to pathogenesis, therefore, it is essential to realize that rhegmatogenous retinal detachment is not related exclusively to retinal breaks but is the result of a complex interplay involving the sensory retina, the vitreous body, the retinal pigment epithelium, and the choroid. In the entire sequence of what may be described as the "detachment disease," there are many variables that must be considered, and many forms of the disease may be presented to the ophthalmologist.

Dr. Curtin commented on the more advanced stages of the detachment disease in his description of the pathologic changes that occur in the detached retina. In addition, he reported on the retinal morphology and other characteristics observed in eyes that had undergone successful detachment surgery.

All the material obtained from laboratories of pathology and even from extensive studies of autopsy material leaves certain gaps in the overview of the sequence of events that occur when the retina becomes detached, remains detached, and is then reattached. Some of these gaps can be filled by experimental studies, and, indeed, one of the highlights of this meeting was a discussion by Dr. Machemer and Dr. Kroll of experimental retinal detachment in the owl monkey. With this experimental approach, they were able to study the succession of events that caused the detachment and to view at close range the degenerative changes that occurred in the detached retina. They outlined changes in the inner portion of the sensory retina, changes in the outer segments of the rods and cones, and changes in the pigment epithelium.

Of particular interest were the alterations in the outer segments of the rods and cones. These outer segments degenerated when the retina was detached and appeared to regenerate when the retina was surgically reattached. Significantly, these observations of outer segment degeneration and regeneration are corroborated in various ways by previous work done by Dowling at Johns Hopkins, Young at UCLA, and Kuwabara and Friedman at Harvard. In essence, the experimental studies of Dr. Machemer and Dr. Kroll, as well as those of other workers cited, indicate that retinal detachment is associated with degeneration of the outer segments of the rods and cones and that if retinal reattachment is achieved regeneration of the outer segments probably occurs to a remarkable extent. Thus, studies of autopsy material, surgically enucleated eyes, an experimental model of retinal detachment, and a variety of basic laboratory investigations can be drawn together by means of *systems analysis* to form an overall concept of rhegmatogenous retinal detachment—including its pathogenesis, pathology, and morphologic response to surgical correction.

Clinically, the "detachment disease" may be encountered at any one of many stages; that is, it may be encountered when a detachment seems imminent, when the detachment is localized, or when it is progressive. Each of these clinical situations was reviewed in this meeting, but prophylactic therapy was not extensively considered. There seemed to be agreement, however, that in a complex disease such as retinal detachment a decision concerning the wisdom of performing prophylactic therapy must be based on an evaluation of every pertinent factor. Specifically, there must be evaluation of the patient as a whole, the history of the opposite eye, and the size, shape, degree, and location of the pathologic condition for which prophylactic treatment is being considered. Even after these factors are evaluated, it is evident from the discussion that certain members of the panel are far more likely than others to apply prophylactic treatment. There is a spectrum of opinion on this subject, just as there has been for a number of years past.

When faced with a progressive, extensive retinal detachment, all members of the panel agreed on the necessity for treatment and on the objectives of the treatment. All agreed on the basic principle of careful localization of retinal breaks and other areas of focal retinal pathology. All agreed on the wisdom of a scleral infolding or buckling procedure, although there was discrepancy in the actual form of the infolding and in the materials used. Both segmental and encircling procedures were described, and materials employed included silicone rubber, silicone sponge, cadaver sclera, gelatin, and plantaris tendon. In essence, there was a range of surgical practice that had in common the basic principle of indentation of the sclera over areas of focal pathology.

Another common element in all the descriptions of retinal detachment surgery was the use of some form of therapy to achieve a reaction involving the sensory retina, the pigment epithelium, and, obviously, the choroid. There were extensive discussions by Drs. Meyer-Schwickerath, Schepens, and Norton regarding photocoagulation, diathermy, and cryotherapy. From these discussions, it was evident that with proper care and skilled application any one of these three general modes of treatment could be applied in a wide variety of circumstances. There were, however, indications that under certain circumstances one or the other method was the treatment of choice. Without attempting to be comprehensive, one can state that photocoagulation is the treatment of choice when there is need for a localized reaction in the posterior segment of an eye with clear media. Diathermy may well be the procedure of choice when an immediate, rather sticky reaction is desired, such as in the treatment of extensive retinal dialysis. Unfortunately, diathermy causes scleral necrosis, which is a factor weighing against its use. Cryotherapy is the procedure of choice for creation of a reaction through full-thickness sclera and when a procedure is to be carried out transconjunctivally.

The relase of subretinal fluid during surgery for rhegmatogenous retinal detachment was also employed by all members of the panel. Because the indications for this are relative, no hard and sharp guidelines were presented by the speakers. Interestingly, however, all members of the panel seemed to concur that this is the most precarious part of the surgical procedure or, as one panel member put it, "the part in which things are under least control." Consequently, subretinal fluid was released only when it appeared absolutely necessary.

From a practical standpoint, there was some indication that drainage of subretinal fluid was carried out less frequently when sponge material was applied to the scleral surface than when more solid material was used. In terms of drainage technique, a number of practical suggestions were given—all designed to prevent the complications of retinal incarceration, vitreous loss, and choroidal bleeding.

The results of retinal detachment surgery were described primarily by those members of the panel who discussed the various surgical procedures. On the whole, reattachment was described in over 90% of large series of random or unselected cases. Visual function was surprisingly good, even after macular separation in some cases. Moreover, there was an important trend toward the reporting of long-term follow-ups rather than, as was customary in the past, the reporting of observations during the 6 months or 1 year after surgery. In effect, with good immediate results, the surgeon is now able to give increasing attention to long-term results.

Apart from these generalizations in the surgical management of retinal detachment, there was extensive discussion of certain particularly difficult therapeutic problems. One of these was giant retinal breaks—retinal breaks extending over a quadrant or more of the eye. These were classified in general terms as (1) related to lattice degeneration of the retina, (2) dialysis-type breaks, (3) breaks associated with a rolled-over edge, and (4) immobile breaks with a rolled-over edge and with some adherence of the edge to the remainder of the retina. Though generally useful, this classification needs to be further defined before results from different centers can be truly compared.

There are great differences in the management of giant retinal breaks. In various centers, procedures such as movements of the head; use of the inverted position of the head; injections of air, saline, and silicone into the vitreous cavity; retinal diathermy; retinal cryotherapy; and even retinal incarceration are employed. For evaluating these procedures, the results reported by different speakers cannot really be compared because of the great diversity of cases treated, the methods employed, and the technique of reporting results. Clearly, experimental models, such as the collie dog used by Dr. Freeman and the owl monkey described in this meeting by Dr. Machemer and Dr. Kroll, can be of great value in supplying objective and truly comparable data on different methods of treating giant retinal breaks.

Intravitreous surgery was discussed during several phases of the symposium. All members of the panel seem to have employed, on occasion, intravitreous saline injection. A number have employed intravitreous air injection, several have introduced scissors of various types into the vitreous cavity to divide a membrane or strands, and at least two members of the panel have injected liquid silicone into the vitreous cavity.

Intravitreous silicone injection, according to Dr. Meyer-Schwickerath and Dr. Okun, was indicated only when other methods were unsuccessful and there was preretinal membrane formation or a giant retinal break. Moreover, Dr. Okun employed this material only when attempting to save vision in a patient's sole remaining eye. The technique of intravitreous silicone injection incorporated the passage of a needle through the pars plana into the vitreous cavity, slow injection assisted by a 3-ring syringe or a pump when preretinal membrane was present, and placement of the material into the funnel located posterior to the main body of the formed vitreous. This placement represented an effort to use the silicone to separate the preretinal membrane from the retinal surface.

The results of intraretinal silicone injection reported by both Dr. Okun and Dr. Meyer-Schwickerath were quite comparable. Both reported that about a third of the patients treated by this technique achieved retinal reattachment.

Traumatic retinal detachment was described by Dr. Schepens. His comments were directed to its pathogenesis, management, and results. Of practical importance were his statements regarding the interval between the trauma and the onset of retinal detachment. In a large series of patients, this interval was in some instances extremely short, but in approximately 20% of the patients it was greater than 2 years.

During the final portion of the symposium, attention was given to diabetic retinopathy. This subject was appropriate because diabetic retinopathy, by virtue of its incidence, predictable increase, and associated vision loss, is probably the greatest single problem of our profession.

At present, patients with diabetes mellitus are encouraged to maintain optimum medical control of their disease. All too frequently, despite this control and all other general medical measures, diabetic retinopathy develops and progresses to a stage that necessitates consideration of photocoagulation, pituitary ablation, or retinal detachment surgery. The indications for each of these procedures are not entirely clear from the data available at this time. Surely, photocoagulation is most effective when performed rather early and when the treatment is relatively expensive. Applied late, when the disease is far advanced, retinal photocoagulation may be deleterious. Pituitary ablation is generally performed when photocoagulation is contraindicated or when the retinopathy progresses despite photocoagulation and other measures.

When diabetic retinopathy progressed to the stage of retinal detachment, Dr. Okun advocated retinal detachment surgery. For selected cases with retinal breaks and progressive detachment or with extension of a traction-induced detachment into the macula, he recommended scleral buckling procedures.

Finally, apart from the general subjects, this symposium revealed several trends that, in my judgment, are of great significance to students of the retina—and that includes every ophthalmologist. First, there is a trend to move from the purely qualitative to the quantitative. For example, it is no longer appropriate to refer to conditions such as lattice degeneration of the retina or therapeutic chorioretinal reactions simply as entities. The former must be defined, as done in the symposium, in terms of degree, extent, and position. The latter, although incompletely studied to date, must be quantitated to describe therapeutic chorioretinal adhesions induced by diathermy, photocoagulation, or cryotherapy in terms of the strength of the adhesion and the rate at which this strength develops.

Second, there is a general trend to move from the empirical to the experimental. Evidence of this trend came from the use of an experimental model of giant retinal breaks by Dr. Freeman and the experimental model of rhegmatogenous retinal detachment by Dr. Machemer and Dr. Kroll. Without question, these experimental models can provide valuable information regarding structural alterations in the detached retina and the relative merits of different methods of therapy.

Third, there is a significant trend to shift from short-term to long-term evaluation of the results following retinal detachment therapy. In essence, this means that, with generally satisfactory immediate results in the vast majority of patients, it is now appropriate to consider the long-term results of retinal detachment surgery.

Fourth, there is an important trend for retinal surgeons to move from the restricted field of rhegmatogenous retinal detachment to the more general subject of retinal detachment as a whole. For example, ophthalmic surgeons are giving increasing attention to the management of retinal detachment secondary to uveal inflammations, ocular tumors, and diabetic retinopathy. Thus, the retinal specialist of the future will need overall knowledge of retinal anatomy, biochemistry, and physiology, in addition to an understanding of the mechanical aspects of the retina and its reattachment.

These trends combine with the foregoing *systems analysis* of the subject material to summarize this scientific assembly. Intellectually and—as a reflection of gracious New Orleans—in diverse ways, this symposium has been a rich and rewarding experience.

Round table discussion

Question: Many years ago when only simple end alignment was done and you switched from direct to indirect ophthalmoscopy examination, by how much did your rate of success increase?

Dr. Schepens: My rate of success increased by over 20%.

Question: With regard to aging and the formation of lattice degeneration, are newer lesions usually anterior to older lesions?

Dr. Straatsma: Really, there are two aspects to this question. The first inquires about the relationship between age and lattice degeneration. In this regard, it's pertinent to note that lattice degeneration can be extremely extensive in terms of the area of involvement early in life—well, in the first decade. Therefore, from material that has been seen in the pathology laboratories, there seems to be no true relationship between areas of involvement and age. I think it is interesting that Dr. Byer came to the same conclusion in his clinical study of lattice degeneration.

The second aspect is an inquiry regarding the relationship between the stage of lattice degeneration and the anteroposterior position of the lesions within the eye. Generally, the more advanced lesions are more posterior. In addition, the more posterior lesions are more prone to develop the complications of lattice degeneration, notably tears along the margin. Surely, there are exceptions, but the more posterior lesions are more prone to develop the total mechanical picture that leads to retinal breaks.

Among the panel members, there may be different opinions, and if there are, I'd be pleased to hear them.

Another question is as follows: In lattice degeneration, is the formation of a new lesion possibly related to the edge of a progressing vitreous detachment? The answer to this is no. We often find multiple rows of lattice degeneration in anteroposterior distribution with no relationship to the edge of a vitreous detachment. In fact, there can be two or even three rows of lattice in a very young individual who may not have any gross posterior detachment of the vitreous.

The third question is: Why do tears not occur at the anterior edge of lattice lesions, even though visible vitreous condensation and potential traction occurs all around?

Well, I think the tearing that occurs in conjunction with lattice is the result of a combination of factors, including vitreous traction, the exaggerated attachment that

334

exists between the retina and vitreous, and the thinning of the retina that occurs within the process. Actual rupture occurs when all three factors are in precisely the right proportion, and they are more likely to reach this proper proportion at the posterior edge of the degeneration. That's the first place the tear occurs; then there is some relaxation of the more anterior attachments simply as a result of that ripping of the retina.

Dr. Schepens: What is your practice in prophylactic treatment of lattice degeneration with and without holes and holes present without a flap? Does anyone have a comment on that? Dr. Straatsma, would you like to comment on this question?

Dr. Straatsma: I'll be glad to start a discussion. I'm sure there will be many who will add to it.

The problem is one of selection. There is ample evidence that both holes and the general condition of lattice degeneration are far more prevalent than retinal detachment. Consequently the ophthalmologist must select from this group of abnormal findings those conditions that are likely to go on to retinal detachment. In doing this, I think it is essential to use every available clue. This means that the ophthalmologist must gain as much information as possible from a review of the family history, the sequence of events in the opposite eye, and the general findings—such as cataractous changes, vitreous alteration, and chorioretinal reaction—in the eye in question. Then he must consider the location of the retinal abnormality—that is, superior versus inferior, temporal versus nasal—and the type of retinal lesion that is present. From the discussion this morning, however, it is evidently not enough simply to diagnose a retinal hole or lattice degeneration. This must be qualified in terms of the size of the hole and the degree or stage of the retinal degeneration. Is it relatively early, or its it relatively advanced? Even the ophthalmologist can't always know the stage or degree of retinal degeneration; he should at least attempt to evaluate the situation and move from the purely qualitative into the quantitative area.

On the basis of these factors, the physician must decide whether a case should be treated prophylactically or not treated. Obviously, this is not a clear-cut answer, but there is no definite answer. Too many factors are involved, and I think it's a foolish person who tries to use one or two simple guidelines to resolve a complex question.

Dr. Meyer-Schwickerath: I would like to say that one of our main guidelines in regard to prophylactic treatment is the history of the first eye. This means that we mainly submit fellow-eyes for prophylactic treatment which come under our care. And we are more likely to do prophylactic treatment in fellow-eyes than in eyes without detachment even if we find a rather late stage of equatorial degeneration. As you know, the different factors, which have just been mentioned by Dr. Straatsma, have come together at the same time. You may find a fellow who lost one eye 30 years ago at an early age who never was treated. You look at his fellow-eye, and it has severe equatorial degeneration. But if you look at this retinal area with a slit lamp, you may find this retinal area completely free of adhesions of the vitreous. In such a case, in regard to the risk of prophylactic treatment, I would not perform a prophylactic cauterization. But if this patient had come to me 30 years earlier, besides the operation of the detachment, I would have done prophylactic treatment in his second eye. It is quite safe to perform prophylactic treatment in the second eye. Why? Because it is rare, as everybody who does detachment work knows, that a detachment may occur in both eyes at the same time. It means it is extremely rare that the different factors that have to be ready to trigger off a detachment are present at the same time in one eye as well as in the second eye. I do hope that I made myself understood.

Mr. Hudson: I first want to thank you for the opportunity of being allowed to join the panel. I think that one of the factors that ought to be taken into account is a continued view of the eye that is under observation; and although one might look at an eye and say, "This eye does not require treatment now," if it is kept under observation, assuming that it is feasible to keep the eye under observation at frequent intervals, you may decide that changes are occurring which make you change your mind. And I think that it has to be borne in mind that an eye that doesn't require treatment today may easily require treatment in 2 or 3 months' time. We are now, ourselves, using cryotherapy increasingly, instead of photocoagulation in prophylactic treatment, and I think we shall have to await a good deal more experience before we can express a view as to which is the least damaging in producing prophylactic effect. I think the thing one must remember before starting to treat an eye, particularly in its temporal half, is the possibility of macula lutea disease, which has been mentioned in the papers at this meeting. And although it is not a frequent complication, I think that if you are starting with an eye with six-fifths or six-sixths vision you will want to be extremely careful before you apply any treatment that is likely to cause deterioration in the vision.

Dr. Schepens: I wish to stress two points. First, I agree with Dr. Meyer-Schwickerath when he insists on the importance of vitreous traction. Slit lamp microscopy is a better method to study vitreous traction than is ophthalmoscopy. The other point was discussed at the International Congress of 1958.[1] I reported that of 517 cases of subclinical retinal detachment no more than 158 (30.6%) were treated prophylactically. None of the other 14 members of the panel agreed with this conservative attitude. Today, I would say that probably no more than 20% should be treated prophylactically. Because photocoagulation and transconjunctival cryoapplications are so easy to apply, surgeons tend to use these modalities too freely on cases which need no treatment.

Dr. Cockerham: I agree with the other panelists who have mentioned findings in the vitreous. I have been impressed with slit lamp findings associated with areas of lattice degeneration which can sway you toward or away from treatment. After you have some experience in examining these lesions, you can estimate how dense and taut the bands of traction are on the margins of the lattice. Also, you may see irregular plaques of tissue in the vitreous just over the lesions which could be portions of partial-thickness retina that may have torn loose. The edges may even be involved in a very slight localized retinal detachment even though there is no break. I think one can come to have a feeling as to how dangerous a lattice lesion or group of lesions may be.

---

[1]Schepens, C. L.: The preventative treatment of idiopathic and secondary retinal detachment, Acta XVIII Concilium Ophthalmologicum 1:1019, 1958.

Dr. Okun: I would just like to restress, once again, what Dr. Meyer-Schwickerath said about the second eye of patients who have already demonstrated the tendency to detach their retinas, with breaks secondary to the lattice degeneration. Unfortunately, even with careful follow-up examinations and adequate warnings concerning symptoms associated with fresh retinal breaks, we are not always able to treat the retinal tear before it has gone on to a frank retinal detachment. I have the impression that not infrequently the tear and the detachment occur within a very short time of one another, if not simultaneously. Areas of lattice degeneration always contain an overlying pool of liquefied vitreous which may enter the subretinal space at the same time the area of retinal degeneration breaks open. Since these breaks tend to follow the margins of the zone of degeneration, extensive areas of degeneration tend to produce very large breaks frequently associated with rolled posterior margins and large vitreous hemorrhages. Because this type of retinal detachment carries a poorer prognosis than do cases with simple tears and minimal degeneration, particularly if the first eye had retinal detachment secondary to this type of change. I have had the unfortunate opportunity of having watched five patients go on to retinal tears and detachments in their untreated second eye. In each of these instances, I could look at a previous drawing and say, "Oh, I had seen that area of lattice degeneration before it broke down." Areas of lattice degeneration showing large amounts of pigmentation and chorioretinal atrophy are less predisposed to retinal tears and detachment than those showing minimal chorioretinal reaction; but, in the second eye of patients who have had the type of detachment described above, I, personally, elect to treat most of these cases prophylactically. I am more concerned about vitreoretinal degenerations in the second eye than I am with long-standing frank retinal tears.

Question: We have been told that 6% of autopsy eyes have lattice degeneration; 12% of autopsy eyes have holes without detachment, and about one hundredth of one percent of the population develops retinal detachment. Therefore, one must look with disfavor upon prophylactic treatment. Question: What percentage of patients with true holes develop retinal detachments? And the question they would like you to discuss is to compare that to the morbidity when cryo is used as a prophylactic modality.

Dr. Schwickerath: We know from a paper of Collier Atuchel that about 40% of holes in the upper half of the retina within 10 years lead to retinal detachment. This is a fact. Of course, these holes are not the same holes that are found very close to the ora serrata in these eyes, as stated very nicely by Dr. Straatsma. These holes are not dangerous in regard to retinal detachment—at least not as long as it is in a phakic eye. So in regard to the overall number of holes which we find clinically in the average population, I would like to go back to our cataract patients who are carefully observed in regard to retinal holes and equatorial degeneration. The frequency of equatorial degeneration in phakic eyes is, in our material, between 3% and 4%, and the frequency of holes is about 2%. We usually, which means if there is no other contraindication, treat these cases after we have performed the cataract operation.

Dr. Straatsma: This relates closely to the earlier question on prophylactic treatment. I think this repetition means that many are disturbed by the fact that there is no one-to-one ratio between retinal breaks and detachments. As Dr. Schepens said earlier, perhaps we have overemphasized the importance of breaks. Now, we must put retinal breaks in their proper perspective. The comments Dr. Schepens made earlier and the comments of Dr. Meyer-Schwickerath contribute to this perspective, as we mature our concept regarding the significance of retinal breaks. In effect, it is not enough to say a retinal break is present, we must consider the entire ocular status and attempt to select retinal breaks that are likely to lead to retinal detachment.

Dr. Okun: I just want to stress one point that Dr. Meyer-Schwickerath touched upon, the precataract extraction fundus examination. Many recently aphakic patients show retinal detachments secondary to retinal breaks or limited detachments which were obviously present prior to cataract surgery. These are eyes which show demarcation lines or a ring of pigment around the break or on the choroid corresponding to the site of the break. It would be much wiser to treat areas of lattice degeneration, retinal breaks, and areas of limited retinal detachment before the cataract is removed rather than to wait until the full-blown detachment occurs, 4 or 5 weeks following surgery.

Mr. Hudson: I think it is difficult to work from statistics on to a practical working basis but, we have found from experience that if the flat retinal tear we see is preceded by a history which could be that of a vitreous hemorrhage, the incidence we get of detachments following tears associated with vitreous hemorrhage is sufficiently high to make prophylactic treatment the right procedure. This also means, of course, that if you get a patient with a vitreous hemorrhage in which there is no history of systemic disease, our view is that we should treat him as an inpatient and wait for the vitreous hemorrhage to clear, which it seems to do more quickly with inpatient treatment; and there is an extremely high incidence of retinal tears associated with this type of hemorrhage.

Dr. Schepens: It should be remembered that the paper of Collier Pischel, which was referred to by Dr. Meyer-Schwickerath, describes retinal breaks found by direct ophthalmoscopy. Therefore, breaks found were relatively posterior and easy to see. Such a fact cannot be compared to the findings of Dr. Straatsma in autopsy eyes, where most of the retinal breaks noted were so small and peripheral that they could not have been detected in vivo by direct ophthalmoscopy. Rutnin and I found about the same number of retinal breaks in normal living subjects as Dr. Straatsma did in autopsy eyes.* Our findings were without vitreous traction. These breaks seal off spontaneously in the course of time. Older subjects tend to develop breaks which are the result of vitreous traction. Once more, it should be emphasized that the mere presence of a small peripheral retinal break is not sufficient reason to perform prophylactic treatment.

Dr. Curtin: I think that, as ophthalmologists, when we are examining a patient, there are two kinds of breaks that we see clinically, which Mr. Hudson mentioned but didn't say so specifically. The first is one that is a symptomatic break versus an asymptomatic break. And if we have a symptomatic break, then we can probably

---

*Rutnin, V., and Schepens, C. L.: Fundus appearance in normal eyes, IV. Retinal breaks and other findings, Amer. J. Ophthal. **64:**1063, 1967.

assume we are now dealing with recent history and the course of management we are going to propose is going to be from a point that is in the early stages of this disease. If we see an asymptomatic break, then there has probably been a long period of time in which this has been there, and since nothing has been deleterious to the eye up to this point, we don't go in and disturb the equilibrium in that eye. And so, just looking at Dr. Straatsma's statistics and whenever I want to make educated guesses, I always bet on what I think is going to be the winning side and I look at those statistics especially when I see asymptomatic breaks in an eye.

Dr. Schwickerath: I would not like to put too much emphasis on the term "symptomatic" or "asymptomatic" because from a statistical study of René Dufour in Lausanne we know that quite a number of typical horseshoe-shaped tears related to equatorial degeneration are present without symptoms. However, the question of symptoms with a tear are very important in regard to prophylactic treatment, because many tears are found at the moment when the patient has the first symptoms. He comes up with floaters, with hemorrhage, and he goes to his doctor. The doctor recommends prophylactic treatment. Prophylactic treatment is performed on Monday, and on Wednesday the patient has a detachment. And the doctor says, "Well, his detachment was triggered off by the prophylaxis." This is not true in many cases because this detachment was on the way. And in these cases, which have symptoms, we rather prefer to wait 1 week, with the patient in bed, before we do our prophylactic treatment to be sure the retina is as long attached as the coagulation needs to become a scar.

Dr. Foos: I'd like to bring up a basic point. And I'm glad to hear Dr. Schepens using the generic term "retinal breaks." I think we've got to distinguish between retinal holes and retinal tears. We now know enough to do this, at least as pathologists looking at autopsy material; I think we're dealing with a different entity, with a different pathogenesis, and I merely want to make this basic point.

Dr. Freeman: Walter and I have been working out an editorial on this very topic. We have been going through the literature and statistics, and it seems to me that probably the best treatment for the patient is to draw and not quarter him in most cases.

Dr. Norton: I have a question here that is directed to Dr. Schepens, Dr. Okun, and me: Would we please summarize the criteria and indication of employing the encircling band in scleral buckling procedures? I think this was done, but it obviously didn't get across during one of the lectures or maybe several of them. But just briefly, I think all of us, and they will have a chance to speak for themselves, would probably agree on massive vitreous retraction—that this has been the only thing that has been useful to date in reattaching these retinas. If I find equatorial traction or vitreous traction that tends to be all the way around the globe, I would certainly want to put a 360-degree band in. When I encounter localized traction, I think about it, but the hole and other factors determine my decision. I like a 360-degree band when I'm dealing with an aphakic case that has a very moth-eaten ora, all the way around, especially when I have trouble interpreting where and what are retinal breaks. I do not feel this is necessary in an aphakic case that has a perfectly normal-looking ora and has a simple tear. I also like the encircling procedure in cases with multiple breaks that involve multiple quadrants, say three quadrants. I think with multiple breaks in one quadrant I don't feel any necessity to go for a 360-degree band. But, if there are multiple breaks in three quadrants, I just find it easier to put a 360-degree band around and to cover those breaks than to start worrying about individual treatments.

Dr. Okun: And I might add to that—we usually resort to an encircling procedure in patients in whom a segmental buckle has been tried but has failed because of the formation of a new break secondary to vitreous traction in an area not treated. Otherwise, I think that Dr. Norton has covered our indications very well.

Dr. Schepens: I use a circling element in the cases described by the previous two speakers. I do not use a segmental buckle for multiple breaks, except when a study of the fundus by slit lamp microscopy reveals an absence of visible vitreous traction. In general, I lean toward using a circling element in all cases showing preoperative signs (by ophthalmoscopy or by slit lamp microscopy), indicating that there is a risk of recurrence. I tend to use a circling element in nearly all cases of aphakic, fixed folds and in eyes showing retinal breaks with rolled edges or breaks with extensive lattice-like degeneration. I also use a circling element when the sclera is thin, as a segmental buckle tends to flatten out in this case because it is maintained in place by scleral sutures which must necessarily be superficial. In cases of reoperation, I also prefer using a circling element. In segmental buckles, I always use an absorbable gelatin implant. This type of operation is particularly indicated in young patients with few or no signs of vitreous traction.

Mr. Hudson: The only place where I think I'd divert from Dr. Norton is that we regularly use an encircling procedure in aphakic detachments because we find in our experience that if we do use a segmental procedure we're apt to find that we have a recurrence. In fact, our recurrence rate is low in aphakic detachment since we have been using an encircling procedure.

Dr. Okun: We classify retinal detachments in our aphakic patients as either "aphakic" or "phakic" in type. The aphakic type shows many small peripheral breaks frequently secondary to elevated ora bays, small anteriorly displaced rosettes, or tiny peripheral flap tears. The "phakic" type shows one or more typical flap tears, usually equatorial or pre-equatorial in location. The ora serrata in these patients appears normal. While examining this type of patient, you think, "Well, this could just as well be an eye with a lens." Our success rate with local procedures in these phakic-appearing cases has been as good as in those eyes which are truly phakic.

Question: Even though a segmental buckle, Custodis type, does seal a hole, would it be better to use a primary 360-degree band to prevent redetachment due to continuous vitreous pull?

Dr. Norton: Well, I think that 10 years ago we might have answered this yes; this is what our thinking was—that you needed to have a 360-degree element to reduce the intraocular volume and maintain it at that level. But all of us had experience with infected sutures, implants eroding inward with the polyethylene that forced us to take out these elements. I think we learned what happened when we took them out. If the retina was fully attached both anterior and, of course, presumably posterior to the element, then we could take these out without much concern of their redetaching. The problem occurred when they had a detachment anterior to the buckle, and then when we took out the element, we could get into trouble and would have to reoperate them. Next we started using segmental procedures in face of what we called vitreous traction and found that it had worked very well and had stood up over a long period of time. We are talking now *not* about the severe cases, with organization in the vitreous and traction everywhere, but just localized traction in these cases. I think that a segmental buckle is adequate. I would also like to say that a lot of people have the idea that an eternal silicone rubber sponge implant put in without drainage of fluid will last a period of only 1 to 2 months. We'd be glad to have them visit us, and we would be glad to show them patients 3 years postoperative that have a big buckle although fluid was never drained. So these do last for a long time, and I think they reduce the traction at least enough so that a firm adhesion forms and you don't get into trouble.

Dr. Schepens: This subject could lead to a long discussion. A definite answer will not be available until more data is available. My experience is different from that of younger panelists. In 1950, I started with segmental buckles, both episcleral and intrascleral, and went on from there to circling procedures. The main reason was that if a lasting buckle was necessary it had to include a circling element. Occasionally, the ridge caused by a segmental buckle will last for years (17 years is the longest I have observed one), but in many cases it lasts for months only.

There are a number of cases where a circling element is not necessary and a segmental procedure is sufficient. In these cases, why couldn't we use a spongious, nonabsorbable, and easily sterilizable material which can imbibe antibiotics and has low antigenicity? With such a material there is little chance of precipitating an immediate infection and none to cause late complications such as erosion or delayed infection. I favor using gelatin for this purpose because it swells postoperatively, causing the buckle to increase for about 3 weeks. Disappearance of a gelatin buckle is the rule after about 6 months.

An external nonabsorbable spongelike material is sometimes hard to cover with orbital tissues and not infrequently becomes exposed through a conjunctival dehiscence. Although the silicone sponge is claimed to be of the closed-cell type, body fluids can be expressed from an implanted sponge, indicating that some of the cells must communicate. Such dead spaces will make any infection intractable. Because its surface is not smooth, the sponge tends to stick to underlying tissues. Silicone sponges occasionally cause erosion, and when they do, their irregular surface may stick to the choroid. In such a case their removal is often followed by choroidal rupture and vitreous loss.

Dr. Freeman: Speaking of segmental buckles, it just happens that I would like to show four slides. Dr. Schepens mentioned gelatin as an absorbable implant. We have been using gelatin now as an absorbable implant for, I guess, about a year. The slide will show you; it comes sterilized from Upjohn Company, and it comes in sheets of 0.5 mm. in thickness and 0.75 mm. in thickness. And the good thing about it is that you can cut it into any shape or size that you want and insert it into a pocket in the sclera, and it produces a very good buckle. As it absorbs intraocular fluids, only those fluids surrounding the globe, it increases in size and makes a very smooth buckle and tends to seal very tightly a horseshoe tear. (Could you show the first slide, please?) This is a sheet of Gelfilm, pigskin gelatin, sterilized, and it is, as I've said, a half a millimeter in thickness and easily cut. It has to be hydrated— it is dehydrated at the factory and then hydrated before surgery. (Next slide.) Here is shown where it is being inserted in a pocket in the sclera. This will produce a buckle for anywhere from 2 to 6 months, and then it is spontaneously absorbed. (Next slide.) There are two ways of using it—in a pocket as you see here or in a tract.

Dr. Okun: While we are on the subject of segmental buckle, we see that it can be produced in many different ways, and my experience has been exactly the same as Dr. Norton's in terms of permanence of the episcleral buckle; it will remain as long as the suture will remain, and if you take a long suture bite of 6 or 7 mm., this suture is not prone to cut through the sclera. Many of our segmental episcleral infolding procedures still show their internal bulge 3 years later. Now, when one stuffs a pocket, regardless of what one stuffs it with, in most cases it will disappear after 3 months. We have used solid silicone, silicone sponge, sclera, and tendon. Many materials can be used. I think that the two questions which come up are (1) How important is it for the infolding to remain permanent? (2) Which is the safer procedure to perform, the episcleral or the intrascleral?

In answer to the first question, I have become impressed that the permanency of the reattachment is more dependent on the complete and adequate closure of all of the breaks than it is on the residual shape of the globe. Most flap-type tears show enough posttreatment atrophy of the flap that it has either pulled free into the vitreous or the major vitreous traction-producing strands have degenerated enough so that very little residual traction remains. Even if some traction remains, well-placed chorioretinal scars appear to be strong enough to result in permanent closure. Recurrences have been rare, following removal of either encircling elements or episcleral segmental elements, provided all breaks had been well sealed preoperatively. Likewise, very few recurrences of retinal detachment have been attributed to the gradual loss of infolding effect which is seen with segmental intrascleral pocket procedures.

The episcleral segmental buckles utilizing the silicone sponge and cryotherapy have made it unnecessary to drain subretinal fluid in many cases that would have required drainage had they been done with an intrascleral technique. Elimination of this potentially dangerous step adds to the safety of this procedure.

Dr. Schepens: In relation to what was just said, I think it important to seal not only the retinal breaks but also those areas which may become breaks at a later date. This may be even more important than the permanency of a buckle. A statement to which I take exception is that if a scleral pocket is filled with absorbable material the nature of the material is not important. I believe it essential to use a material that is easy to sterilize, has low antigenicity, can imbibe antibiotics, and is easily available.

Mr. Hudson: I'm interested that no mention had been made in doing segmental procedures of actually burying the hinged flap that one produces if one does a scleral resection. I hesitated to mention this until someone talked about making a scleral pocket because I had a feeling that any sort of scleral surgery was becoming unpopular. But it is possible, with suitable sutures, to bury the scleral flap to produce a much deeper indentation than one can get with an ordinary buckle and as deep an indentation as one can get with some synthetic material. And, we still use this as a method of getting a permanent and reasonably deep buckle. I'd like to support what Dr. Schepens said about the cellularity of the silicone rubber sponge materials. We have found specifically that if we use them more than once, that is, if we use a piece of material and keep the remainder of the material and resterilize it, any attempt to sterilize it by any form of heating renders it absorbent, and, therefore, if it is used after it has been resterilized, it should be done in ethylene oxide gas.

I would like to add that, because not all of you might be aware of what type operations will be predominant in foreign countries, about 50% of the retinal detachments we operate on are operated with a full-thickness scleral infolding and subsequent photocoagulation, thus avoiding using any type of foreign body in the eye. I prefer this operation, especially in those cases in which we have a high myopia, because this scleral infolding reduced the amount of myopia and the patients usually are very lucky about it.

Dr. Okun: The next questions are: How do you treat, how do you decide when to treat diabetic retinopathy, and what exactly is the aim of the treatment? Exactly what do you aim the treatment beam at? And also, do you have fluorescein in the vessels while you are treating?

The first time we see a diabetic patient a complete baseline ophthalmologic examination is performed. This includes a fundus drawing of each eye, fundus photographs, and classification of the severity of disease in each eye. We do not treat nonproliferative retinopathy, with one exception: occasionally areas of hemorrhagic activity and microaneurysms just outside the macular region are coagulated in an attempt to decrease macular edema and exudation. This has resulted in improved visual function in several cases. A patient with Grade I or II proliferative retinopathy, who has never bled into the vitreous, receives a baseline examination as described and is then followed periodically, initially at 1-month intervals. As soon as we have become convinced that this disease is progressing and not regressing, we undertake therapy. There is another group that we prefer to treat at the time of initial visit, and that is the group that has recently experienced a bad vitreous hemorrhage. If the bleeding site can be located and if the media is clear enough for light treatment, the site of leakage is coagulated. If there remains doubts as to the site of origin of the vitreous hemorrhage, we wait for the hemorrhage to clear. Following a day or two of bed rest with the head elevated, we can sometimes spot an area of neovascularization or proliferation with a little preretinal blood aiming toward it. We coagulate these areas because we have become impressed that these are the sites of origin of recurrent hemorrhages. We try to avoid excessive photocoagulation whenever there is blood in the vitreous. However, when the vitreous hemorrhage clears, we will then complete the treatment of that eye.

What is your treatment beam aimed at? We treat all areas of surface neovascularization and hemorrhagic activity, carefully avoiding direct treatment to the large veins and the macula. I like to treat all four quadrants at one sitting, with most of the therapy placed within five disc diameters of the disc. In this way, as many as 250 lesions may be placed during the initial treatment. I don't photocoagulate the periphery because diabetic changes are minimal peripheral to the equator.

Question: Do you treat with fluorescein in the vessels?

Dr. Okun: I have not had a great deal of experience with fluorescein in the vessels while treating. I certainly do not see any necessity for fluorescein when the vessels are on the surface of the retina because the heat generated in the pigment epithelial zone is enough to coagulate these vessels. However, in those eyes in which the major source of hemorrhagic activity is the intravitreal fibrovascular proliferations, or proliferations directly off the disc, fluorescein diffusing into these membranes allows them to be light coagulated. We have tried to treat these areas with the aid of intravascular fluorescein injections. There is visible shrinkage of these membranes as the light strikes them, but it is practically impossible to completely devascularize them. As I stated earlier, I am somewhat concerned about shrinkage of these membranes for I have seen retinal detachment occur shortly after such therapy. Likewise, we do not have adequate therapy for the neovascularization that occurs on the disc, except that occasionally treatment elsewhere in the posterior pole results in regression of the neovascularization in the region of the disc.

Question: Did the photocoagulation done in the posterior pole influence any of the changes elsewhere in the eye?

Dr. Okun: Yes, we have frequently observed the retina change from an edematous pale yellowish or greenish color to a perfectly dry retina with a healthy-appearing red reflex following photocoagulation of hemorrhagic zones near the posterior pole. We have also noticed neovascularization undergo sclerosis and obliteration in areas not directly treated, but I am not certain that this is not a spontaneous change unrelated to the light treatment. Maximal therapy, as has been described, frequently results in a generalized decrease in the distention of veins and an increase in the amount of sclerosis of new-formed capillaries. This type of therapy can be likened to a debridement of unhealthy tissue, with resultant improvement in the appearance of the remaining tissue.

Question: Is the laser as effective as the photocoagulator in the therapy of diabetic retinopathy?

Dr. Okun: I have had no experience with the A.O. laser. I have had some experience with the Optics Technology laser and I do not feel it is effective in the therapy of proliferative diabetic retinopathy. It will eliminate some microaneurysms, but it does not effectively eliminate surface neovascularization. Perhaps, I haven't used it enough. The laser lesions are very fine lesions, with maximal effect limited to the choroid and external retinal layers, and for this reason I much prefer the Zeiss photocoagulators. We use both the West and East German Zeiss models. The photocoagulator after Meyer-Schwickerath is the one that most of you are accustomed to; the photocoagulator after Comber, manufactured by Zeiss-Jena, has an indirect binocular observation system, the optics of which are excellent. The exposure time is very short and not subject to control; therefore, the degree of coagulation is controlled only by the intensity setting. This is a slight disadvantage which is compensated for by the improved optics.

Question: In diabetic retinopathy, are the retinal lesions that are treated sites of bleeding, arteries, or veins, or are neovascularization sites treated by photocoagulation?

Dr. Okun: I try to treat the areas of neovascularization on the surface of the retina. I try to be very careful not to place any lesions directly across veins, for I have seen severe bleeding follow acute vein occlusion. I have approached veins very closely many times, since the majority of these tufts of neovascularization do originate on the edges of veins, but I am very careful not to hit the vein itself. I don't mind coagulating over arteries for I've never seen trouble come from that. In general, I prefer to use a large amount of photocoagulation, enough to produce a certain degree of retrograde optic atrophy. This seems to be beneficial.

Question: If you have a 34-year-old Caucasian woman with progressive diabetic retinopathy and with recurrent vitreous hemorrhage from a vascular proliferation from the disc, can photocoagulation technique be utilized?

Dr. Okun: Photocoagulation is not too effective in this type of case. Many times the neovascularization which accompanies these stalks are on the nasal side. Photocoagulation of these neovascular stalks while they are coated with blood can be effective in obliterating the neovascularization which accompanies the fibrous proliferation. We have not been very effective in obliterating the neovascularization while the vessels are filled with fluorescein. Again, one must be warned about the possibility of inducing a retinal detachment secondary to photocoagulation-induced shrinkage of these membranes. I am not too enthusiastic about undertaking photocoagulation treatment in this type of case.

Question: How extensive and what modality of treatment is used when buckling diabetic retinal detachment?

Dr. Okun: We have used various modalities. I have been impressed that the people who have done extremely well for a long period of time have been those who have received what we would consider today an excessive amount of diathermy therapy. They have fairly high, atrophic buckles. The traction on the proliferans appears fairly lax, and there has been cessation of bleeding. What we use today is the combination of all types of buckling procedures. If there is a break too close, then we usually accomplish this with an intrascleral plombage, frequently accompanied by an episcleral encircling buckle. However, if there are no breaks, I usually create a lamellar undermining in the meridian of greatest vitreous traction. This area is pretreated, usually with diathermy, and then a fair amount of sclera placed into this bed. A silicone band is then used to encircle the globe.

Question: Would you explain why diabetic retinopathy is usually unilateral in cases of unilateral myopia, or unilateral in asymmetrical carotid disease?

Dr. Okun: In cases of unilateral carotid occlusive disease, there seems to be less retinopathy on the side in which the carotid occlusion occurs. The reason for this still remains speculative. In cases of carotid occlusion, there is less vascular inflow to the ipsilateral eye; this may favorably affect the pressure within the abnormally fragile diabetic capillaries and result in less leakage. Now, in myopia there is some degree of retinal atrophy and optic nerve atrophy. Perhaps this leads to a decreased nutritional demand, less arterial inflow, and less venous stasis, with a decreased tendency for subsequent neovascularization. How have these observations affected our method of treatment? One could go on to speculate that perhaps there is improvement in the metabolism of the retina in areas which are left untreated. By eliminating zones of leakage, in which the local metabolism is impaired, perhaps there is a factor "X" that is being eliminated, leaving residual retinal tissue that is relatively healthy. This is all entirely conjecture. These hypotheses are certainly worthy of future investigation, but until more basic knowledge becomes available, we must continue to make careful observations and empirically direct our therapy in a way that appears to be beneficial to the patient.

Question: Since there are many times no holes and you have relaxed the vitreous traction with your buckle, why is it not possible to omit drainage of subretinal fluid and allow it to absorb?

Dr. Okun: We now have two patients with diabetic traction detachments which we have buckled without drainage of subretinal fluid, and the fluid has absorbed in both of these cases. These were both treated with episcleral buckles. Remember, however, that these were fairly long-standing detachments and it did take about 2 or 3 weeks for the macular area to dry up. The patients we prefer to operate on are those who have very recently detached a macula, and in these cases we prefer to drain subretinal fluid and flatten the macula as soon as possible. We are planning to evaluate the effect of scleral buckling on retinal detachments not yet involving but threatening the macula, and we do not plan to drain subretinal fluid in these cases. In cases of rhegmatogenous retinal detachment treated without drainage of subretinal fluid, the macula is usually the first area to flatten. However, in a diabetic detachment, the primary vitreous traction is central, and even though this traction is relieved by producing a buckle at the equator, this area is still the last zone to become flattened when scleral buckling is performed without drainage of subretinal fluid.

Question: Would a scleral buckling procedure perhaps provide an additional protection in altering blood flow to areas involved with diabetic retinopathy?

Dr. Okun: If this does, it may do it via a retrograde degeneration of some nerve fibers, with compensatory decrease in retinal blood flow. The only blood flow that a scleral buckling procedure might be interfering with would be anterior choroidal flow, both peripheral and retrograde, and I don't think that this is the mechanism. I think that the primary protection from a scleral buckling procedure is in terms of relieving vitreous traction. Some additional help stems from the fact that there is sometimes induced atrophy of the optic nerve with associated decrease in arterial flow. Again, this is purely speculative; we first make the observation and then we attempt to explain it.

Dr. Norton: I have a specific question to ask as to how our group treats diabetic retinopathy, and I am not going to repeat what Dr. Okun has just gone through. There are a few little things that are worth remembering. I can remember the first diabetic retinopathy patient I treated when I first got the photocoagulator in 1959 and we did treat a series of patients, just treating one eye. It interested me at that time that a lot of people were saying that this is the worst thing that you can do with diabetic retinopathy. You may remember that Graham Clark said that you treat these patients and they bleed, and they do very badly, and that photocoagulation is contraindicated. It's interesting to see that we have swung a little bit the other way. In regard to the patients that we treated in one eye in 1959 and 1960 and have an opportunity to follow—we do not have a big series—I can only tell you that the results would not impress you. It is amazing to me how the untreated eye has done so well in so many of those patients—that was because we were treating early diabetic retinopathy. At the present time, I can come to no conclusion that is worth anything from those studies.

Coming into proliferative retinopathy, I think that essentially we do what Dr. Okun said he does. It is interesting that we now have a fellow with us who spent 6 months with Dr. Okun, so I asked him one day, "How does our method of retinopathy differ from Dr. Okun's method?" And he said, "Well, Dr. Norton, I think you both do about the same thing. You both cover big areas of the retina; there is only one difference," he said, "Dr. Okun goes along the arteries, and you go along the veins." I am sure that we both do it as a result of profound judgment. Dr. Okun is worried about going over the veins and I straddle the veins as I move along with the photocoagulator. Now, I don't hit them so they occlude, but I do straddle the veins, and it is strictly imperative; I have no . . . I don't even want to get off into the reason for it—the moon isn't full yet. We do not treat . . . neovascularization on the disc. Dr. Paul Wetzig does and has shown some very impressive results. At this moment, I believe the important aspect is extensive destruction of more critical retina with the intent of "causing" arrest of the progress of the retinopathy. In the case of diabetic maculopathy, I don't think there is any question that the pictures shown to you this morning by Dr. Schwickerath represent the disappearance of the maculopathy following photocoagulation. We have similar pictures of one eye, with the other eye left untreated; it is very impressive. I think that the big problem is that we usually wait so long that the retinal changes have become permanent while the exudates and edema may disappear, but because the visual acuity does not improve much, it may be that we have to treat these patients earlier. Then you get into all the problems of trying to control the observations.

Don Gasser in our group is enthusiastic about treating the detachments associated with diabetes similar to Dr. Okun's method. The only difference is that we do not put any treatment under the band if there is no break. All we do is put a band 360 degrees around, drain fluid, and pull it up as high as we can. There are some very impressive results with this technique, but there are some bad results also. Bleeding is a complication especially when the eye is soft. Just a word on pituitary ablation. I think that none of us really know where any of this is leading us. But, I do think it is fair to say that the interest in pituitary ablation that existed, let's say 5 years ago or 8 years ago, has definitely decreased now. I personally have stopped recommending pituitary ablation, and I don't have sound reason one way or the other. But 2 years ago, Dr. Curtin, myself, and Mr. Justice went up to Cornell Hospital Medical Center (New York). We got back 24 patients that Dr. Ray had done hypophysectomy on for fluorescein angiography. One thing we can say is that hypophysectomy in no way influences the permeability of the retinal blood vessels to fluorescein. These patients all behaved just like every other diabetic and leaked fluorescein brilliantly. I think that some cases impressed us that they might have done a little better than we would have expected, but there were an awful lot of cases that did not have very much useful vision. We did not feel at the time that the results were good enough to justify our recommending patients to go on with pituitary ablations. So at the moment, I am left with only photocoagulation. I do think it will help neovascularization on the retina; I think it will help maculopathy; I think the buckling procedure when the retina is detached with organization in the vitreous is worthwhile. But I do think that at the present moment photo-coagulation is still in an experimental stage. As I told Dr. Straatsma earlier, it's sort of like treating cancer with surgery—it's the best we can do at the moment, but as soon as somebody comes along with anything worthwhile, it's going to be terminated.

Mr. Hudson: There are one or two points that emerge from this. I'd like to take Dr. Okun's speculation a little bit further with regard to the so-called factor "X" because Franceschetti many years ago advised equatorial diathermy treatment in cases of Eales' disease in an attempt to cut down the venous congestion. The possibility here is that improvement in this is due to reducing the amount of anoxic retina and therefore the oxygen demand of the retina and, as Dr. Okun has already pointed out, the need for a large circulation is decreased. This was taken a step further, in a way, by Redmond Smith, who thought that he could reduce the liability of a patient with a central retinal vein thrombosis to neovascularization and particularly to thrombotic glaucoma if he treated the case early enough. But in both these situations and in diabetic retinopathy we are speculating. But these three things have something in common, and it is possible that the treatment of diabetic retinopathy with photocoagulation is just another nonspecific way of reducing the oxygen requirement of the retina. As far as pituitary ablation is concerned, I think that in Great Britain, certainly, it has a significant mortality and a high morbidity because your patient is never quite the same after he has been treated; they are dependent on steroids and things like that to keep them going. It makes the life of the diabetic perhaps more complicated. I've always felt, and this is a purely personal point of view, that if you allow the retinopathy to advance to the stage where some people undertake pituitary ablation you've gone past the point where it is likely to be beneficial. Although it may not lead to an improvement in the eye, it's possible that if it were done earlier it might have cut down the speed of the development of the retinopathy. My own feeling, and I think the feeling in Great Britain generally, is that pituitary ablation has a very small part, if any, in the treatment of these cases in view of its mortality and its morbidity.

Dr. Straatsma: We can all agree on the uncertainties associated with pituitary ablation. I feel it would be improper to leave the discussion so one sided, however, because there is evidence now that the procedure can be done with extremely low mortality, extremely limited morbidity, and with preservation of vision, or actual improvement in vision in about 75% of properly selected cases. The number of patients who fulfill the general medical and ophthalmologic criteria and will undergo this treatment is limited, but I think the treatment is an important part in the overall approach to this disease. The technique of pituitary ablation employed at UCLA was developed by Dr. Robert Rand. The procedure is performed under local anesthesia with a cryoprobe that is passed through the nasal passages and inserted into the anterior lobe of the pituitary. Careful control of the probe placement is achieved with a stereotaxic technique, and both visual field and ocular motility are tested as the cryoreaction is being created. Obviously, the procedure must be performed very carefully. Details of cryohypophysectomy are currently in press in the annals of internal medicine.*

---

*Brown, J., and Straatsma, B. R., et al.: Diabetic mellitus, current concepts and vascular lesions (renal and retinal), Ann. Int. Med. **68:**634, Mar. 1968.

Dr. Schepens: It is interesting but confusing to hear so many different opinions on the treatment of diabetic retinopathy. One thing is obvious: nobody really knows what the treatment of choice is. From the standpoint of indications for treatment, one can divide the cases into three broad categories: (1) intraretinal changes including aneurysms, new vessels, and small hemorrhages, (2) proliferation of new vessels in the vitreous cavity, on the posterior surface of the hyaloid, and (3) spontaneous fibrosis of the angiopathy. Blindness may occur in the third stage by retinal detachment or vitreous hemorrhage, both resulting from traction by the fibrosed strands.

Cases amenable to photocoagulation include the first category. Before using photocoagulation, it is essential to examine the eye by slit lamp microscopy in addition to ophthalmoscopy with complete fundus drawing and fundus photography. This is the only way to determine the existence of retraction of the vitreous gel. If retraction is present and new vessels are already visible by slit lamp on the hyaloid, then photocoagulation may not be indicated as it may precipitate further retraction of the vitreous gel, secondary retinal detachment, and vitreous hemorrhage. If bleeding is present in the vitreous, a complete study of the fundus and extensive and repeated medical studies are needed. The decision to operate must be based on the prospects of visual recovery in those patients whose life expectancy is fairly good. Failures may result from a failure to depress sufficiently the pituitary function or from inadequate selection on the basis of fundus changes. I agree that today the easiest and safest method is probably destruction of the pituitary by cold. It should be remembered that the cold type of treatment simply stimulates fibrosis of the retinal angiopathy which is a process occurring naturally in a certain number of cases.

Once the angiopathy is fibrosed it may cause rhegmatogenous or nonrhegmatogenous retinal detachment and vitreous hemorrhage by traction. During the past 10 to 12 years, I have done a number of scleral bucklings in hope of improving this type of retinal detachment. My findings were that visual results were poor and that after a few months the retinal detachment recurred.

Dr. Cockerham: Dr. Schepens, I would like to add one point concerning the fundus drawing of diabetics. We should never use scleral depression because there have been a few cases that have bled significantly. I think this is the only condition where we avoid scleral depression.

Dr. Kroll: Dr. Schepens, I wish to register a mild protest against attempting to photocoagulate retinal neovascularization, with the hope of sparing the nerve fiber layer. After all, the very vessels you want to photocoagulate are lying on the internal limiting membrane, which is adjacent to the nerve fiber layer and most of the heat generated in photocoagulation is generated in the pigment epithelium.

Dr. Schepens: If it were necessary to close the retinal vessels by photocoagulation, then many of the cases described as successes should really have failed because all sizable abnormal vessels were intentionally avoided. It is not certain that photocoagulation should close any retinal vessels immediately. We simply do not know how this treatment works. When weak spots of photocoagulation are done around the posterior pole and no sector defect occurs in the visual field, it must be that many blood vessels and many optic nerve fibers are spared by this treatment.

Dr. Okun: I'm sure that some of the optic nerve fibers are not spared; however, as Professor Meyer-Schwickerath has stated and as we have reported, repeated visual field studies on these patients have revealed primarily discrete scotomas and not nerve fiber bundle defects. Initially, there may be large defects, but as the edema of the acute lesion subsides, the nerve fiber defects become less prominent and finally disappear. That is not to say that an excellent visual field might not pick an occasional nerve fiber defect, but the fact remains that most patients are not bothered by the results of this therapy. Some very intelligent people who have had uniocular therapy have had difficulty recalling which eye received the photocoagulation. These are complete scars. Histopathologic examinations of the type of scars produced in these patients show the nerve fiber layer at least partially destroyed.

Dr. Norton: I'd just like to say two things. One about the scattered photocoagulation: I've been on a couple of panels where the same thing has been said that you knock out the field even though you have knocked out the diabetic retinopathy. All I can say is that I thought the same thing before I did it too. Anyone who says it really hasn't done it, because it's amazing to me how the patient can have his whole fundus peppered with photocoagulation scars such as Meyer-Schwickerath showed and yet function quite well.

Now on hypophysectomy: We're not going to settle this. It is now 13 years, at least. I don't recall if it was 13 or 14 years since the first one was done in this country for diabetic retinopathy. I think it is interesting that a procedure as traumatic and as serious as hypophysectomy is, any way it is done, has been carried out on countless patients. I don't know, but there must be at least a thousand patients in this country alone. And after 14 years' experience we still do not know its value. It clearly shows you that this is an extremely complex problem.

Dr. Okun: When we see patients whom we don't think we can help with photocoagulation or on whom we have tried photocoagulation and feel that we are being ineffective, we have, for want of something else to do, advised pituitary ablation. Although we do not have a very large series, I have been very much impressed by the changes that I have seen in some of these eyes. These were eyes that were progressing at a very rapid rate, and if this progression continued, blindness would have occurred within a short period of time. The rapid sclerosis of large zones of neovascularization we have documented in some of these cases and the improvement in their retinopathy had to be related to the surgery.

Now I think that one of the major stumbling blocks in the evaluation of past efforts to treat this disease has been in the lack of a uniform system of classification of the retinopathy. Moreover, much of the pituitary surgery has been done without expert ophthalmologic follow-up. I agree with Dr. Schepens' description of the ideal initial work-up. In addition, I would include visual field studies. I would like to stress that these studies be repeated at a minimum of 3-month intervals after therapy has been instituted. As has been stated, the late fibrotic changes can and do occur even after the vasculopathy has been eliminated. As I stated earlier, I feel that traction-induced retinal detachments and hemorrhages respond better to a scleral buckling procedure than to any other means of therapy.

Question: You alluded to a detrimental effect of the light used in indirect ophthalmoscopy and to the incorporation of a filter in the new ophthalmoscope. Would you elaborate?

Dr. Schepens: The basic work in this area was done by W. Noell, T. Kuwabara and E. Friedman. They have shown that animals exposed to high levels of illumination show irreversible changes in their rods and cones. Such changes are temperature dependent, more damage being done at higher temperatures. Raising the temperature of the retina by 1 or 2 degrees centigrade may be a decisive factor in the causation of permanent damage. When the retinal temperature is raised, the level of illumination needed to cause damage in rabbit and monkey retinas is not far from the level used in indirect ophthalmoscopy, when the patient's pupil is fully dilated. Heating of the retina can occur by looking at the same area, with the indirect ophthalmoscope, for longer than 10 to 15 minutes. I think, therefore, that if we perform indirect ophthalmoscopy with a strong light we should filter out all the infrared rays which are not useful to fundus illumination. If we consider only those infrared rays which can penetrate the eye (between 8500 Å and 12,000 Å), they represent over 50% of the total energy emitted by the ophthalmoscope bulb. So-called heat-absorbing filters are not efficient in eliminating these radiations because they absorb part of the infrared rays only. Interference filters are much preferable for this purpose. Another practical point is that if a patient has a fever prolonged examination of his retina with a strong light is a hazard.

Dr. Kroll: I'd just like to comment that one of the really fascinating things about the work of Kuwabara and Gorn, which recently appeared in the Archives of Ophthalmology (vol. 79, p. 69), is that if one subjects rats to ordinary fluorescent lights for 24 hours a day and cools the cage so there is no elevation in the temperature, the retina in the region of the outer segments will rapidly begin to degenerate. It is not only the intensity and temperature of the light but also prolonged exposure to ordinary light at ordinary temperatures which can inflict retinal damage.

Dr. Straatsma: In this conversation, we're seeing a perfect example of the close relationship between pure science and practical application. We in ophthalmology are becoming concerned about these external segments, and it's important to know that in all of the species studied so far these very vital external segments of the rods and cones are undergoing a constant process of formation and destruction. This is not a static system; it is a dynamic system. If frogs, mice, and rats are given amino acids and other protein precursors, these appear within a very few hours in the outer portions of the inner segments of the rods and cones. If these are tagged with radioactive material, they can be traced progressively from the inner portion of the outer segments all the way to the outer portion of the outer segments. This work was done at UCLA by Dr. Richard Young, and it establishes the fact that there is a constant replacement and regeneration of these outer segments. I think this concept is an important aid in evaluating the extremely valuable findings presented by Dr. Kuwabara and Dr. Friedman in Boston and is very helpful in analyzing and further interpreting the excellent results reported here by Dr. Machemer and Dr. Kroll.

Dr. Norton: This is a fairly practical question, and I know a lot of people would like the answer too. It's directed not only to me but to the panel too, and I think that everyone on the panel who has an opinion should give it, because it's going to mean the purchase of equipment.

Which cryo unit is regarded as the most functional?

I would say at this point in history that, for me, I like the Linde unit the best.

Now, that's based on 4 years of sweat and toil and hardships, so you get to have an emotional involvement with it. I like the unit, but I certainly would not recommend it for anyone to buy. The next one in history development is the Frigitronic unit and I think this is a good unit; I think it probably can do all you need to do—I'm just talking as far as retinal surgery now—you're going to have to worry about cataract probes. The major disadvantage is that you have to buy the coolant in cans and, therefore, if you have trouble with delivery or something like that, it may not be feasible for you. Coming to the third commonly available unit—the Amoil unit—I must admit that this does seem to me to be the nicest to use. I can just tell you the nurses in the operating room by far put this as no. 1. I do have that little reservation I talked to you about Tuesday, about control, so the temperature doesn't always go down to minus 70.

At this time, you'll have to decide for yourself between the Frigitronic and the Amoil, as far as I am concerned. I think they are both good. I'm sure that better and smaller units are going to come along.

Does anyone else want to speak for these units? There are a couple of others that are available, but I've had no experience with them. Maybe somebody could talk on the Worst unit or the Thomas unit. I've not had any experience with them, so I can't talk about them.

Mr. Hudson: We, of course, have a predisposition to use the Amoil unit because it is more accessible to us. We have used a nitrogen coolant in the Rubenstein instrument, and I think an advantage of an instrument that doesn't begin precooled in this way is that you can indent the sclera and then look inside and then turn on the cold. I feel, from my own point of view, that what I require in an instrument is a high degree of reliability, rapid or reasonably rapid cooling, ability to reheat, and evidence as to what temperature you are using if you are using the detachment probe. Our experience is that the Amoil unit has provided these features, and also the cataract probe can be controlled by controlling the input pressure of the instrument. As you know, the coolant is easily accessible. There are ways of making it not work by disregarding some of the warnings on top of the instrument, and the chief one of these, of course, is that the coolant used is liquid carbon dioxide but is used in gaseous form. In other words, you've got a liquid carbon dioxide reservoir, and the only important feature is that this should be kept vertical so that you get nothing but gas into the machine. I feel that any instrument that will provide the features that I have mentioned should be pretty good.

Dr. Okun: We have the three units that Dr. Norton mentioned. The unit that I use most often is the Amoil unit. However, I find this unit a bit too cold for an eye with a staphyloma, even after turning it down. So, I use the Frigitronic unit for that. Then again, if I have to lower the temperature to $-100°$ C., either for very posterior treatment or for retreating over a scleral patch, I resort to the Linde unit. For the average ophthalmologist who can afford just one unit, the Linde unit would be the unit of choice because it would allow you to reach any temperature. However, for ease of operation, and so on, the Amoil unit is the one that has given us the least difficulty.

Question: Has the new American Optical monocular indirect ophthalmoscope been of any help in detachment work and at the operating table?

Dr. Cockerham: I have had very little experience with this instrument. However, I am convinced the binocular indirect ophthalmoscope worn on the head is greatly superior in all aspects of retina work because it frees both hands for scleral depression, provides stereopsis, and has brighter illumination.

Question: In retinal detachment cases, do you examine the peripheral retina with the 3-mirror Goldmann prism routinely?

Dr. Norton: No, I don't. I have gone through this phase though. And you know, I think it's a good thing, but the thing I learned most from it was how well I could see holes with the binocular indirect ophthalmoscope. The thing that amazed me the most was that when I would look with the 3-mirror lens and see these holes I really would have trouble finding them if I didn't know where to look, and I had to examine with the binocular indirect first to know where to look, then I could find these holes with the contact lens. It amazed me how small these holes were that I had been able to see with the indirect. So I think that, from the point of view of finding holes, I am perfectly willing to contend that if you spend 30 minutes just looking with a Goldmann lens, in addition to your binocular indirect ophthalmoscope, you may pick up something additional. After all, if you spend 30 minutes more examining the patient, you could do so. But I think it's fair to say that with a binocular indirect ophthalmoscope you can find most of the breaks. It would be very unusual to miss one. And certainly, the reverse I do not think is true. If you have to do one or the other, the binocular indirect is the one to do.

Dr. Schwickerath: Just say that this is exactly the same answer which Professor Goldmann gave 1 year ago to the same question.

Dr. Okun: It's encouraging that everybody is coming to a similar conclusion concerning the methods of examination. When we use a microscope, we have found that it is best to start by scanning the entire field at a low power; when we locate suspicious or interesting areas, we study these at higher magnification. The biomicroscope with slit beam and contact lens gives us both the magnification necessary for more careful study of retinal pathology and allows us to learn more about the vitreous. At the present time, we have a retina fellow with us who has trained in Switzerland. He is very competent with the Goldmann 3-mirror contact lens and is now becoming very competent with the binocular indirect ophthalmoscope. We have frequently compared findings, mine with the indirect ophthalmoscope and his with the 3-mirror prism. Most of the time we come out about even. But I hope that by the time he leaves that he will feel that he will want to use both, just as I feel that I should use both. But certainly if I were equally adept with both and had a choice of only one, I would choose the binocular indirect stereoscopic ophthalmoscope.

Dr. Cockerham: I agree with the previous statement that the indirect ophthalmoscope used with scleral depression is by far the best way to look for retinal breaks. However, I do not think it is as good as the Goldmann 3-mirror lens is for observing the vitreous body. For this reason, I feel that the use of both methods provides the best evaluation of a case.

Dr. Okun: I would like to reiterate what was mentioned yesterday by Dr. Cockerham in the examination of the eye that there are certain times when the 3-mirror prism is rather indispensable. And if you do not find a break, especially in an eye that has had previous diathermy, and the bed underneath the hole is not red from the choroid but there is pigmentation or white from the sclera where there has been choroidal atrophy, the 3-mirror Goldmann prism is of great importance in finding a hole. Just recently, this helped me considerably in one case.

Dr. Cockerham: One trick to remember is that if you can't find the hole with ophthalmoscopy and are suspicious as to where it may be, find the detached posterior hyaloid face with the slit beam and follow it to where it attaches to the retina. Then, if you follow that line of attachment along the retina, you sometimes can find a very small hole or at least a suspicious area that you will want to treat.

Question: On the basis of your electron-microscopic studies, what do you think the internal limiting membrane of the retina consists of?

Dr. Kroll: Well, this has been well shown by the studies of Ben Fine. The internal limiting membrane is actually a basement membrane consisting of collagen and glycoproteins. It is the basement membrane of the Müller cells of the retina. These Müller cells extend through the entire thickness of the retina, and they rest at one end on the internal limiting membrane, much as the pigment epithelium rests on its basement membrane, which is part of Bruch's membrane.

Dr. Machemer: I would just like to add a little bit to the answer of Dr. Kroll. You probably have in mind that wavy appearance of the posterior side of the retina. And it's easy to understand when a retina like this reattaches, the order of the outer segments will not be as well as if a flat detachment, the flat outer part of the retina, will attach. So that there will be in some areas a compression of outer segments, and this will result in a vision that is not as good as it could be. Also we observed in older detachments that the older they were the better were the results. Naturally, I tried to show you the best I could find. There are eyes, and obviously they have had very wavy retinal detachments, again, which did not settle that well, so that there were tiny left-over folds, and again, this will result in deterioration of vision. So, from our experience, I would say it is good to reattach as soon as possible.

Question: What is the histopathologic explanation of day blindness after successful reattachment?

Dr. Kroll: As you recall, exposure of the retina to light results in bleaching rhodopsin in the rods, and iodopsin in the cones, to retinine and rhodopsin, and retinine and cone opsin. The recovery from this requires structurally normal outer segments of photoreceptors and contact between these photoreceptors and the pigment epithelium. Day blindness, therefore, could be due to a poor recovery of the bleaching process of rhodopsin or cone opsin. Why? Well, there are two possibilities. There might be residual subretinal fluid still separating the detached retina from the pigment epithelium. This is true in detached retinas and it also could account for poor recovery from bright light in central serous retinopathy. The other possibility is that there has been poor outer-segment reformation, and therefore there is poor reformation of rhodopsin and iodopsin and, therefore, poor recovery from the stress of light.

Question: Could the macrophages in the retrolental space in retinal detachment be migrating pigment epithelium cells?

Dr. Kroll: Yes, they very well may be. In order to identify a macrophage possibly as a migrating type, one has to observe what is in its cytoplasm. The normal pigment epithelium in the owl monkey contains at least three inclusions: (1) the dark melanin granules, (2) the lighter (aging pigment) lipofuscin granules, and (3) the myeloid bodies. The lipofuscin granules are nonspecific; they are found in many cells, so we can't count on them for identification. The myeloid bodies resemble phagocytized outer segment material, so we can't rely on them. However, the melanin granules in the pigment epithelium are fairly specific, and fortunately, we have a way of telling the difference between a phagocytized melanin granule and a melanin granule that is primary in a cell. In the normal pigment epithelium, there are single melanin granules, each one surrounded by an individual membrane. In a phagocyte, melanin is usually present as a group of granules and the whole group of them are surrounded by a single membrane. There is a difference between a single granule which normally occurs in a pigment epithelial cell and a phagocytized bag of granules in a macrophage. We have found in several of these macrophages single melanin granules surrounded by a single membrane. It is therefore possible, in fact it is likely, that some of these macrophages do derive from pigment epithelium.

Dr. Machemer: And after some time we were astonished to observe something that we hadn't seen before. And I want to cite, first, the work of Friedman and co-workers that was published some time ago where they made flat preparations of different pigment epithelium and human eyes and animal eyes. And what they found was that in animal eyes, you very often see double-nucleated cells. But interestingly enough, in the human eye, at least in their picture, there is no double-nucleated cell of the pigment eptihelium. And they don't put much emphasis on that. Now, what did we find in the retinal detachments? We suddenly found cells that had huge nuclei. When does a cell have huge nuclei? It either has a high metabolic activity and thus needs an increase of DNA, or it prepares to divide.

The next picture shows such a cell. We think this could represent an amitosis, a cell that is going to divide.

Next you see pigment epithelium cells with double-nuclei, and they occur rather often. And then you might remember one of the pictures shown this morning that very often so-called macrophages were just overlying the pigment epithelium in the detached retina and they actually might derive from divided cells when these cells with the double nuclei have divided their site. So there is a possibility that the macrophages found in the subretinal space and later in the vitreous may derive from the pigment epithelium.

Dr. Machemer: I have a question, or actually three, concerning our experimental retinal detachments. The first is: Did you do histologic stains to study for the presence of vitreous detachment or the role of vitreous degeneration in the production of retinal detachment in the owl monkey? I was waiting for that question, and I will show you some slides that give our present idea. We want to be very careful because we are not the ones to say what hyaluronidase is doing. We can just observe and some of our findings correspond to what I did previously in rabbits. Rabbits have a very gel-like vitreous and it is much easier to see what is happening in their eyes. Very similar findings, I thought, I could see in the eye of the monkey. As you know, the vitreous consists of a framework of collagen fibers and within these fibers there are huge molecules of hyaluronic acid. Once hyaluronidase is injected into the vitreous, these molecules break down; they get smaller and water is liberated. You see that the collagen framework begins to collapse, and in an even further stage the hyaluronic acid molecules are liberated and the collagen fibrils have collapsed so much that fibers are seen now. In a rabbit you can see fibers; in a monkey, not. Now what do we think happens when we do our procedure? It is very difficult to photograph the normal vitreous and to stain the normal vitreous in an owl monkey because (1) the vitreous is very liquid, and (2) it stains very faintly, although you try to stain it very intensely. But you may be able to see that there is quite a thick layer of cortex which is intact and which lies over the retina. This slide shows a normal eye. This is a semischematic drawing of the full eye, and the dots correspond to intact vitreous. We think that the cortex of the intact eye, which has a rather firm structure and is not destroyed by the histological work-up, is rather thick and overlies the retina.

Now what happens when we destroy vitreous? I use now for the first time the word "destroy." I wanted to avoid that in my paper. We aspirate and reinject vitreous, and what happens probably is that hyaluronidase makes the collagen framework break down, fibrils collect to make fibers, and now, when we aspirate the vitreous, we pull on fibers—on thick threads—and it is much easier to get intact cortex from the retinal surface. And we think that is the point in the retinal detachment—that the retina is free from vitreous.

And I come now to the second question on this paper. They asked me why I didn't report about controlled injection of saline without hyaluronidase. We did that. And it is astonishing how unsuccessful these injections were. You don't get a detachment. Our explanation for that is that although you produced a retinal hole and you had a surrounding detachment the retina spontaneously reattached within 2 days, even 1 day. And I think it has something to do with the elasticity of the collagen framework. Now, let us say it very mechanically that it wants to get back in its original position. I can't explain it better. This next schematic drawing is of an eye in which we did hyaluronidase injection, together with aspiration and reinjection. And you see that now the cortex is much thinner and that there are areas where there is no vitreous. No vitreous, in our sense, means that there is left on the retinal surface only the outer hyaloid membrane. You can't differentiate histologically between hyaloid membrane and internal limiting membrane, at least it is very difficult. The next photograph will show you the difference between the two parts of the eye. This is at the ora serrata, and you see the retinal part of the vitreous is destroyed because the high content of protein has made it visible, and you see these are all crumbs. The anterior part, the vitreous phase, is still intact, and you see the fine filaments and the very good structure on that. And when you look at areas that show good destruction, it's not all over the retina; you get the opinion that actually the cortex was destroyed during our procedure.

The third question is: Did you study the vitreous with contact lens and slit lamp before and after injection?

We did, and we tried. It's not so easy because all the instruments that are available are for human eyes, and we are not yet at the stage that we have our own instruments just for monkeys. But our impression is that the normal vitreous doesn't show much. But as soon as you destroy vitreous, you see a lot of floaters; it's floating around, it's very liquid. You see vitreous strands and they are mainly in the anterior part of the eye and some of them a little bit more posterior. You can't see the vitreous cortex, but I admit I may not have been careful enough to do that. This has to be done in the future. You can't do everything at once. Thank you.

Question: Does allergy or autoimmunological factors play a part in the pathology of retinal detachment?

Mr. Hudson: I take it that the questioner means "Is retinal detachment an autoimmune disease?" I think that my answer to that is that I know of no evidence that it is. At the same time, I think that one does get what may be allergic or inflammatory type of reaction which produces a condition in the eye which is clinically a retinal detachment; and in the few cases of this that I have seen, one has an anterior segment uveitis of mild degree associated with a shallow retinal detachment, in which a scattered fine-pigment proliferation occurs underneath the retina over quite a large area, and we find that these cases are not associated with any retinal tear, and that, given a course of systemic steroids and time, or both, the condition resolves, leaving the eye with good visual acuity. These are the only ones I think might have an allergic etiology. I would be interested to know what the experience of other panel members has been with this.

Dr. Kroll: I'm glad I passed that question on.

Question: The first one: It is said that the distance from the ora serrata to the limbus is 7 to 8 mm. Your measurements were less. Why the discrepancy?

Dr. Straatsma: The most important surgical landmark in the anterior segment of the eye is the posterior border of the limbus. This is the border that corresponds internally to Schwalbe's line and externally to the junction between translucent limbal tissue and opaque sclera. Knowing that this is an important surgical landmark anteriorly and that the anterior border of the limbus varies a great deal, we used this posterior border of the limbus, corresponding to Schwalbe's line, as the starting point for the measurements I quoted to you earlier this week. This probably accounts for our measurements being approximately a millimeter less than those in the conventional texts.

Question: Are occlusions of small peripheral arterials in the retina or choroid responsible for any retinal holes or detachment?

Dr. Foos: Well, I really have no specific statistics to give on this, but I think I am on firm ground in saying that, certainly, vascular insufficiencies predispose to and exaggerate degenerative conditions. I don't think they specifically cause holes, at least not the holes I described, insofar as usually two thirds of them occur intact and in rather thick peripheral retinas. Only one third occur in areas of cystoid degeneration, and one can't have retinal detachments, at least in this regard, without the retinal holes preceding it. I think that they do form the predisposing complex but not specifically.

I have one other comment to make relative to something said previously. I preface this by saying I want to congratulate Dr. Machemer and Dr. Kroll on their work because I think it is something that has needed doing for a long time and I think they are well on their way to giving us some specific information.

I want to make one comment relative to animal work: I think we need to use animal work in getting some of the information, but, again we have to be careful.

The first two slides I will show you are animal material—simians—about midway in the primate group.

This is the right picture and it shows a tamarin—a simian—and notice the light-colored band in front of the ora serrata, extending about midway or almost two thirds of the way to the base of the ciliary processes. In a dark individual, this represents the anterior portion of the vitreous base. Notice how wide and uniform it is.

The next slide shows a galago—a prosimian—and I want you to notice specifically that the retina has been taken off to expose this dark band extending to and behind the equator, that I believe corresponds to the posterior portion of the vitreous base.

These next specimens are youngsters—this, in fact, is a newborn—autopsy material, with the retina on.

Next is the small sclera of that eye, a newborn. Notice the pigmented band with the retina removed from the ora serrata corresponding to what I believe is the posterior portion of vitreous base.

Next shows the relatively uniform pigmented band transilluminated.

I want to make only one comment relative to those illustrations: I think we are really dealing with a modification of the vitreous base which has put us at an evolutionary disadvantage. So we're seeing shrinkage of vitreous base. I think it's not only predisposed to retinal degeneration, including tears, but it has also complicated all the heroic efforts that my surgical colleagues have talked about today. Thank you.

Question: Why do you feel that the pigment at the pigment layer of retina is responsible for the chorioretinal adhesion?

Dr. Curtin: I'm not sure it is completely responsible, but in examining eyes after photocoagulation and cryotherapy, there definitely seems to be either regeneration of this layer, or else it is not permanently damaged when the therapy at least is rather moderate and to a similar degree but perhaps not so complete in diathermy. You can still see this layer there at the interface of the choroid and the retina. I think it probably plays an important part in the adhesion of the retina to the underlying choroid.

Question: In surrounding a large retinal break by cryotherapy, how can the surgeon be sure that it is well sealed off at the end of the procedure? Do the members of the panel make all of their cryoapplications under ophthalmoscopic observation, or are some of them made by directly observing the sclera?

Dr. Okun: I personally make every application under direct viewing, with one exception, and that is in reoperations where there may be a very necrotic sclera. Elevation of the intraocular tension definitely occurs while the eye is indented with the cryoprobe, so care must be taken not to rupture the globe with a weakened outer coat. The reason for observing each lesion is that the time required for a freeze to reach the retina in different areas is extremely variable. Also, the chorioretinal location of a lesion does not always correspond to the location of scleral application. Cryocoagulation differs from photocoagulation in that a watertight seal with cryo requires contiguous lesions. Therefore, one must remember where the previous lesion has been placed because it is very hard to find these effects in the retina after the freeze has thawed. My end point has been the first sign of whitening of the retina in fairly flat detachments. In bullous detachments, my end point has been the first sign of whitening of the underlying choroid.

Question: What are the specific indications for prophylactic treatment with cryoapplications and with photocoagulation?

Dr. Schepens: When the lesions to be treated prophylactically are anterior to the equator, transconjunctival cryoapplications are used. If they are located at the equator or posteriorly and if the media are clear and the pupil widely dilated, photocoagulation is preferred. When technical difficulties are encountered, I do not hesitate to switch from cryoapplications to photocoagulation or vice versa as the case may indicate.

Question: It is said that cryo, substituted for diathermy, practically eliminates the scleral abscess when a silicone sponge is firmly placed over a treated area of the sclera. Do you know if cryo has reduced or eliminated the chronic orbital granuloma which occurs about the sutures and implants in an occasional case? What is the incidence of this complication with diathermy and with cryotherapy?

Mr. Hudson: I think probably what the questioner means when he speaks of the abscess caused by diathermy is the scleral necrosis that one gets following the use of diathermy or of excessive diathermy. And I think that the fair answer to this is that if diathermy is not used in excess there is not as much scleral damage as would cause anything resembling an abscess, but with cryotherapy, scleral damage is very, very restricted, and as you have seen from Dr. Curtin's histologic preparations, there is evidence that there is virtually no scleral damage with cryotherapy and this has been borne out by work done by Harvey Lincoff, so that the amount of scleral necrosis that you get with silicone sponge is certainly related to the underlying treatment, and I would think that it is minimal with cryotherapy. It does, of course, depend to some extent upon how tightly you do suture your implant onto the sclera, and I think that pressure necrosis can occur even with silicone sponge in these circumstances. In the relationship between the use of diathermy and cryotherapy in relation to chronic orbital granuloma, I think that the answer is that the chronic orbital granuloma is related to the surgical technique, rather than to the application of any form of treatment to the sclera and choroid, and that it is not associated with a particular method such as diathermy or cryotherapy. I'm not surprised not to get any more opposition from any other members of the panel, so I'll go on to the next one.

Question: It is said that cryo, substituted for diathermy, practically eliminates scleral abscess when a silicone sponge is firmly placed over a treated area of the sclera. Do you know if cryoapplications have reduced or eliminated the chronic orbital granuloma which occurs about the sutures and implants in an occasional case? What is the incidence of this complication with diathermy and with cryotherapy?

Dr. Schepens: I agree entirely with Mr. Hudson's last statement that whether it be cryoapplication or diathermy the incidence of chronic granuloma is the same. This fits with our experience. Chronic granuloma is invariably tied with either one of two conditions: infection or sterile abscess caused by a silk suture. It does not seem to be influenced by the use of cryoapplications or diathermy.

Question: Do you observe that cryotherapy results in more exudative reactions of the choroid than does diathermy? How can this be minimized?

Mr. Hudson: I think the degree of exudation in any method of producing choroidal retinal inflammation is dependent upon the application of the treatment rather than the type of treatment itself. It has been brought out in several of the papers at this meeting that what we are trying to avoid is excessive treatment to produce choroidal retinal reaction, so that we make a reaction which produces fine and scattered pigmentation but not the gross degree of scleral atrophy which you have seen in some of the pictures. I think that probably the exudative reaction you get, either with diathermy or with cryotherapy or, for that matter, with light coagulation, depends upon the intensity of the application, to a great extent, and that the way of avoiding excessive choroidal exudation, which appears as if it were a shallow detachment away from the area of treatment depends upon using the right amount of diathermy for the right length of time and not using excessive cryotherapy, as has been emphasized by Dr. Norton, and equally with light coagulation. I would certainly subscribe to Dr. Norton's view that there is a greater breadth of safety with cryotherapy than there is with diathermy. Even in eyes in which the cryotherapy has perhaps been excessive, I have not seen the development of a secondary retinal tear along the edge of the treatment, which happened not infrequently if diathermy were used excessively.

Question: And the final question on this: Do you have to be concerned with the long ciliary arteries and nerves in treating over them with cryoapplications as much as diathermy?

Mr. Hudson: This really takes me back to the last answer again because I have never really avoided using light diathermy over the long ciliary vessels, but I think it would probably be fair to say that the likelihood of permanent damage to the vessels is less with cryotherapy than it is with diathermy. At the same time, one might consider whether the question shouldn't have been asked as to whether division of the medial and lateral rectus muscles was more damaging to the anterior circulation of the globe than the use of either diathermy or cryotherapy on the vessels themselves, and I think that Dr. Harrell Pearce in Baltimore has a point in doing as little muscle detachment as is possible or as is consistent with the fact of doing a detachment operation.

Question: In segmental cryosurgery without drainage of subretinal fluid, do you have an average number of days after which a firm adhesion will not occur?

Dr. Norton: I do not know the exact time that tissues cease being "sticky" or how long the pigment epithelium remains "sticky," so that if the settling doesn't occur in 24 or 48 hours, will it be "sticky" enough to form a firm union? It would be nice to know the answer to this question, and I think we'll be able to find it out with the experimental model we have. But, at this moment, we don't know the answer. I have arbitrarily worked on the premise that if it isn't in contact in 5 days then I will add photocoagulation to supplement the treatment. If there is an area of retina flat around the break, then nothing is necessary. But if there is a layer of fluid around the hole at the end of 5 days, I will apply photocoagulation to reactivate the irritation.

Dr. Okun: I've had a moderate amount of experience in this line and I have handled these in a very similar way. However, there were three patients who did not have contact between the buckle and the break at the tenth day, but it was very close and there was still some fluid. These three were discharged and on their return visit 4 days later, the break was perfectly sealed. However, this is something that we can't usually wait for. We have been doing supplemental photocoagulation on patients on the fifth or sixth day. Once again, I think that perhaps I wait longer than the others. We have done over 100 cases of episcleral segmental procedures with full-thickness cryo and no drainage in which the breaks were still open at the close of surgery. The great majority of these are sealed on the first postoperative day (approximately 70%). Approximately 20% will become sealed on the second or third day. This leaves only about 10% that we remain concerned about. If the implant is improperly placed, the break will not be closed. This diagnosis can be made by observing that the choroidal bulge is malplaced. Reoperation and replacement of the sponge will usually seal the break without the necessity of drainage of subretinal fluid.

Question: On postoperative care—when does the average detachment patient go back to work?

Dr. Norton: We usually try to discharge the patient from the hospital between the fourth and fifth day. We then see them in 1 week, and if they look good at that time, It tell the patients to stop their medications and that they can return to work usually within 3 weeks' time. Now, there are some patients who are very anxious to get back to work, and I tell them, "You can resume normal activities at the end of 3 weeks." They say, "Well, Doctor, does this mean I can get my hair set? I can read a book?" I say, "You may resume normal activities." The problem you run into is would you let a patient who is very anxious to go back to work go back sooner? And I don't hesitate to let them go back at the end of twelve days, plus or minus, depending on how the retina looks. I think there's an adequate union at that time. I wouldn't let them go back to boxing, but I am talking about ordinary work. Now, you run into the other problem which is brought up here, and that is insurance forms requesting information concerning the length of partial and total disability. How many days do you allow them on the insurance forms? I don't think that the patient should be penalized for coming to me because I tend to mobilize them earlier than others and try to urge them to go back to work sooner than others. I try to adjust to the personality of the patient. If I know some patients are going to create a problem about returning to work, I tell them they ought to go back to work at 4 weeks. And then, of course, at 4 weeks they can't possibly go back to work, and I say, "Well, you know you should have been able to go back to work now, but I'll tell you what: we'll give you 2 more weeks on the insurance policy." And they're so delighted that they take that, and then you don't have any further problem, so I end up giving them 6 weeks if they really want it.

Question: Can you give us a reference to a comprehensive publication or interpretation of fluorescein fundus angiography?

Dr. Norton: The only book—I mean, there are lots of publications on this that are available to you—the only monograph that I'm aware of that is presently in print is Donald Gass's monograph on the diseases of the macula, which I think covers the macula section very well. Dr. Vessing, who works with Dr. Meyer-

Schwickerath, has a book which he tells me will be out in 1 week in Germany on angiography and it will be translated in this country by Gunther von Noorden and it will be published here by Mosby.

Question: According to the pathogenesis of retinal detachment, the farther the retina is separated from the pigment epithelium, the worse is the pathologic outlook. How far should the diathermy or cryosurgery be applied around the hole to get the best result?

Dr. Machemer: I think this is easy to answer because experience has shown how these lesions have to be treated. Follow the rule as little as possible and use as much diathermy as necessary. When you have a small hole, just use one coagulation and you can reattach the retina. When you have a large hole, a complicated case, you have to use more. But I think it is not dependent on whether there are heavy changes in that area (of the retina) that will overlie the coagulated pigment epithelium.

Question: How do you localize large tears with bullous detachments, and how do you judge whether the hole is likely to be lined up with the buckle once the retina is flat?

Dr. Straatsma: In very bullous detachments, there may be a problem viewing the actual indentation of whatever device is on the external surface, but if it is possible to view the external indentation, I think it is quite reasonable to line this up properly with the break, even though it cannot be brought into direct contact with the break itself, and use this as the guide for placement of the scleral buckle. One other thing may be helpful: A large number of retinal breaks are associated with a small amount of pigment change corresponding to the original position of the retinal break before it pulled away; use this as a precise guide for localization.

Dr. Norton: In localizing a break with a highly elevated detachment, usually I utilize the tip of the probe as I see it, looking through the hole of the detachment; usually if you are looking carefully, you can see it elevate and you will have an idea that your retina will fall probably a little bit anterior to where you would like it to, and I use this as my posterior mark for my localization. When I plant an implant after doing something such as this, you realize that the margin of error is greater, then I probably will plant a little larger implant. If after fluid has been drained and the retina has fallen back in place and it is not quite in the place were I would like it, I usually use a piece of Silastic sponge to put the hole in proper relation to the buckle.

Dr. Cockerham: I think one point that can be helpful in localizing the position of a tear, so far as its distance behind the ora is concerned, is to relate the edges of the tear to the blood-vessel pattern of the retina. If you can see that your tear is related to a relatively large vessel, you can find a vessel in a similar part of the eye where there isn't detachment and estimate to some extent how far back you are going to have to go by the size of the vessels you are working with.

I should add one other thing: If the hole is large, then frequently the anterior side of the retina is closer to the underlying choroid and it is easier to localize this; then you can utilize this side and you will have some idea of the total size of the hole, looking at it, and you can use this as a little bit of an estimate and a guide, as to where you put your posterior mark if you've sort of overestimated the full width of the hole.

Dr. Schwickerath: I would like to explain shortly our technique in these cases in which localization by pressure from the outside fails. In these cases, we like to transfer a high bullous detachment into a shallow one. We perform a puncture with electrolysis in the area of the high bullous detachment and inject saline from 6 o'clock if the hole is at 12, and the other way around. After this, when the retina has settled over the puncture, the eye remains hard and we start localizing again.

Question: Another question here is a bit apart from lattice. What is the best means for handling a large, single, horseshoe break just behind the equator, in the superior temporal quadrant, which is associated with quadrant detachment, which on drainage fish-mouths, and drainage without incarceration results only in obtaining liquid vitreous, and there is no settling of the retina?

Dr. Straatsma: There are three things that can help in this problem: The first is to extend the buckle and the treatment an adequate distance posteriorly, because frequently by doing this it is possible to eliminate the open fish-mouth appearance of the retinal break. As the initial step I would follow, both the treatment and the buckle would be extended posteriorly. The second measure is to create a less steep margin at the posterior edge of this buckle to further decrease the tendency toward fish-mouthing. This can be done by releasing some of the scleral sutures and injecting material into the vitreous. If some contact can be obtained between the retina and the buckle by these procedures, I'd be inclined to stop the operation at this point and, subsequently, to use photocoagulation to bring these tissues farther into apposition. This is done by progressive step-by-step photocoagulation from the posterior margin of the buckle toward the margin of the retinal break. Perhaps Dr. Meyer-Schwickerath will comment on that. I believe he first described this method some years ago.

Dr. Okun: I would like to make just one comment on this, because I don't see this problem very much anymore. This was described as a large superior temporal retinal break with a quadrant detachment. I believe that the therapy of choice here is cryotherapy with full-thickness scleral infolding which omits drainage. When you try to drain subretinal fluid in these relatively small detachments with large breaks, you drain all of the vitreous out of the eye. I've seen formed vitreous come through the break and into the drainage sites, thus distorting the break and making it even more difficult to close. The simple Custodis procedure with full-thickness cryo has converted this type of case from a nightmare to a simple successful procedure.

Dr. Schwickerath: I agree with Dr. Okun, with one little exception. I would, in these cases, recommend what I describe as a two-step operation, for one reason. Well, first to explain again what it is—I would put the episcleral material in the area of the hole and then, as Dr. Okun said, forget about the case. But I would not do the cryo first. Why? Because if the retina does not settle, it may happen that you have already done a coagulation and you get an atrophy of choroid in this area and it will be more difficult to re-treat this case. Now, if it doesn't settle and you haven't done cryosurgery, you don't have to blame yourself for not doing the cryosurgery because the cryosurgery does not improve the tendency for settling of the retina; we know that there is a physical factor which causes it. If you go in 3 to 7 days later, when the retina is on the buckle, and you then perform photocoagulation, you will be sure that the retina has settled; and if it has not settled, you have to blame something else for being wrong in your operation.

Question: Short of scraping of the epithelium from the cornea, what measures have the panel members found helpful in maintaining corneal transparency during surgery?

Mr. Hudson: I think there are several things that can be done in a very simple way: The first is to avoid anything that irritates the cornea during the period prior to surgery. We try, whenever possible, to avoid extensive examinations or dilating the pupil vigorously, with Neo-Synephrine particularly, as well as other medications during the 24 hours prior to surgery, if the examinations can be done earlier and the surgery is going to be delayed. So, in effect, the cornea is not in an irritated state. In addition, I think the simple instruction to the patient to simply keep the eyes closed after the start of preoperative mydriasis is a helpful thing. This again will prevent the superficial punctate staining that will follow the use of Neo-Synephrine particularly in aphakic patients.

The third precaution, of course, is to avoid exposure to the eye during anesthesia—whatever type of anesthetic is used. Again, use the precorneal sponge, of the type that has been described—a small hat or ring of Gelfoam is helpful in keeping it moist—and, finally, I think that the use of infrared filters in the operating room lights and probably in the near future in the ophthalmoscopes, will help to avoid the dryness of the cornea. So I think, in effect, all of these factors, plus the amount of looking and time of the operation, are important in maintaining corneal transparency. There may be other comments.

Dr. Schwickerath: I would like to add that it is important to have a good assistant to irrigate the cornea between the times of ophthalmoscopy; and secondly, we have found that Neo-Synephrine of higher concentration than 2.5% is dangerous for the cornea in this regard, and we found that any topical anesthesia of the cornea is also dangerous.

Dr. Freeman: Can we have, I think it's slide no. 4? The question is: Why wasn't photocoagulation used as a means of treating this giant break? This is the giant break that the question was asked about. Well, in answer, no, I wouldn't use light coagulation. Notice that the retina, the posterior retinal flap, is detached and in this eye there is a considerable amount of vitreous traction. No. I'd do a scleral buckling—not photocoagulation alone.

Dr. Okun: In his therapy for rolled-over retina, I'm not sure that I understand yet whether Charles (Schepens) uses positioning and incarceration first, air without incarceration first, or air with incarceration first. I would also like to know what percentage of success was achieved in the cases of giant tears with rolled-over posterior flaps. The overall success rate of close to 50%, of course, does not apply to this more unfavorable group of giant tears. Giant tears with minimal detachment or inversion carry a much more favorable prognosis than those that are folded over and fixed in this position. My best results have been in those cases which are more favorable to begin with. These cases usually respond to a procedure which utilizes a wide but shallow buckle, intravitreal air, and positioning. Now I have seen failures in this technique, and I agree that when there is a failure in this technique then you wish you had incarcerated. But could it possibly be that the cases that we succeed in with incarceration are also the same cases that we would have succeeded in had we used air without incarceration?

Dr. Schepens: We try incarceration alone when the retinal flap can be mobilized by preoperative exercise, and we try an air injection first when the flap cannot be mobilized either preoperatively or during operation. The reason for using intentional incarcerations even if an air injection is successful in bringing the flap in apposition with the choroid is that postoperative cases of giant retinal break have a marked tendency toward fixed retinal folds and massive preretinal retraction. Retinal incarcerations have helped us prevent a number of recurrences and late failures.

Dr. Norton: I'm not sure that it's good to spend the bulk of the audience's time on such a difficult subject as giant retinal breaks. It's obvious that none of us really know the best way to treat them. To me, these cases boil down into two types. There is the type in which the folded-over retina is relatively mobile. I don't mean it must be so mobile that you can get it flat before you enter the operating room by standing the patient on his head or some such manipulation. But they are relatively mobile—they will unfold from the 6 o'clock position to that of coming into the vitreous cavity straight at you. I think that this type has a very favorable prognosis when you treat it with air. I'll come back to what I mean by "favorable" in a moment. Then you have the type which will not unfold and there's organization in the vitreous. The vitreous is attached to the folded retina; the retina is immobile. No matter what position you put them in or how you move their head, the retina remains fixed. I think these are the very unfavorable cases and, in my hands, are mostly inoperable. I think this is where intravitreous surgery of the various types that have been discussed here will have to be employed. Now, coming back to the type in which the flap is mobile, in which some mobility is evident. When it's 180 degrees to 230 degrees, I can truthfully say that we have yet to have one that we have not been able to unfold with air, that is, unfold after they leave the operating table. Now, does that mean we have cured them? No. Because there is a second component to this disease and that is vitreous shrinkage. This comes on anywhere from 2 to 4 weeks postoperatively, the retina will often tear in one or another area, and usually you are then dealing with a small break rather than a giant break, but with vitreous changes. At this point, I treat them like I would any other detachment which has vitreous changes and a small break. I do a buckling procedure corresponding with the break. Now, when I first started doing this, I used diathermy, and since I did a lot of diathermy in the area of the bed of the folded retina (I did it with a lamella undermining, a very wide undermining), I found it much more profitable to put in an encircling band at that time. Even though I didn't pull it up tight—just to have it in place so that when and if I had to reoperate—I didn't have to take down the undermining that was there; I could just take the band and pull it up tighter or put in another piece to accommodate for it. However, now that I use cryotherapy, I don't put in the buckle, and if I have to go back in, I can do a segmental procedure or a 360-degree implant, depending on what I want to do. I really have found this very useful. I do know that when Hal Freeman called me to ask how we used air, because they wanted to start using air in the treatment of giant breaks, one of our former fellows was in Boston and I suggested he assist Hal, and subsequently I learned that even though the retina unfolded they did proceed to incarcerate. I think all of us will agree that a complication we try to avoid every-where else in retinal surgery shouldn't be embarked upon as an elective procedure if we can avoid it. I know from my own experience you do not have to incarcerate these cases. They don't return as giant breaks when they fail. They only tear in one little area, and we then treat them as a small break. So to me, and as I say, we're not going to settle this thing, to me it's just not logical to purposely perform a complication that we try to avoid in better than 90% of cases.

Mr. Hudson: Well, we in England have, of course, had a limited experience in these cases because they aren't extraordinarily frequent, and so far as the flaps that do not roll over are concerned, we have done a proportion of our cases with low indentation procedures and have had the same, I hope, limited success most people have. We have tried posture with the rolled-over flap, and we find that this is the most helpful preliminary step toward the operative procedure.

Dr. Cockerham: I would like to make a point about incarcerations. The term "incarceration" may have a bad connotation to some because they envision the accidental one with its large radiating folds and extraocular prolapse of retina and vitreous gel. We must remember the intentional incarceration is executed with control and is always very small. In Boston, I have seen many of these which appear as small dimples of retina where it is stuck in the choroid. Indeed, they may be so small as to be difficult to see with the indirect ophthalmoscope. These are sufficient to hold the retina to the choroid.

Question: Have you reason to think that planned retinal incarcerations as recom-mended by Dr. Freeman and your group affect the visual result in giant break surgery?

Dr. Schepens: No. Statements indicating that this technique affects adversely the visual result have been based, as far as I know, on speculation and not on factual evidence. Let us remember that our technique consists in making a tiny choroidal perforation—so tiny that the incarcerated retina often fails to form a star-shaped retinal fold. This incarceration is obtained by using the force of gravity and pressing gently on the globe. No adverse visual results have been observed in Boston.

The incarceration procedure described this afternoon is entirely different from that recommended by our group. Trying to hook the edge of a retinal flap with an instrument and to incarcerate it forcibly into a choroidal perforation is, in my opinion, a maneuver fraught with danger.

Question: What is your experience with air injection in the treatment of giant breaks?

Dr. Schepens: Air injection was first recommended by B. Rosengren.* It is fairly easy to perform correctly and works well in favorable types of giant retinal breaks. Why don't we do more air injections and limit ourselves to adding the necessary chorioretinal reaction? Experience has shown that with giant breaks, there is no room for errors because the first operation is that which has by far the best chance of success. With each reoperation, preretinal organization and retraction progress,

---

*Rosengren, B.: Air injection in retinal detachment, Acta XXI Concilium Ophthalmologicum (Brittanica) 2:1212, 1950.

making success less likely. Even air or saline injections in the vitreous causes intra-ocular irritation, resulting in greater fixity of the inverted retinal flap.

Each operation for a giant retinal break is started, expecting the worst. The patient is placed on the giant break table, which does not mean that we will operate on him upside down but it gives us the latitude to do so, should it become necessary.

With a case showing an inverted retinal flap, we have tried using air injection as a first step without incarceration and we have also tried intentional retinal incarcerations without air injection as a first step. At the present time our procedure is as follows: We determine preoperatively the mobility of the retinal flap by positioning and exercise. If the flap can be mobilized before operation, then we turn the patient in the prone position and incarcerate the retina without air injection because air makes subsequent opththalmoscopic observation more difficult and less accurate. If attempts to incarcerate the retina fail, we inject air in prone position and try again to incarcerate the retina, with the additional help of the air bubble. If it is impossible to mobilize the flap preoperatively, then air injection is used as the first step.

I should like to comment on the statement made this afternoon that the last thing to do in the treatment of a giant break is to perform a scleral buckling. It was in 1958 that I first observed that the flap of a giant break tended to roll off a high scleral buckling, and this observation spurred my interest in positioning and exercises. For the past 10 years we have advocated doing a low but wide buckle in giant retinal breaks. A high buckle tends to push the retinal flap against the posterior hyaloid, and I suspect that it is the hyaloid which rubs the retinal flap off the buckle.

Another comment concerns exercises: I am afraid that the audience may have been confused because some speakers did not differentiate between fact and speculation. The speculation is that exercises as described may precipitate an increase or development of giant breaks in either of the patient's eyes. However, I know of no documented report indicating that this was ever observed. We have never seen inverted flaps of giant retinal breaks get worse as a result of logically directed exercises, but we know that exercises may affect adversely equatorial horseshoe breaks.

Question: How many cases of giant breaks has your group operated on?

Dr. Schepens: Between 1947 and 1961, 90 eyes with giant retinal breaks were operated on; between 1962 and 1966, 72 eyes with a giant break were operated on; in the past 10 months (December 1966 through September 1967), 42 eyes with a giant break were operated on. Our total experience, therefore, is well in excess of 200 eyes operated on for giant retinal breaks.

Question: If you excluded all giant tears due to an inferior temporal dialysis, or a traumatic dialysis, what are your anatomical results with remaining true giant rolled-over retinas?

Dr. Schepens: In the past 10 months, 42 eyes with giant break were seen and *all* were operated on. Of these, none were due to an inferior temporal dialysis, thus leaving 34 cases of true giant rolled-over retinas. A reattachment was obtained in 15 of these 34 eyes (44%).

Question. A patient with a 180-degree giant tear has a small amount of subretinal fluid. A production of a suitable buckle causes a rise in the intraocular pressure to 50. How do you lower the intraocular pressure?

Dr. Okun: We'll handle the first question first. This isn't too complete, but we'll of course assume for the first part that no drainage of subretinal fluid has been performed up to this point. Well, with a very small amount of subretinal fluid and a pressure of 50, the question also doesn't state what type of buckle was performed. Let us assume that the buckle was a segmental episcleral buckle and the giant break is now in contact with the episcleral buckle. I would not hesitate to leave this eye at a pressure of 50, provided the view of the central retinal artery reveals that there are no pulsations in the artery itself. If there are pulsations in the artery, I would simply wait until the pulsations cease. If the pressure is above diastolic, I would take down enough of the buckle to restore the retinal circulation; if it is an episcleral buckle, I would remove a suture or two, or if it is an encircling buckle, I would loosen it. I would not be very happy about putting an encircling buckle on the 180-degree giant tear, with a pressure of 50, if this elevation of pressure were obtained by tightening the encircling buckle. However, if the pressure were raised by pulling up on the sutures which secure the implant, then I think I would not hesitate to leave it at 50. If this were a giant 180-degree tear which had only a small amount of fluid to begin with and if the fluid did not extend posterior to the equator, then I would not have put a buckle in to begin with. I would have used photocoagulation and cryo to wall it off. This barrier must be very wide, approximately four disc diameters wide.

Question: What are the latest concepts of cause and significance of "white with pressure" and "white without pressure"?

Dr. Schepens: White with pressure covers two entities. The first is trivial and shows the type of white with pressure which moves when the depressor is moved. It is always slightly ahead of the location where pressure is applied. This is a normal finding, which is more marked in infants and is found in practically all deeply pigmented fundi.

The second entity called "white with pressure" has a geographic contour and does not change in shape when the observer displaces the pressure. This finding is also frequent in normal fundi. In pathological cases, it may result from a traction on the internal retinal layers or from atrophy of the external layer of the retina; it may be the late result of peripheral uveitis, after the exudates have absorbed. In the latter case, I think that the white with pressure is due to retinal edema or to a small accumulation of exudative fluid under the retina.

White without pressure is the nearest thing to a very flat detachment. In my opinion, it results either from atrophy of the outer retinal layers, accompanied by traction on the inner layers, or from a very flat retinal detachment.

Dr. Okun: I've always had the feeling that white with pressure, while it connotes some change in the structure of the retina, is largely the result of a change in the optical properties of the retina. I think that retinal edema sometimes appears as white without pressure. However, there can be just enough retinal edema so that the retina is still transparent when viewed directly without pressure, but when the sclera is depressed and the retina examined somewhat more obliquely, this apparent increase in thickness causes the retina to lose its transparency. I think that atrophy of the retinal layers which signifies a decrease in thickness usually does not produce white with pressure. The most significant white with pressure is that which occurs at the edges of areas of vitreoretinal degeneration where there is condensation of the vitreous. Again, these zones appear white because these thickened areas are being examined obliquely. Does anyone else want to comment on that?

Question: What setting and time exposure for the photocoagulator are being used to coagulate conjunctiva vessels and tumors as shown in this morning's lecture? And another one—has anyone had an explosion of a Xenon bulb, either in or out of the machine?

Dr. Schwickerath: To answer the second question first: in the first year there were several explosions, but they have all, as far as I know, been inside the machine and not outside, and nobody has been injured as far as I know.

Question number one: The time on surface coagulation is approximately the same time as that on the fundus. We do not like to go over one of 1.5 seconds. We judge the tumor, which usually is very similar to that of diathermy.

Question: Is there a greater incidence of reaction to silicone sponge than to solid silicone?

Dr. Curtin: I have not seen enough cases of this pathologically to evaluate it, and judging from reoperation, I would say probably not. But, I think that Dr. Okun had far more experience in reoperations. *(Laughter)*

Dr. Okun: Much obliged.

Dr. Curtin: But that was not meant . . . I meant he has had more experience in seeing eyes that had been operated on previously as his series is much larger than mine. Perhaps he can say something about the external differences. I don't have the pathological material.

Dr. Schwickerath: We are using both materials parallel. And we don't find much difference.

Dr. Okun: We had very little difficulty with infection by the episcleral sponge; we haven't had very much difficulty with the solid pieces, either. I have preferred the solid pieces for intrascleral surgery and the sponges for episcleral work. I don't think the solid piece gives the proper type of push for an episcleral procedure without drainage. I have been very much surprised by the comments which I have heard from people who are having difficulty with infections in these sponges. There must be something really different about the way they are sterilized, the way they are used or the way they are covered because this has not been a big problem.

Dr. Norton: Before I start answering the questions I have here, not too many, I would just like to comment a little bit on this question of infection that's been brought up. And I agree with what Mr. Hudson has said about the fact that it is probably not due to the modality you use but to a break in technique at the time of surgery. There are two observations, though, that I think you have to keep in mind. I don't see how we can ignore, unless somebody repeats the work and refutes it, the study that the fourth-year student at Cornell did with Dr. Linkoff, in which he took rabbits' eyes and did the exact same procedures in two sets of animals. In one he froze the sclera and put in a Silastic sponge implant, Custodis type; in the other he diathermized the sclera and put in a Silastic sponge implant. In these two comparable groups, he did one additional thing, which is what Mr. Hudson is referring to as a break in technique. He introduced *Staphylococcus aureus* on the scleral surface. In the rabbits that had received cryotherapy and an implant, infection did not occur. In those that received diathermy treatment, infections occurred in a high percentage. I can't give you the figures offhand, but there was a very significant difference between the two groups. Now, this is an artificial situation, but it is exactly what Mr. Hudson is referring to—it's not the technique, it's the contamination that occurred—and it does seem logical that if you have necrotic tissue from diathermy, or from having made incisions in the sclera, and so on, the sclera may well get infected. Also, our own clinical experience has been a reduction in the number of infections that we've had since we've been using cryo versus diathermy. I can't disagree with what Mr. Hudson said. I think he's absolutely right; we must try to keep the field from getting contaminated during surgery.

Question: Dr. Norton, have you treated hemangiomas with cryotherapy, and have you treated vascular tumors and other retinopathies, such as hemoglobinopathy, with cold, and if you have, could you comment on the results?

Dr. Norton: Yes, we've treated some vascular lesions. We've not treated any hemangiomas with cryo. All the hemangiomas that we've had were very posterior lesions, and they lend themselves very nicely to photocoagulation. In other vascular diseases, though, we have treated with cold. For example, some of the adult Coats's disease cases that we showed. I showed you a man that we treated with cold and he did very well. I treated a woman who got an exudated detachment just like the patient I showed you with the angioma of the retina, the von Hippel lesion that developed a detachment within 5 minutes from the time we applied photocoagulation. This woman with cryo did the same thing, but the detachment was absorbed and she is doing fine. Dr. Curtin treated a patient with what we've called Eales' disease. Victor, how is he doing? Were you able to destroy the vessels?

Dr. Curtin: He is still under evaluation. He certainly had a lot of pigmentary reaction. He does not seem to have progression of this disease, since he was treated. But he has some change probably in the macular region; his vision is not significantly altered according to tests, but he notices a change in the central vision. His other eye, which has disease, has been observed, and there probably has been slight regression and increased exudation. His worse eye was the first one treated.

Dr. Norton: I would like to comment on one other patient. We've had one angioma of the retina that we froze—that Dr. Kasner froze—and the angioma still persisted. Dr. Kasner photocoagulated the angioma, and the lesion went away. There is some doubt in my mind whether we waited long enough between the various therapies to evaluate the effect, but suffice it to say that this is one case that failed with cryo but did respond to photo.

Dr. Schwickerath: The comment of Harvey Linkoff to this problem was that vascular structures with capillary size responded well to photocoagulation whereas those with larger size, to cryosurgery, but those with still larger size, better to photocoagulation.

Dr. Okun: Dr. Norton probably recalls that I put a call in to him once because I was having a great deal of difficulty eliminating all the telangiectatic areas in an eye with a von Hippel tumor. I asked him at that time if he had ever used cryo on these. As a result of that talk, we have subsequently treated three. Each of these had had previous treatment with photocoagulation. The lesions had become sugar-coated and the telangiectatic vessels on the surface resisted further photocoagulation treatment. These eyes maintained a certain degree of exudative detachment, and the larger feeder vessels remained dilated. Each of these eyes had responded favorably to cryotherapy. The telangiectatic areas have decreased dramatically; in one case, there was a transient hemorrhage into the vitreous.

Dr. Straatsma: I'd like to depart a moment from the "which way do you treat them?" and think more generally about von Hippel's disease. All of us, I am sure, see patients with this condition and our obligation goes beyond the treatment of the immediate retinal lesion. I think there is an obligation to look for the disease in other members of the family—particularly siblings—because it is known that about 25% of these patients have familial factors. By finding the disease at an early stage, you may treat it more effectively and do great service by saving vision in that family. Moreover, once a patient with von Hippel's disease has been treated, he should re-main under observation for two reasons: first, he may develop new retinal lesions, and second, he may develop a full-blown von Hippel-Landau disease, in which there are central nervous system changes, which may not become evident until 10 or more years after the onset of the adverse ophthalmic picture.

Question: Has the use of alpha-chymotrypsin decreased the incidence of aphakic detachment?

Dr. Schwickerath: We do almost all our cataract patients with alpha-chymo-trypsin, and as far as we have followed up our cases, the incidence of detachment has not decreased.

Question: A 79-year-old monocular phakic patient with epithelial downgrowths, vision dropped fom 20/100 to light perception because of an inferior detachment with a horseshoe-shaped tear. What to do?

Dr. Schwickerath: G.O.K.—you know that—God only knows! But I would like to comment on that because it is a one-eyed patient for whom I would try to excise the epithelial downgrowths under the operative microscope. In spite of the fact that I have recommended treatment with photocoagulation, I would nowadays rather try to get a whole excision of the cyst under the microscope under 10× magnifica-tion. This has not been possible before without a microscope, I would say. And secondly, if this is successful, I would say it is worthwhile to treat that detachment in the usual way.

Question: What is the highest level you would consider leaving intraocular pressure?

Dr. Okun: This depends entirely upon how the intraocular pressure became as high as it is. At this point, I want to make a little statement about intraocular air. Air is extremely compressible, so the tension which is measured in an eye filled with air may be read falsely low by Schiøtz tonometry. It becomes even more important to view the central retinal artery after air injection than with any other material. I have seen the central retinal artery occlude while the pressure measured 50 mm. Hg Schiøtz after the use of intravitreal air. However, the pressure comes down very rapidly in these cases. If I see the central retinal artery completely occluded, I take down the buckle as fast as I can, loosen it, and try to get the tension normal. If it is elevated because of an excessive injection into the vitreous, I try to remove the excess. This is done with a larger needle than one used for the injection. We usually inject through a no. 300 needle. However, I prefer a no. 24 needle for removal of the excess. Occasionally, we will do an anterior chamber paracentesis. I do not recall who stated that they did not like to do paracentesis on aphakic individuals. Dr. Norton tells me that he did. I don't like to do that either and prefer to get out from where it went in. Adjusting the height of an encircling buckle is not very easy. A suggestion has been made that one must never increase the tension in the eye as measured by Schiøtz tonometry by more than 5 mm. Following adequate subretinal fluid drainage, in many of our aphakic patients the intraocular tension becomes so low that it is not measurable by Schiøtz tonometry. Pulling up on the sutures may raise the tension a little, but sometimes even after you do that, the eye is still too soft and you have to go ahead with an intravitreal injection in order to avoid too high a buckle with its accompanying radial folds. In cases of this type, I have found it very useful to mark the length of the band while it is in position before subretinal fluid drainage. After drainage the band is shortened 4 to 6 mm., and the rest of the volume lost through drainage is made up with an intravitreal injection. If this technique is observed, the buckle will not be too high. While I'm injecting saline, I adjust the tension by means of Schiøtz tonometry and try to end up with a pressure of 20. At this point, one can gauge the height of the buckle and predict that it will be slightly higher the next day with very little change over the next 6 weeks. There are some instances, however, when you might have to end the procedure with tension a little higher than 20, particularly when you elect not to drain subretinal fluid. I think that if one pays very careful attention to the height of the buckle, as related to the intraocular tension at the close of the procedure, a good estimate can be made of the final height of the buckle.

Mr. Hudson: I was interested in what Dr. Ed Okun said about this. I think there is more in this problem of intraocular pressure and central retinal artery patency than would be evident from what he said, because one gets obstructions of the central retinal artery during retinal detachment surgery, from my observation, in cases in which you would not anticipate it with tension of the order of 30 mm. Hg—and this is not related to a drop in the blood pressure, the general blood pressure connected with the anesthesia. And I think one not only has to think about what the central retinal artery is doing the last time you look at it on the operating table; the question is, what is it going to be doing in an hour's time back in the ward? It is possible during this period, if the patient has had a normal blood pressure during the operation, he may have a transient low blood pressure which will result in central retinal artery inadequacy and maybe later a central retinal artery occlusion. I feel that although one is doing a tremendous amount of retinal surgery one may be able to be a little bolder about the retinal circulation. I think the people who do a more limited amount of this type of work should bear in mind the possibility of the central retinal artery obstruction occurring postoperatively. One can always find the odd case in which, in one's own experience, this sort of thing has happened. Mine was an important director in London who had his retinal detachment operation and I looked at his retina the following day and I looked all around it—it had been perfectly all right at the end of the procedure—and the peripheral retina was flat and I commented that I thought the eye was looking very well and he said, "Well, it may look very well to you, but I can't see a damned thing!" When I looked at the central retinal artery, it was obstructed and there was edema at the posterior pole. I think this needs to be taken with a certain amount of caution.

Dr. Okun: I agree with Mr. Hudson in that there are patients who do occlude their central retinal arteries with a normal intraocular tension. However, I'm not sure that there is anything we can do about these individuals; some come into our office never having had a retinal detachment procedure. There may also be a rare individual whose central retinal artery may be affected by temporary subocclusive pressure elevation. Nevertheless, if in the process of producing a scleral buckling procedure without drainage of subretinal fluid the intraocular pressure is temporarily raised to 50, what I propose is that we simply relax a little bit and wait for it to come down. As long as the central retinal artery remains open, I have seen no harm come from this. We have followed the tension in these patients after they have gone back to their rooms and found that it returns to normal or subnormal and remains that way, provided the angle is adequate.

Dr. Schwickerath: We dare to wait 12 minutes with an occluded central artery. We are carrying a very careful record on the time when the retina can do without the supply of the central artery. After 12 minutes we have never seen a definite defect in our cases. We see quite a number of cases in which the elevation of tension is so high that the central artery is completely occluded; because if you do a scleral infolding or scleral section, you like to close it. Now, it is very difficult to predict how much you have to infold or to include, and therefore we take the tension and we look at the central artery. In none of these cases have we seen the occlusion of the central artery. However, I have seen three cases of other types of surgery in which retrobulbar injection was given with adrenaline and which developed central artery occlusion.

Dr. Norton: I think just for historical purposes you might be interested in this: When I first visited Professor Custodis, I asked him how did he arrive at the idea of putting something in the coat of the wall of the eye to push it in against the retinal break. He said he noticed that immediately after diathermy operation, the eye was very hard, and so he followed the tension of all of his patients postoperatively hourly. He noticed that they very promptly dropped down much below what the pressure was in the fellow-eye and that it stayed low for several days. With this in mind, he then sewed into the scleral wall Polyviol material, which pushed the pressure way up. I didn't see him do this, but other people who have been there have seen him tie up the sutures and look in and see the artery occluded. He then goes into the next room on another case and comes back again and ties it up a little tighter, and so on. He did this when he was trying to avoid drainage of fluid. Now, I certainly wouldn't advocate that. I don't like to leave an artery occluded. However, I think it is interesting that this drop in pressure following retinal detachment surgery has been well known for a long time and that it was the thing that stimulated Professor Custodis into putting something into the coat of the eye.

Dr. Kroll: To give an idea of some of the time factors involved in closing off the central retinal artery, we recently have been working with an experimental model of central retinal artery occlusion in monkeys, in which we can put a suture around the central retinal artery, pull the loop of the suture, and completely shut off the central retinal artery. Now we find with this model that the ERG B wave, that is, the wave that is associated with normal function of the inner retinal layers, begins to decrease at anywhere from 6 to 25 seconds and that this B wave is extinguished in all the animals by 120 seconds. Then, if we keep the central retinal artery closed, we find that between 2 and $3\frac{1}{2}$ hours occlusion results in irreversible change in the retina, both by ERG and by electron microscopy. So we would say that in the monkey, at least, one can occlude the central retinal artery completely for a relatively limited period of time before permanent damage is done.

Question: What is the highest level of intraocular pressure you would consider leaving the operating table with?

Dr. Schepens: No higher than 20.

Dr. Schwickerath: About 90% of our operative patients leave the operating table with an intraocular pressure between 40 and 50, and we have never seen any harm in this. We checked them in the first half hour and 1 hour after the operation, and they all went down in about 15 minutes to a normal pressure, except in those cases in which the vitreous was normal, which means in cases which had young patients with traumatic detachments.

Dr. Norton: I think the level at which you leave the intraocular pressure does vary with the procedure you are doing. If you elevated the pressure due to an encircling element, I think I agree with Dr. Freeman, that it would be unwise to leave that pressure high. However, if you are dealing with a segmental element or if you used an air injection into the vitreous, I think you can leave the pressure high, and your criterion is the central retinal artery pulsating. This you can observe. The pressure may be 40, but the artery is in good condition; then I think you can leave the pressure. I certainly would not try to jeopardize the eye by lowering the pressure in those circumstances. But, in an encircling procedure, I am much more careful to leave the eye normotensive.

Dr. Freeman: A patient with 180-degree tear has a small amount of subretinal fluid. Production of a suitable buckle causes a rise of intraocular pressure to 50 mm. How do you lower the intraocular pressure?

Lowering of the intraocular pressure could be done with 500 mg. of intravenous Diamox. If that doesn't do it, you can perforate the anterior chamber and let off fluid there.

Question: Does the panel have any suggestion in helping clear massive vitreous hemorrhages?

Dr. Norton: Well, we have a good medicine—we call it tincture of time.

Dr. Schepens: With regard to the importance of pathologic vitreous in retinal detachment surgery, would you comment on subtotal or total vitreous replacement in an attempt to remove pathologic tissue and protect the retina?

If the pathologic vitreous is removed, it could be replaced either by an absorbable or a nonabsorbable transparent substance.

Nonabsorbable vitreous substitute

Because of our bad experiences with silicone oil, we cannot recommend it as a vitreous substitute. First, a membrane tends to grow around the intravitreous silicone bubble. Second, and even more important, silicone oil is definitely toxic to the ganglion cells and the rods and cones of rabbits and monkeys. Not only did P. F. Lee observe damage to these cells in microscopic sections, but he also noted that the ERG was depressed after injections of silicone oil in the normal eyes of animals.* These animal experiments fit with our clinical observations in 14 patients in whom a silicone injection was followed by retinal reattachment, but visual results were much poorer than expected.

Absorbable vitreous substitute

For the past 12 years, one of my associates, E. A. Balazs, has attempted to produce a reconstituted vitreous made up of human collagen gel reinforced with hyaluronic acid. This work has not yet led to satisfactory clinical applications, but efforts continue actively in this direction. At this time, therefore, I would not consider replacing diseased vitreous with anything, except saline solution or air.

Question: What are your results with silicone injection?

Dr. Cockerham: We have recently reviewed 100 consecutive cases of silicone injection, of which 14 had anatomically successful results. Four of these successes were "partial successes," meaning there were fixed folds posterior to the buckle with a small amount of subretinal fluid which involved less than 30 degrees of the fundus. We were able to follow about 40 cases postoperatively. Almost all of these cases developed membranes around the silicone bubble, especially if they were followed by about a year. The membranes thickened with time, and many became completely opaque with new blood vessels in them. In the early stages, the slit lamp was usually necessary to detect these membranes. These findings tend to corroborate what Dr. Watzke reported recently in some 30 cases.

I would like to make another point concerning silicone injections. We have been surprised in a number of cases which in the immediate postoperative period and for a considerable period afterward appeared with ophthalmoscopy to be successful. The retina appeared attached, showing a good red reflex and a clear choroidal pattern. However, careful examination with the slit lamp and 3-mirror contact lens proved some of these apparent attachments to be total or extensive flat retinal detachments. I think that the globular shape of the silicone bubble presses the detached retina into a smooth contour which is transparent. I was interested that in the discussions of silicone injections by Dr. Schwickerath and Dr. Okun no mention was made of postoperative slit lamp follow-up. I wonder if they have had any similar experiences.

Dr. Okun: We have studied 10 eyes which were enucleated and we have found fine membranes in some of these eyes. These unsuccessful cases enable us to examine these membranes under great magnification, and the findings of such slight membrane formation has been encouraging. We study all patients who have had liquid silicone procedures with the slit lamp, and when possible, we take slit beam photographs of pertinent findings. Dr. Cibis has published several excellent slit lamp photographs showing the anterior vitreous and its relationship to the silicone globule. Certainly it would be inconceivable that a patient could have 20/50, 20/60, 20/70,

---

*Lee, P. F.: Personal communication.

or 20/100 visual acuity and have a very dense membrane or a great deal of fluid under his retina. Let's not forget that we're all talking about patients who, in our judgment, would have been blind without the liquid silicone procedure. We have all observed dense membrane formation in eyes not subjected to liquid silicone. As a matter of fact, the very eyes that we choose to perform liquid silicone procedures on frequently have dense membrane formation to begin with. These membranes may have continued to enlarge and become vascularized even without liquid silicone. In Dr. Watzke's series, only 1000 cs. liquid silicone was used, and one third of his cases were treated with fluorosilicone, a type of silicone which appears more liable to foamy breakdown. The characteristic of the lighter (1000 cs.) silicone explained some of his late complications. We have not noted this complication with the more viscous no. 360 medical fluid.

I have been asked why I limit the use of liquid silicone to essentially one-eyed people. Since liquid silicone has been shown to lead to ocular complications in a large percentage of patients, especially when malpositioned within the eye, we have felt that it was unwise to risk these complications in the therapy of an eye which probably wouldn't be used. This refers to patients who have one good eye not threatened by retinal detachment such as is seen in uniocular traumatic retinal detachment. This brings us back to the philosophy of how hard we should work to save a second eye. However, if the other eye already has had retinal detachment or appears threatened by the same, these patients are considered as liquid silicone candidates. As our techniques continue to improve and we observe less in terms of complications, we will swing back to treating patients who still have one good eye.

Question: Has vitreous transplant still a place in detachment surgery? If not, what caused it to be discontinued?

Dr. Schepens: Injections of stored human vitreous were first used by Norman Cutler, and the method was popularized 10 to 15 years ago by Donald Shafer. Unfortunately stored human vitreous is barely more viscid than water and results obtained with it did not appear to be superior to those following injection of saline solution. Personally, I prefer using a saline solution rather than stored vitreous because it is more convenient.

Question: Is there a way to predict which vitreous will shrink after a successful detachment operation, and in case you say yes, how would this influence your surgical procedure?

Dr. Schepens: It is difficult to predict. The history of the fellow-eye may be helpful because massive preretinal retraction is often bilateral. My clinical impression is often fooled in this respect, as massive preretinal retraction does occur when I expect it least and it sometimes fails to develop in eyes where I fear it. If I anticipate its development, I make a wider and higher buckle and use stronger diathermy applications than usual.

Dr. Okun: When we reviewed our cases that had developed vitreous shrinkage with massive preretinal fibroplasia, we not infrequently found that this condition had already set in prior to the first procedure, although not in its full-blown extent. Preretinal membranes had already formed, fixed folds were present, and the breaks showed rolled-over posterior edges. These are the cases which are most apt to develop massive preretinal retraction. Occasionally, we were very much surprised to see an eye that looked very good, both pre- and postoperatively, but that suddenly developed this condition. I suspect that a transparent membrane may have been missed in these cases. In those cases in which we suspect an impending preretinal retraction, we elect to do an encircling buckle in an attempt to offset the vitreous traction which is already present. We have seen less preretinal retractions since we have stressed the concept of the minimal amount of surgical trauma to do the job.

Question: What is the present status of microscopically controlled total vitrectomy (excision of the vitreous)?

Dr. Norton: I think most of the audience was probably in Chicago at the academy meeting and have heard prior presentation on vitreous surgery. I would just say that this is still an experimental procedure. I think Dr. Curtin showed you a woman that we did in 1962 with a membrane in the middle of her vitreous and there certainly was a dramatic result in that case. I think that in amyloid patients, who have no other cause, who have only light perception vision, and to whom we have no other way of giving sight this has been a useful procedure. To us, it is the only way that has ever been achieved successfully in restoring sight in these patients. The sad thing is having to take out a clear lens. But, I do think this is an approach that is going to be used in the treatment of a lot of diseases that we consider untreatable today.

Question: Please explain again how you obtain a single bubble with air injection.

Dr. Norton: The only thing I can say is that, to me, the most important thing is having everything dry: have the syringe dry, the air dry, and the needle dry. And you then put the needle through the wall into the vitreous cavity and inject under direct view so that you know that the needle is in the vitreous cavity, and then as soon as you've got a significant bubble, keep the needle tip in the bubble. If it's in the bubble, it will expand the bubble wider and wider. Once you've got a single bubble, it's not a problem at all to look through it. You've only got to understand that things are minified. The only problem is that if you aren't cautious and lucky and use a wet syringe you will get a lot of little bubbles, then it does create a problem in viewing.

Question: What criteria do the panelists use to abandon attempts at reattachment—abandon meaning when do you quit?

Dr. Schepens: Several elements must be considered. The two basic factors are, first, the extent and fixity of the retinal folds and, second, the status of the visual function. For instance, it is nowadays still impossible to reattach the retina of an eye with completely organized massive preretinal retraction. Also eyes with no light perception do not, in most instances, recover any vision after reattachment, and those with bare light perception have a very poor chance of recovering useful vision. In this respect, however, the status of the fellow-eye is important; if one deals with a patient's only functioning eye, more extensive efforts at reattachment must be made. Recovery of a vision limited to hand movements or even light perception is useless to an individual whose fellow-eye is good, but such recovery means a great deal to a patient whose alternative is total darkness. Another important factor to be considered is: What are the dangers involved in operating? For instance, a long operation with poor chances of recovery should not be performed on an individual who may be unable to stand a general anesthesia of long duration.

In any case, it is always indispensable for the surgeon to try putting himself in the patient's shoes before giving him final advice.

Dr. Norton: I do think there are two different people we have to think about: There is the ophthalmologist out in practice who is doing a few detachments. I would think that he would hesitate to tell a patient that his retina is inoperable. I think he ought to have it seen by somebody who is doing a lot of detachments to make that final decision. On the other hand, I think that those of us who are in retinal centers tend to get carried away with reattaching the retina and forget about the patient. We have all seen patients who, to the best of anyone's ability to judge, had no potential for useful sight but have undergone further retinal surgery for re-attachment. I really question the wisdom of this. On the other hand, I think that if we are going to make progress in this somebody has to do some experimental work. At the present time, whether you like it or not, this is what we have to do. So those of us who are in the retinal institutions have to sort of balance these two elements. I personally know I have operated on patients who I felt "down deep" had no hope, and they ended up with no hope; I had put them through an operative procedure that perhaps with better judgment, I wouldn't have done.

Question: Can you mention some of the criteria you use to decide when to advise that a patient not have further surgery—financial considerations aside?

Dr. Norton: I think we did discuss it in the panel discussion the first day. I don't think our opinions have changed. If you've done the five preceding operations, you're much more likely to quit than if the patient has had five operations done elsewhere and then comes to you. I think that a lot depends upon your emotional involvement with the patient. So I would just say that, in general, so long as you think that there is potential for vision, useful vision, and the patient is willing to go along with you and you think your stomach can take it, then I think you ought to try. Once you have reached the conclusion, however, that the patient will not get useful vision out of the eye, I think you just have to face the fact that this is it. You should start educating the patient by introducing him to the Council for the Blind, etc. I think there comes a time when this has to be done.

Dr. Schepens: I agree with what was just said, with one additional note. There are a number of ophthalmologists who don't seem to realize that useful vision in one-eyed patients is very different from useful vision in the fellow-eye when one eye is seeing and the other not seeing. It makes a world of difference to many patients to have just light perception or hand movements in one eye versus nothing. And there it might be completely unjustified to work to get light perception to one eye when the other eye has 20/20, except if one has indications that the eye will turn out bad also. But, there I think we should remember that what is useful vision for these poor patients is a level of vision that we, as the seeing, would not consider as vision at all. To them it may mean a great deal and we should remember that.

Dr. Straatsma: We have talked about this question on 2 days and it bothers me a little, because I think it is the wrong way to put the question. It implies that "quitting" is a unilateral decision by the ophthalmologist and really it is not. In practical terms, the situation is usually best resolved if the ophthalmologist analyzes the medical situation and presents it fairly to the patient. The physician and the patient then arrive at a joint decision regarding management.

Dr. Kroll: The question is: There are many things that affect the prognosis for future visual acuity in patients with retinal detachments, for example, site, size of hole, presence of fixed folds, and so on. But timewise, what is the maximum amount (2 weeks, 2 months) one can wait before operating?

Well, at one end of the spectrum I learned something last year: I examined a one-eyed lady with a retinal detachment of 8 years' duration. She had had three unsuccessful attempts at reattachment by retinopexy with diathermy. She had never had a scleral buckling. The retina was very thin and her visual acuity was questionably accurate light projection. I showed the patient to Dr. Norton and asked him whether this patient was operable, and he said, "You have nothing to lose." So I operated and was fortunate enough to have a successful result. The patient's acuity now is hand motions. She cannot quite count fingers, but this vision is very valuable to her because she can see the furniture in the house and not fall over it. That's 8 years, at the maximum, that I have personally seen an improvement in acuity. The visual result was not spectacular, but nevertheless it was useful vision. Now in regard to the work that we showed yesterday—it seems to me that it is rational to regard a retinal detachment as a little more of an emergency procedure than we have thought. If, as we saw yesterday, some photoreceptors are dying in a detached retina, one really has little to gain by postponing surgery unless one is waiting for hemorrhage to clear or for fluid to reabsorb so that the surgery could be done more easily. But, my personal recommendation, now, would be to operate as soon as is reasonably possible.

New Orleans Academy of Ophthalmology
Midwinter Convention
February 11-16, 1968

OFFICERS

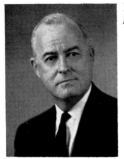

N. Leon Hart
President

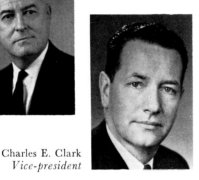

Charles E. Clark
Vice-president

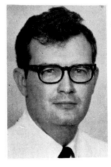

James McComiskey
Secretary

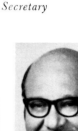

Julius Finkelstein
Treasurer

EXECUTIVE COMMITTEE

 Horace B. Dozier
 E. L. Leckert, Jr.
 C. L. M. Samson

COMMITTEES
Condolence

 H. B. Strauss, Chairman
 Hartwig Adler
 Wilfred Finkelstein

Exhibits

 George Ellis, Chairman
 Robert Azar
 Miles Friedlander
 George Dimitri
 Porter Puryear

Finance

 Julius Finkelstein, Chairman
 Thomas C. Naugle
 W. McD. Boles
 Harry Caplan
 Horace B. Dozier
 Robert E. Schoel

Historian

 Charles E. Clark, Chairman
 J. William Rosenthal
 M. C. Wilensky

Host

 Robert A. Schimek, Chairman
 Harry Caplan
 Robert Azar
 Frank Boswell
 J. William Rosenthal

Liaison

 J. Wm. Reddoch, Jr., Chairman
 Frank Boswell
 Anthony Failla
 C. L. M. Samson

Meeting rooms

 Oliver H. Dabezies, Chairman
 Miles Friedlander
 Hilliard Haik
 Betty Jean Wood

Membership

    M. C. Wilensky, Chairman
    Marie Stanbery
    George Dimitri
    A. Failla
    Earl Sonnier

Program

    James H. Allen, Chairman
    W. McD. Boles
    Monte Holland
    E. L. Leckert, Jr.
    James McComiskey
    J. Wm. Reddoch, Jr.

Publications

    J. Wm. Rosenthal, Chairman
    James H. Allen
    C. L. M. Samson
    Robert A. Schimek
    Robert E. Schoel

Publicity

    Robert J. Cangelosi, Chairman
    Robert Azar
    Shelley Faines
    A. F. W. Habeeb
    Robert Long
    J. Wm. Reddoch, Jr.

Registration

    Joseph Rumage, Chairman
    Julius Finkelstein
    Charles Clark
    Bonnie Adair
    Robert Long

Members of the
New Orleans Academy of Ophthalmology, 1968

Active members

Adair, Bonnie L., *Gretna, La.*
Adler, Hartwig M., *New Orleans, La.*
Allen, James H., *New Orleans, La.*
Anthony, Moss L., *New Orleans, La.*
Azar, Robert F., *New Orleans, La.*
Baldone, Joseph A., *Houma, La.*
Beatrous, F. Theo, *New Orleans, La.*
Blakeney, C. C., *New Orleans, La.*
Boles, Wm. McD., *New Orleans, La.*
Boswell, H. F., *New Orleans, La.*
Brock, Joseph R., *Metairie, La.*
Cangelosi, Robert Joseph, *New Orleans, La.*
Caplan, Harry B., *New Orleans, La.*
Clark, Charles E., *New Orleans, La.*
Clark, Wm. B., *New Orleans, La.*
Cohen, Sam Charles, *New Orleans, La.*
Cox, Charles L., *New Orleans, La.*
Dabezies, Oliver H., *New Orleans, La.*
Diaz, Walter P., *New Orleans, La.*
Dillon, Thomas K., *New Orleans, La.*
Dimitri, George J., *New Orleans, La.*
Dozier, Horace B., *New Orleans, La.*
Ellis, George S., *New Orleans, La.*
Failla, Anthony, *New Orleans, La.*
Farrington, Nolley Craft, *New Orleans, La.*
Ferry, John Francis, *New Orleans, La.*
Finkelstein, Julius, *New Orleans, La.*
Finkelstein, Wilfred, *New Orleans, La.*
Friedlander, Miles, *New Orleans, La.*
Gaines, Shelley Rice, *New Orleans, La.*
Gooch, John B., *New Orleans, La.*
Habeeb, Albert F. W., *New Orleans, La.*

Haik, George M., *New Orleans, La.*
Haik, Hilliard M., *New Orleans, La.*
Hanley, J. Roeling, *New Orleans, La.*
Hart, N. Leon, *New Orleans, La.*
Holland, Monte G., *New Orleans, La.*
Lea, Martha Ellis, *Marrero, La.*
Leckert, Edmund L., Jr., *New Orleans, La.*
Long, Robert A., *New Orleans, La.*
McComiskey, James, *New Orleans, La.*
McNeil, David Lee, *New Orleans, La.*
Naugle, Thomas C., *New Orleans, La.*
Pinschmidt, Norman Wm., *New Orleans, La.*
Pollard, Joel B., *New Orleans, La.*
Puryear, G. Porter, *New Orleans, La.*
Reddoch, Joseph Wm., Jr., *New Orleans, La.*
Rosenthal, J. W., *New Orleans, La.*
Rumage, Joseph P., *New Orleans, La.*
Samson, C. L. M., *New Orleans, La.*
Schimek, Robert A., *New Orleans, La.*
Schoel, Robert Edward, *New Orleans, La.*
Sonnier, Earl, *Gretna, La.*
Stanbery, Marie, *New Orleans, La.*
Strauss, Howard B., *New Orleans, La.*
Tedesco, Joseph Alexander, *New Orleans, La.*
Tuman, Walter C., *New Orleans, La.*
Wilensky, M. C., *New Orleans, La.*
Wood, B. Jean, *Gretna, La.*
Zoller, Harry, *New Orleans, La.*

Associate members

Abraham, Robert K., *Encino, Calif.*
Ackermann, Kurt, *Louisville, Ky.*
Anderson, Wm. Banks, Jr., *Durham, N. C.*
Anderson, Wm. D., *Ft. Carson, Colo.*
Anhalt, Edward F., *Winnipeg, Canada*
Arnold, Charles O., *Denver, Colo.*
Austin, Frederick L., *Great Lakes, Ill.*
Bade, Craig, *Victoria, Texas*
Bailey, Joseph C., *Murfreesboro, Tenn.*
Baller, Robert Stuart, *Norfolk, Va.*
Barker, Arnold G., Jr., *Shreveport, La.*
Barton, Seth H.
Beale, John P., Jr., *San Francisco, Calif.*
Beasley, J. O., *Spartanburg, S. C.*
Bernstein, Howard N., *Bethesda, Md.*
Berry, Juanedo, *San Diego, Calif.*
Beaudette, Robert P., *Raton, N. Mex.*
Binion, Warren, *Ft. Worth, Texas*
Bishop, David W., *Oklahoma City, Okla.*
Blocker, Donald Russell, *Lake Charles, La.*
Bond, John Benjamin, *Nashville, Tenn.*
Born, John H., *New York, N. Y.*
Bounds, George William, Jr., *Nashville, Tenn.*
Bourgeois, James Francis, *Houma, La.*
Bowers, Robert G., Jr., *Temple, Texas*
Braverman, Sheldon P., *San Antonio, Texas*
Breffeilh, Louis S., *Shreveport, La.*
Brown, Charles R., *Texas City, Texas*
Bunting, Richard Fry, *Richmond, Va.*
Burnham, Charles J., *Birmingham, Ala.*

Butler, Richard G., *Dearborn, Mich.*
Byer, Norman Eugene, *Torrance, Calif.*
Byers, Jerome, *Dallas, Texas*
Campbell, Lamar M., *Birmingham, Ala.*
Casanova, Thomas H., *Crowley, La.*
Cheskes, Albert, *Toronto, Ont., Canada*
Chickering, Donald H., *Warren, Ohio*
Childers, Melvin Davis, *Charlotte, N. C.*
Clark, Douglas H., *Lumberton, N. D.*
Clark, George H., *Indianapolis, Ind.*
Clarke, William M., *Montgomery, Ala.*
Clevenger, Charles E., *Pensacola, Fla.*
Cook, Raymond C., *Little Rock, Ark.*
Cooper, Jack C., *Dallas, Texas*
Corcoran, Geo. B., Jr., *Springfield, Mass.*
Cosgrove, J. W., Jr., *Little Rock, Ark.*
Coutler, William Harold, *Brooks AFB, Texas*
Cox, Morton S., *Ann Arbor, Mich.*
Cross, J. B., *Little Rock, Ark.*
Crosswell, Hal H., Jr., *Columbia, S. C.*
Cultron, F. T., *Salina, Kansas*
Curtis, James L., *Danville, Pa.*
Deer, Philip J., Jr., *Little Rock, Ark.*
DeHaven, C. Roger, *Tyler, Texas*
de Juan, Eugene, *Mobile, Ala.*
Delgado, Robert E., *Orlando, Fla.*
Deters, Curtis F., *Chicago, Ill.*
Deweese, Melvin W., *Memphis, Tenn.*
Dicksheet, Sharad K., *Westland, Mich.*
Dismukes, Henry M., *Mobile, Ala.*
Doughman, Donald James, *Iowa City, Iowa*
Dugan, Robert B., *Erie, Pa.*

Dukes, T. Earle, *Lakeland, Fla.*
Dumas, Jean, *St. Joseph, Quebec, Canada*
Eckley, Robert, *Temple, Texas*
Edward, Wm. O., *Albuquerque, N. Mex.*
Edwards, William C., *Louisville, Ky.*
Eggert, James F., *Oakland, Calif.*
Eigner, Edwin H., *Cleveland, Ohio*
Evans, Fred S., *Pensacola, Fla.*
Fairfax, Kenneth T., *Geneva, N. Y.*
Faulk, Wallace H., *Nashville, Tenn.*
Faulkner, Gerald P., *Kailua, H. T.*
Ferwerda, James, *Kenosha, Wis.*
Filar, Alfred A., *Baltimore, Md.*
Fisackerly, James S., *Biloxi, Miss.*
Fjordbotten, Alf. Lee, *Arlington, Va.*
Ford, Donald P., *Houston, Texas*
Fox, Brent, *Columbus, Ga.*
Freilich, Dennis Byron, *New York, N. Y.*
Fritch, John M., *Lafayette, La.*
Fulmer, John M., *Little Rock, Ark.*
Gahagan, Lawrence O., *Dallas, Texas*
Galas, Stanley M., *Ft. Lewis, Wash.*
Gettelfinger, Ralph A., *Louisville, Ky.*
Gilligan, John H., Jr., *Alexandria, Va.*
Gimbel, Howard V., *Calgary, Alberta, Canada*
Golden, John J., *Chicago, Ill.*
Green, Carl Alexander, *Tuskegee, Ala.*
Green, Ray L., *Plainview, Texas*
Greenberg, Richard S., *Omaha, Nebr.*
Griffin, Carlton C., *Lafayette, La.*
Grisham, Richard S. C., *Bartlesville, Okla.*
Gutow, Richard F., *Denver, Colo.*
Hagler, William S., *Atlanta, Ga.*
Hall, James, *South Bend, Ind.*
Hall, Marvin, *Marshall, Texas*
Hamilton, Ralph S., *Memphis, Tenn.*
Hammeke, John Cleo, *Leavenworth, Kan.*
Haney, Lawrence O., *Colorado Springs, Colo.*
Harper, John Yerkes, *Port Arthur, Texas*
Harper, John Y., Jr., *San Antonio, Texas*
Heath, William D., *Oklahoma City, Okla.*
Heatley, John, *Mexico City, D. F., Mexico*
Hertzog, Francis Carl, *Long Beach, Calif.*

Heyner, Frederick John, *South Field, Mich.*
Hirsch, Lucien, *Plainfield, N. J.*
Hitz, John B., *Milwaukee, Wis.*
Howard, Jed Lee, *Houston, Texas*
Humeke, John W., *Ada, Okla.*
Humphreys, John A., *Denver, Colo.*
Hudson, James Ralph, *London, England*
Hutson, Clare Frederick, *Madison, Wis.*
Ide, Carl H., *Columbia, Mo.*
Isaeff, Wayne B., *Oceanside, Calif.*
Jackson, William Edward, *Denver, Colo.*
Jimenez, Tim B., *Manila, Phil. Is.*
Jucker, James L., *Abilene, Texas*
Kanter, Yale C., *St. Paul, Minn.*
Kasner, David, *Coral Gables, Fla.*
Keith, Frank K., *Port Arthur, Texas*
Kemper, Robert A., *Cincinnati, Ohio*
Kerstine, Richard S., *Cincinnati, Ohio*
Key, Charles B., *Dallas, Texas*
Kimbell, Paul, *Denver, Colo.*
Kirkland, Theo. N., *Birmingham, Ala.*
Kleinfeld, Jerome, *Albuquerque, N. Mex.*
Knowled, Wm. F., *San Diego, Calif.*
Koons, Jess W., *Liberal, Kan.*
Kraft, James E., *Tulsa, Okla.*
Kraushar, Marvin Frederic, *Minneapolis, Minn.*
Kreshon, Martin John, *Charlotte, N. C.*
Kubitschek, William Ralph, *Denver, Colo.*
Lahey, Duane D., *Denver, Colo.*
Lansche, Richard K., *La Jolla, Calif.*
Lawaczeck, Elmar, *Birmingham, Ala.*
Lawrence, G. Allen, *Nashville, Tenn.*
Lawson, Edgar C., *Charlottesville, Va.*
Lerner, Leonard H., *Detroit, Mich.*
Levin, Joseph M., *Cincinnati, Ohio*
LeVine, Jerome Edward, *Baton Rouge, La.*
Lidster, Donald Kenneth, *Redding, Calif.*
Lieberman, Warren, *Coral Gables, Fla.*
Locke, John Craig, *Montreal, Canada*
Loftis, John R., *Longview, Texas*
Lowe, Percy E., *Houston, Texas*
Lowrey, James R., *Clearwater, Fla.*
Luedde, Harriet, *St. Louis, Mo.*
Manigan, Thos. P., *Memphis, Tenn.*
Margo, R. E., *Weslaco, Texas*
Mason, Gordon L., *Johnson City, Tenn.*

Matheus, Charles G., *Yuma, Ariz.*
Mattis, Robert Dean, *St. Louis, Mo.*
McCaffery, James M., *Glendale, Calif.*
McCallum, George C., *Eugene, Oregon*
McEwen, Stanley R., *Fort Smith, Ark.*
McGarry, H. Isabelle, *Evanston, Ill.*
McGowan, Bernard Lawrence, *Belmont, Mass.*
McKenna, Thomas J., *Johnstown, Pa.*
McKinzie, James W., *Ventura, Calif.*
McLain, Patrick Gene, *Vicksburg, Miss.*
Meaders, Robert H., *Pensacola, Fla.*
Membreno, Mauro G., *Panama, Rep. of Panama*
Miller, Robert J., *Sunnyvale, Calif.*
Mims, James L., Jr., *San Antonio, Texas*
Mishler, Jay E., *Atlantic City, N. J.*
Mixon, William A., *Chula Vista, Calif.*
Mohney, Glenn E., *Port Huron, Mich.*
Montgomery, Daniel Cameron, *Greenville, Miss.*
Moore, E. Lowry, *Meridian, Miss.*
Moorman, Lemuel T., *Denver, Colo.*
Morgan, John Francis, *Kingston, Ontario*
Mortensen, A. V., *Mobile, Ala.*
Murtagh, James Joseph, *Morgan City, La.*
Neely, Robert A., *Bellville, Texas*
Neight, Joseph S., *San Antonio, Texas*
Newsom, Samuel R., *Albuquerque, N. Mex.*
Nicely, Alfred L., *Akron, Ohio*
Nixon, Wm. Robert, *Pine Bluff, Ark.*
O'Connor, Edw. F., *Oak Park, Ill.*
O'Malley, Patrick F., *South Bend, Ind.*
Ottuni, John A., *Green Bay, Wis.*
Padfield, Earl G., *Kansas City, Mo.*
Page, Vernon, *Chicago, Ill.*
Paladino, Frank Paul, *Utica, N. Y.*
Pappas, Stephen S., *Washington, D. C.*
Parker, Bruce W., *Great Lakes, Ill.*
Perraut, L. Edward, *Washington, D. C.*
Pfingast, Harry A., *Louisville, Ky.*
Pistolas, Nicholas G., *Silver Spring, Md.*
Pockley, Edward Waddy, *Sydney, Australia*
Pole, Samuel B., III, *Bridgeton, N. J.*
Prestov, Wm. C., *Lexington, Ky.*
Prewitt, Luland H., *Ottumwa, Iowa*
Priddy, James S., *Shreveport, La.*

Pugh, George B., *Youngstown, Ohio*
Puk, John A., *Cedar Rapids, Iowa*
Reardon, Robert Meighan, *Bloomington, Ill.*
Regan, Charles Douglas James, *Boston, Mass.*
Reed, James S., *Medford, Ore.*
Rencher, Dan M., *Shreveport, La.*
Rich, Richard Budge, *Indianapolis, Ind.*
Ritch, Joseph G., *St. Petersburg, Fla.*
Roberts, Leo J., *Hinsdale, Ill.*
Roberts, Rufus Alston, *Ft. Worth, Texas*
Robertson, Dennis M., *Rochester, Minn.*
Robertson, Wm. Craig, *Gadsden, Ala.*
Rocti, L. Marshall, *Muncie, Ind.*
Rodriguez, Alvaro, *Bogota, Colombia*
Roth, F. Dale, *San Francisco, Calif.*
Rouse, David M., *Mexico, Mo.*
Rubin, Herbert S., *Ft. Sill, Okla.*
Russo, Charles E., *Houston, Texas*
Ryan, John James, *Louisville, Ky.*
Sabates, Felix N., *Kansas City, Mo.*
Sabin, Fred C., *Marquette, Mich.*
St. Dizier, Roger V., Jr., *Lafayette, La.*
Sampson, John Joseph, *Colorado Springs, Colo.*
Schaeffer, E. M., *Springfield, Mo.*
Schwarz, W. J., *Little Rock, Ark.*
Seale, Hubert J., *Abilene, Texas*
Semple, Henry Charles, *Mobile, Ala.*
Serros, Robert N., *Orlando, Fla.*
Shah, Anwar, *St. Louis, Mo.*
Sharrer, Margaret C., *Pittsburgh, Pa.*
Shaver, Robert Paul, *Oklahoma City, Okla.*
Shelton, Philip A., *Hartford, Conn.*
Shepherd, Virgil J., *San Antonio, Texas*
Shusterman, M., *Toronto, Canada*
Sichi, William T., *San Antonio, Texas*
Simmons, John R., *Ft. Sam Houston, Tex.*
Skov, Peter T., *W. Monroe, La.*
Small, Robert Glen, *Midwest City, Okla.*
Smith, Bryant P., *Shreveport, La.*
Smith, Wm. A., *Atlanta, Ga.*
Snip, Russell T., *San Antonio, Texas*
Snowhite, Arthur Bryan, *Marion, Indiana*
Snyder, William B., *Dallas, Texas*
Spalding, Joseph John, *Indianapolis, Ind.*

Spencer, Robt. W., *Tulsa, Okla.*

Spitalny, Lawrence Allan, *Washington, D. C.*

Stahl, Norman O., *Brooklyn, N. Y.*

Stambaugh, James Lee, Jr., *Lexington, Ky.*

Starr, Arthur Gibson, *Denver, Colo.*

Stewart, C. Thomas, *Seattle, Wash.*

Stewart, Robert B., *Springfield, Mo.*

Stern, Sheldon D., *Detroit, Mich.*

Stewart, Landis C., *Adrian, Mich.*

Stiernberg, Douglas D., *Texas City, Texas*

Street, Herbert S., *Decatur, Ala.*

Strong, Leroy E., *Grand Rapids, Mich.*

Sullivan, Paul B., *Etna, N. H.*

Swearingen, David C., *Shreveport, La.*

Sykes, John H., *San Antonio, Texas*

Tabb, Wm. Granville, Jr., *Atlanta, Ga.*

Taylor, Coleman, *Amarillo, Texas*

Thel, Henry Charles, *Aliquippa, Pa.*

Thomson, Richard Joseph, *Baytown, Texas*

Thorlakson, Neil F., *Seattle, Wash.*

Thorn, James I., *Wenatchee, Wash.*

Tirrill, Williard Oakes, III, *Nashville, Tenn.*

Tucker, Leonard C., *University Hgts., Ohio*

Tyner, George, *Denver, Colo.*

Robison, James Travis, *Shawnee Mission, Kan.*

Underwood, Dick H., *Kansas City, Mo.*

U'Ren, Harold M., *Portland, Ore.*

Uribe, Luis E., *New York, N. Y.*

Van Heuven, Wichard A. J., *Albany, N. Y.*

Vaughn, Chester A., *Tyler, Texas*

Vygantas, Charles M., *Chicago, Ill.*

Wahl, Joseph, *La Crosse, Wis.*

Wallner, Ernest F., *Milwaukee, Wis.*

Ward, Eugene L., *Gainesville, Ga.*

Watkins, John G., *Little Rock, Ark.*

Watt, Russell H., *Marshalltown, Iowa*

Weaver, Richard G., *Winston-Salem, N. C.*

Weidentaal, Daniel, *Cleveland Hgts., Ohio*

Weinstein, Louis J., *Lafayette, La.*

Weiss, Larry L., *Winston-Salem, N. C.*

White, Ira M., *Sedalia, Mo.*

Wickerham, Earl Phillips, Jr., *Pittsburgh, Pa.*

Widner, Russell R., *Washington, D. C.*

Williams, Van R., *New Orleans, La.*

Wilson, James Richard, *Los Angeles, Calif.*

Wise, James B., *Oklahoma City, Okla.*

Witter, Gordon Lynn, *Redlands, Calif.*

Womack, Wm. T., *San Angelo, Texas*

Wong, Sauki, *Honolulu, Hawaii*

Wootton, James C., *Mesa, Ariz.*

Worlton, James T., *Colorado Springs, Colo.*

Wright, J. R., *Gainesville, Ga.*

Wright, Robert L., *Elyria, Ohio*

Yassin, John G., *Winter Park, Fla.*

Yee, Rafael, *Panama, Rep. of Panama*

Yonems, Harry T., *Columbus, Texas*

Youens, W. T., *Columbus, Texas*

Young, Charles A., *Roanoke, Va.*

Fellow members

Adams, Varia, *New Orleans, La.*
Allensworth, Wm. Burton, *Jackson, Miss.*
Apple, David J., *New Orleans, La.*
Augustat, Edwin Charles, *New Orleans, La.*
Azar, Geo. James, Jr., *New Orleans, La.*
Ballou, Gordon Steely, *New Orleans, La.*
Balunek, Andrew Daniel, *Cleveland, Ohio*
Barton, Arnold, *Los Angeles, Calif.*
Begg, Robert Brady, *New Orleans, La.*
Blahnik, C. L., *New Orleans, La.*
Blankenship, George William, *New Orleans, La.*
Blount, Wilbur C., *Minneapolis, Minn.*
Botero, Alfredo, *New Orleans, La.*
Bradley, Charles K., *New Orleans, La.*
Braunlin, Earl Albert, *Marion, Ind.*
Bridges, William Z., *Decatur, Ga.*
Bryson, Jerry M., *Iowa City, Iowa*
Burton, Thomas C., *Chicago, Ill.*
Carrico, John David, *Metaire, La.*
Chenoweth, Richard Glenn, *Silver Spring, Md.*
Church, Thomas C., *New Orleans, La.*
Coles, William H., *New Orleans, La.*
Couvillion, Glynne C., *Boston, Mass.*
Davidson, Gene Lee, *Monroe, La.*
Davidson, J. David, *Birmingham, Ala.*
Davidson, John Andrew, *St. Louis, Mo.*
Davies, Gerald T., *Arlington, Va.*
Davis, Bradford Leroy, *Houston, Texas*
Dyster-Aas, Kjell, *New Orleans, La.*

Ederington, John B., *New Orleans, La.*
Edwards, David Aubrey, *San Antonio, Tex.*
Ehrlich, Bernard, *Washington, D. C.*
Eifrig, David Eric, *Santa Monica, Calif.*
Fatoni, Michael Leonard, *New Orleans, La.*
Fanelli, Mary Jo, *New Orleans, La.*
Feit, Lawrence J., *Bronx, N. Y.*
Fine, Stuart L., *Arlington, Va.*
Freeman, George Walter, *New Orleans, La.*
Freeman, Jerre Minor, *Boston, Mass.*
Galman, Barry D., *Philadelphia, Pa.*
Garcia, Charles Albert, *New Orleans, La.*
Gershen, Herbert Joel, *New Orleans, La.*
Gilbert, William Steven, *Philadelphia, Pa.*
Glaser, Joel Stephen, *Jacksonville, Fla.*
Goldbaum, Michael H., *Oakland, Calif.*
Goldberg, M. F., *Arlington, Va.*
Gourgett, C. John, *New Orleans, La.*
Grady, Frank J., *New York, N. Y.*
Grizzard, Henry J., *Memphis, Tenn.*
Hafner, John Norris, *Louisville, Ky.*
Hand, Harold Edward, Jr., *Omaha, Neb.*
Harkey, Michael Erin, *New Orleans, La.*
Hayes, Harrison F., *New York, N. Y.*
Healy, William R., *New Orleans, La.*
Hehn, Richard Wm., *Birmingham, Ala.*
Huertel, Quentin C., *Kansas City, Kan.*
Humphrey, William T., *Decatur, Ga.*

Hunter, Allan A., Jr., *Washington, D. C.*
Jacklin, Harold Norman, *Boston, Mass.*
Jahncke, Paul Gene, *Dickinson, Texas*
Jaegers, Kenneth Ray, *Philadelphia, Pa.*
Janes, Charles L., *San Antonio, Tex.*
Johnson, Alvin, *Detroit, Mich.*
Jones, Wirt A., *New Orleans, La.*
Jove, Minaya, *New Orleans, La.*
Judisch, G. Frank, *Iowa City, Iowa*
Kassoff, Aaron, *Albany, N. Y.*
Keatts, James C., *Galveston, Texas*
Kenny, G. S., *Littleton, Colo.*
Kietzman, Benjamin Paul, *Wheaton, Ill.*
Kimball, Nancy L., *Littleton, Colo.*
King, Yum Y., *Little Rock, Ark.*
Kirby, Charles Gentry, *Atlanta, Ga.*
Klein, Lawrence C., *New Orleans, La.*
Knopf, Merrill M., *Jackson, Miss.*
Knowles, Sally Anne, *San Diego, Calif.*
Koller, Harold Paul, *New Orleans, La.*
Krug, James A., *New Orleans, La.*
Langerman, David Walter, *Jefferson City, Mo.*
Laughlin, Kenneth M., *New Orleans, La.*
Lauring, Lewis M., *San Francisco, Calif.*
LeDoux, Harold W., *Shreveport, La.*
Leslie, C. Doyle, *San Antonio, Texas*
Lewis, Norman G., *New Orleans, La.*
Lipsich, Michael Paul, *Oklahoma City, Okla.*
Logan, Neal J., *New Orleans, La.*
Long, William Brenisen, *New Orleans, La.*
Madere, Sherman G., *New Orleans, La.*
Magovern, Malcolm J., *Atlanta, Ga.*
Marsh, Wallace S., *New Orleans, La.*
Martin, Benjamin G., *San Antonio, Tex.*
McDonald, J. Paul, *Lomita, Calif.*
McMahan, John W., *Nashville, Tenn.*
Melvin, Hiram M., *New Orleans, La.*
Metz, Henry S., *New Orleans, La.*
Milira, Calvin M., *San Francisco, Calif.*
Moak, Wilson E., *Washington, D. C.*
Monaco, Benjamin P., *Albuquerque, N. M.*
Nase, Paul Kenneth, *Philadelphia, Pa.*
Nelson, Robert A., *Cincinnati, Ohio*
Nicklas, Thomas O., *Oklahoma City, Okla.*
Pailet, Sanford L., *New Orleans, La.*

Perez, Luis Francisco, *New Orleans, La.*
Perry, Robert James, *Kingston, Ontario*
Petraysyas, Raymond R., *Ann Arbor, Mich.*
Rashid, Richard C., *South Charleston, W. Va.*
Raulston, Kenneth L., Jr., *New Orleans, La.*
Reitman, Howard S., *New Orleans, La.*
Robins, Sherman Arthur, *New Orleans, La.*
Rucker, George D., *Shreveport, La.*
Rue, L. R., *New Orleans, La.*
Sawyer, Norman Marshall, *Atlanta, Ga.*
Schultz, Gerald R., *New York, N. Y.*
Shahidi, Massoud, *Monroe, Wis.*
Sibley, Riley C., *New Orleans, La.*
Sinchai, Pravit, *New Orleans, La.*
Soileau, James Sherman, *New Orleans, La.*
Sollie, Stanley C., *Ft. Sam Houston, Tex.*
Soyars, James Edward, *New Orleans, La.*
Sparks, George Mann, *Madison, Wis.*
Stanford, Gary B., *New York, N. Y.*
Steen, William Hinton, *New Orleans, La.*
Stevenson, Onex Dara, *New Orleans, La.*
Stumpf, Karl J., *New Orleans, La.*
Swearingen, David C., Jr., *Shreveport, La.*
Taleff, Michael, *Cincinnati, Ohio*
Teller, Richard Michael, *Albany, N. Y.*
Tilley, K. Shannon, *Nashville, Tenn.*
Trimbev, Connell J., *Washington, D. C.*
Tull, John W., *New Orleans, La.*
Vidacovich, Richard Paul, *New Orleans, La.*
Waller, John P., *New Orleans, La.*
Welch, James W., Jr., *New Orleans, La.*
Wells, John Anderson, *Atlanta, Ga.*
Wheat, Reginald D., *New Orleans, La.*
White, Stephen Vincent, *Oklahoma City, Okla.*
Williamson, Stoney, *Shreveport, La.*
Winkler, Moseley H., *Charlottesville, Va.*
Wofford, Michael Wesley, *Augusta, Ga.*
Wolchok, Eugene B., *Westover AFB, Mass.*
Wood, John W., *Nashville, Tenn.*
Wunaprapa, Wera, *New Orleans, La.*

Index

A

Acetazolamide, 201
Adhesions
  chorioretinal, and pigment at pigment layer of retina, 358
  between retina and vitreous, 87
Age
  in differential diagnosis
    of hemangioma, 58-59
    of malignant melanoma, 57
  and lattice degeneration, relationship between, 334
Air injection in treatment of giant breaks, 366-367
Alaimo, 31, 32
Allergy in pathology of retinal detachment, 357
Alpha-chymotrypsin in aphakic detachment, 371
American Optical monocular indirect ophthalmoscope, evaluation of, 352-353
Amoils, S. P., 34
Amoils cryosurgical unit, 142, 352
Anesthesia, topical
  in insertion of lens for vitreous cavity examination, 72
  in scleral depression, 47
Angiography, fluorescein, in differential diagnosis of retinal detachment, 56
Antibiotic solutions with silicone implants, 208
Aphakic detachment, alpha-chymotrypsin in, 371
Arlt, F., 29

Arterials, occlusions in small peripheral, in retinal or choroid detachment, 357-358
Artifactitious ghost image, 87
Ascension phenomenon, 74, 75
Astigmatism in examination of fundus periphery, 41
Atrophy
  choroidal, secondary to cryotherapy, 150
  iris, small pupil in, 199
  retinal, 150
Attachments, exaggerated vitreoretinal, 111
Autogenous plantaris tendon in scleral buckling, 189
Autoimmunological factors in pathology of retinal detachment, 357

B

Balazs, E. A., 34
Band, primary 360-degree, versus segmental buckle, Custodis-type, 340-344
Berrocal, Dr. Jose A., technique of, in transillumination, 54
Bietti, G. B., 34
Biomicroscopy
  as aid in planning surgery, 88
  in differential diagnosis of retinal detachment, 53-54
  in retinal breaks, 88
  slit lamp, in vitreous cavity examination, description of, 69-71
  of vitreous cavity, 66; *see also* Vitreous cavity examination
  intravenous fluorescein and, 69

Blindness, day, after successful reattachment, 354

Blood between vitreous body and retina in vitreous detachment, 80

Breaks, retinal, 88
giant
air injection in treatment of, 366-367
current management of, 171-183
planned retinal incarcerations in surgery for, 366
horseshoe, management of, 363
intravitreal surgery with liquid silicone, management of, 291
large, cryotherapy in, 358-359
localization of, difficulties with, 227-228
recording of, 40

Bruch's membrane, 99

Buckle; *see also* Scleral buckling
Custodis-type segmental, versus primary 360-degree band, 340-344
for giant tear, lowering of intraocular pressure for, 368
lowering of intraocular pressure after, 374

Buckling in diabetic retinal detachment, 345

Bullous detachments, localization of large tears with, 362

C

Campbell American Optical laser instrument, 130

Canthotomy during retinal detachment surgery, 227

Capsular remnants after extracapsular cataract extraction, 199

Carbonic anhydrase inhibitors, 208

Case reports of diabetic retinopathy, 297-300

Cataract extraction
extracapsular, capsular remnants after, 199
prior to retina surgery, 198

Cataract formation after intravitreal surgery with liquid silicone, 288, 291

Cataract surgery with round-pupil extraction, small pupil in, 199

Cataracta complicata, 237

Chart, Tolentino, 79

Checkerboard type of mottling in choroid in metastatic tumors, 61

Chorioretinal adhesion, producing of, in special surgical technique, 208

Chorioretinal exudation, recording of, 40

Choroid
exudative reactions of, diathermy and cryotherapy in, 360
hemangioma of, 58-61

Choroid—cont'd
malignant melanoma of, 56-58
mass in, in differential diagnosis of malignant melanoma, 57
occlusions in small peripheral arterials in, 357-358
pigment in
in metastatic tumors, 61
recording of, 40

Choroidal
atrophy secondary to cryotherapy, 150
coloboma, 217-220
detachment, 160, 161
or combined, in differential diagnosis, 52
development of, 229
in differential diagnosis of retinal detachment, 63, 64
malignant melanoma and, 165
serous, and solid lesions, differential diagnosis of, 54
elevation after localized pocket procedure, 192
knuckle, perforation of, 207
loss of pattern in hemangioma, 60
vessels, dilatation and engorgement of, 162

Cibis, P. A., 35

Ciliary arteries and nerves, long, cryoapplications and diathermy in treating over, 360

Clinical correlations of retina; *see* Retina, topography and clinical correlations in

Clinical and experimental study of traumatic retinal detachment, 302-318

Cloquet's canal, 80

Coagulation
of conjunctiva vessels and tumors, 369
xenon-flash, on Comberg instrument, 134-135

Coagulation time, surface, 369

Coccius, A., 28, 29, 30

Cold probe, danger from moving of, 140

Coloboma, choroidal, 217-220

Comberg instrument, 133

Complications
of intravitreal surgery with liquid silicone, 288-290
management of, 290-293
of retinal detachment surgery, 222-234
postoperative, 229-230
previous intraocular surgery in, 224-225
during surgery, 225-226
of silicone injections into vitreous cavity, 237

Compression, photographic recordings of, 312-313

Concave lens for focal illumination, history of, 28-29

Congenital defects in differential diagnosis, 52-53

Conjunctiva vessels and tumors, coagulation of, 369

Connective tissue defect, Ehlers-Danlos syndrome as, 217

Contact lens
  for focal illumination, history of, 28
  Goldmann 3-mirror
    description of, 66-68
    in vitreous cavity examination, 66
    in vitreous cavity examination, description of, 71-72

Contusion
  damage to pig eyes by, 305-309
  of globe, chronic open-angle glaucoma from, 200
  intraocular damage by, experimental observations of, 305-317
  retinal detachment, clinical observations on, 302-305

Cooper, I. S., 34

Corneal
  dystrophy after intravitreal surgery with liquid silicone, 290, 291
  epithelium, edema of, and biomicroscopy of vitreous cavity, 69
  opacifications in complications of retinal detachment surgery, 223
  opacities or lens opacities in preoperative management, 198-199
  transparency during surgery, maintenance of, 364-366

Crock, procedure of, for formation of fusil, 189

Cryoapplications
  and choroidal coloboma, 220
  and diathermy in treating over long ciliary arteries and nerves, 360
  in giant retinal breaks, 179
  and photocoagulation, indications for prophylactic treatment with, 359
  in thin sclera, 215

Cryocoagulation versus diathermy, 193

Cryohypophysectomy, 348

Cryoprobe, vitreous, in giant retinal breaks, 180

Cryosurgery
  development of, 34
  extent of application of, 362

Cryosurgery—cont'd
  segmental, without drainage of subretinal fluid, 360-361

Cryotherapy
  adequate treatment with, 228
  advantages of, 136-142, 150, 153, 195
  in comparison to photocoagulation
    or diathermy, margin of safety in, 137-138
    for retinal detachment, 137
  and diathermy, 142-146, 194, 195
    in exudative reactions of choroid, 360
    pathologic changes following, 147
  disadvantages of, 139-142
  equipment for, 141-142
  and full-thickness scleral buckling versus lamellar undermining, diathermy, and tissue transplantation, 184-196
  incidence of chronic orbital granuloma with, 359
  in large retinal breaks, 358-359
  margin of safety in, 137-138
  in retinal detachment surgery, 136-146
  in treatment of vascular lesions, 370-371
  versus lack of prophylaxis in retinal holes in lattice degeneration, 337-340

Cryotherapy units, evaluation of, 351-352

Custodis, E., 34

Custodis method in reattachment of retinas, 246

Custodis procedure, 136, 165
  in experimental retinal detachment and reattachment, 241

Custodis-type segmental buckle versus primary 360-degree band, 340-344

Cutler, N. L., 32, 33

Cyclogyl in mydriatic mixture, 39

Cyclopentolate hydrochloride, 201

Cystic retinal tuft, 105-106

Cystoid changes in macula of aphakic patient, 56

Cystoid degeneration of middle retina, 95-96

Cystoid spaces in retina after retinal detachment, 276

Czermak, J., 28

D

Day blindness after successful reattachment, 354

Decompression, photographic recordings of, 313

Deformation of pig and human globes by high-speed impact, 309-317
  materials and methods in, 309-311

Deformation—cont'd
photographic recordings in, 309-314
results of, 311-316
Degenerations
cystoid, of middle retina, 95-96, 97
definition of, 90
lattice, of peripheral retina, 114-127; *see
also* Lattice degeneration of retina
paving-stone, 99-101
of peripheral retina
tractional, 103-127; *see also* Tractional
degenerations of peripheral retina
trophic, 90-102; *see also* Trophic degenerations of peripheral retina
senile peripheral tapetochoroidal, 100, 101
360-Degree band, primary, versus segmental
buckle, Custodis type, 340-344
Dehiscences of sclera, 211, 212
de Jaeger, E., 29
de la Hire, 28
Dellaporta, A., 32, 33
Dentate process, 5
Desmarres scarifier in lamellar scleral undermining, 203
de St. Yves, C., 27
Detached retina; *see* Retinal detachment
Detached vitreous, 80; *see also* Detachments,
vitreous
Detachment surgery
criteria for abandoning attempts at reattachment in, 377-379
principles in, 136
retinal; *see* Retinal detachment surgery
shrinkage of vitreous after, 376-377
vitreous transplant in, 376
Detachments
aphakic, alpha-chymotrypsin in, 371
associated with systemic disease in differential diagnosis, 53
bullous, localization of large tears with, 362
choroidal; *see* Choroidal detachment
exudative, with retinal or choroidal vascular disease in differential diagnosis, 53
inflammatory, in differential diagnosis, 52
of muscles during retinal detachment surgery, 227
pigment epithelial, 55, 56
and proliferation, prevention of, in diabetic
retinopathy, 294-301; *see also* Diabetic retinal detachment
retinal; *see* Retinal detachment
vitreous, 80, 87
with collapse of gel, 80
simple, 80, 83

Deutschmann, R., 31, 32, 35
Developmental defects in differential diagnosis, 52-53
Developmental pathology in choroidal coloboma, 217-218
Developmental variation, definition of, 90
de Wecker, L., 29, 30, 32
Diabetic retinal detachment, 319-327
buckling in, 345
discussion of therapy in, 326
indications for therapy in, 322-324
operative procedure in, 324-325
pathogenesis and ophthalmoscopic appearance of, 319-322
results of therapy of, 325-326
Diabetic retinopathy
case reports of, 297-300
changes in treatment of, 295-296
laser in therapy of, 344
photocoagulation and, 294, 347, 348, 349,
350
prevention of detachment and proliferation
in, 294-301
progressive, photocoagulation in, 345
results of treatment of, 296
scleral buckling procedure with, 346-350
sites of treatment of, 344-345
unilateral, 345-346
Diagnosis, differential
of retinal detachment, 52-65
specific problems in, 56-65
techniques of examination in, 53-56
of serous choroidal detachments and solid
lesions, 54
Diagram, conventional fundus, topography
and, 22
Diameters of optic disc, average, 3
Diathermy
advantages of, 193
and choroidal coloboma, 220
in closing choroidal vessels, 207
and cryoapplications over ciliary arteries
and nerves, 360
and cryotherapy
in exudative reactions of choroid, 360
margin of safety in, 137-138
pathologic changes following, 147
extent of application of, 362
in giant retinal breaks, 176, 177
incidence of chronic orbital granuloma
with, 359
lamellar undermining, and tissue transplantation versus cryotherapy and
full-thickness scleral buckling, 184-
196

Diathermy—cont'd
in special surgical techniques for marked fixed folds and massive preretinal retraction, 208
in surgical technique for fixed folds and massive preretinal retraction, 203
versus cryocoagulation, 193
versus cryotherapy, 142-146, 194, 195
Differential diagnosis; *see* Diagnosis, differential
Dilatation and engorgement of choroidal vessels, 162
Disinsertions, procedure for, 188-189
Dislocated lens, small pupil in, 199
Donor sclera in implants for thin sclera, 215
Drainage
of fluid, indications for, 228
of subretinal fluid, 346
cryotherapy in avoiding, 195
segmental cryosurgery without, 360-361
Dystrophy of cornea after silicone injection, 237

E

Edema of corneal epithelium and biomicroscopy of vitreous cavity, 69
Ehlers-Danlos syndrome, 216-217
Eisner, modification of Goldmann's scleral depressor of, 76
El Bayadi, G., 33
Electron microscopy in experimental retinal detachment and reattachment, 258-277
comment on, 274-276
materials and methods in, 258-259
observations in, 259
End point, ease of seeing, in cryotherapy, 138
Endophthalmitis, infectious, 169
Engorgement, dilatation and, of choroidal vessels, 162
Epinephrine bitartrate, 201
Epithelial detachments, pigment, 55, 56
Epithelium, pigment
in experimental retinal detachment and reattachment, 252-255
lamellar inclusion bodies of, electron microscopy and, 274
and retina, 87
Epon 812, 258
Equatorial staphyloma, 211, 212
Equatorial zone of fundus periphery, 39
Equipment for cryotherapy, 141-142

Ethylene oxide gas in sterilization
of contact lens for vitreous cavity examination, 72
of transilluminator tip, 49
Evolution of concepts related to retinal detachment, 27-38; *see also* Retinal detachment, evolution of concepts
Examination
of fundus periphery, techniques of, 39-51; *see also* Fundus, periphery of
methods of
in differential diagnosis of retinal detachment, 53-56
evolution of concepts in, 27-29
contemporary period in, 33-34
early period in, 27-28
modern period in, 28-29
procedure for vitreous cavity examination, 72-78; *see also* Vitreous cavity examination
of vitreous cavity
performing of, 73-78
technique of, 66-89; *see also* Vitreous cavity examination
Experimental observations of intraocular damage by contusion, 305-317
Experimental retinal detachment and reattachment, 239-277
clinical picture in, 240-246
electron microscopy in, 258-277
observations and comment on, 259, 274-276
histology in, 247-256
materials and methods of, 239-246
methods, clinical picture, and histology, 239-257
results and comments on, 242-246
Exposure in complications during retinal detachment surgery, 227
Extracapsular cataract extraction, capsular remnants after, 199
Exudative detachment with retinal or choroidal vascular disease in differential diagnosis, 53
Exudative reactions of choroid, diathermy and cryotherapy in, 360
Eye
abnormalities of, in Ehlers-Danlos syndrome, 216-217
anteroposterior position of lesions within, and stage of lattice degeneration, relationship between, 334
development of, 52
experimental damage to, by contusion, 305-317

F

Fiber-optic light source in transillumination, 54

Fibroplasia, massive preretinal, in complications of therapy, 278-293

Fibrovascular proliferations, preretinal, in diabetic retinal detachment, 319

Fish mouthing, 192

Flare between vitreous body and retina in vitreous detachment, 80

Flat mass, white, mottled, in differential diagnosis of metastatic tumors, 61-62

Fluid; *see* Drainage; Subretinal fluid

Fluorescein
  in differential diagnosis
    of hemangioma, 60-61
    of malignant melanoma, 58
    of metastatic tumors, 62-63
  intravenous, and biomicroscopy of vitreous cavity, 69
  in vessels, 344

Fluorescein angiography in differential diagnosis of retinal detachment, 56

Folds
  fixed, and massive preretinal retraction
    general surgical technique for, 203-208
    problems during surgery and, 201-211
    special techniques for, 208-211
  in tractional degenerations of peripheral retina, 108-110

Foveola, one location and dimension of, 3-4

Frigitronic cryosurgical unit, 142
  evaluation of, 352

Fundus
  diagram of
    conventional, topography and, 22
    preceding biomicroscopy of vitreous cavity, 68
    representation of ora serrata on, 22
    in vitreous cavity examination, 79
  observation of, interference with, 197-200
  peripheral
    examination, 75-77
    horizontal views of, 77
    oblique views of, 77-78
    superior views of, 77
  periphery of
    definition of, 39
    inferior, examination of, 47, 77
    landmarks of, 39
    techniques of examination of, 39-51
      improved scleral depressor in, 47-49
      indirect stereoscopic ophthalmoscopy with scleral indentation in, 39-49

Fundus—cont'd
  periphery of—cont'd
    techniques of examination of—cont'd
      problems in, 41-42
      slit lamp microscopy of fundus in, 50-51
      small-pupil ophthalmoscope in, 43-44
      transillumination in, 49-50
      use of scleral indentation in, 44-47
    upper, examination of, 47
    zones of, 39
  recording details of, 40-41
  slit lamp microscopy of, 50-51
    development of, 28-29

G

Gass, sclera marker of, 140

Ghost image, artifactitious, 87

Giant retinal breaks
  air injection in treatment of, 366-367
  current management of, 171-183
  planned retinal incarcerations in surgery for, 366
  results of surgery in, 182
  surgical technique in, 176-182

Giant retinal tear
  complicated by massive preretinal retraction, 181-182
  lowering of intraocular pressure in buckle for, 368

Giant rolled-over retinas, results of surgery on, 367

Giraud-Teulon, 28, 29

Glaucoma
  associated with retinal detachment, 200-201
  chronic open-angle, from contusion of globe, 200
  in complications of retinal detachment surgery, 224
  late, after intravitreal surgery with liquid silicone, 293
  postoperative, 231
  presence of, in retinal detachment, 200-201
  pupillary-block, 288
  secondary
    after intravitreal surgery with liquid silicone, 290
    after silicone injection into vitreous cavity, 237, 239

Globes, human
  deformation of, by high-speed impact, 309-317

Globes, human—cont'd
   sketches of, in vitreous cavity examination, 79
Glycerin in edema of corneal epithelium, 69
Goldmann, H., 34
Goldmann scleral depressor, 76
Goldmann 3-mirror contact lens
   description of, 66-68
   in differential diagnosis of retinal detachment, 54
   in examination of retinal detachment, 353-354
   in vitreous cavity examination, 66
Gonin, J., 30, 31, 32, 33
Granuloma, chronic orbital, incidence of, with diathermy and cryotherapy, 359
Graphic reconstruction of photographic recordings of high-speed impact, 314-316
Guist, G., 32
Gullstrand, A., 28, 29

H

Haag-Streit model-900 slit lamp
   description of, 66, 67
   in vitreous cavity examination, 66
Heim, H., 32, 33
Helmholtz, H., 28, 29
Hemangioma in differential diagnosis of retinal detachment, 58-61
Hematoxylin-eosin, 247
Hemorrhage
   in differential diagnosis of malignant melanoma, 57
   posterior polar, 55, 56
   retinal
     during intravitreal surgery with liquid silicone, management of, 291
     recording of, 40
   vitreous
     in differential diagnosis, 52
     in Ehlers-Danlos syndrome, 217
     after intravitreal surgery with liquid silicone, 288
     preoperative management of, 197-198
High-speed impact, deformation of pig and human globes by, 309-317
Hildesheimer, S., 32, 33
Histologic features of lattice degeneration, 122-123
Histology in experimental retinal detachment and reattachment, 247-256
   materials and methods, 247
   results and comments, 247

History of first eye in lattice degeneration, 335
Homatropine hydrobromide in mydriatic mixture, 40
Horseshoe break, management of, 363
Hruby, K., 29, 33
Hruby lens
   in differential diagnosis of retinal detachment, 54
   shortcomings of, in vitreous cavity examination, 68
Human globes, deformation of, by high-speed impact, 309-317
Human sclera
   in stuffing out intrascleral pockets, 185, 187
   in techniques of scleral buckling, 184
Hyaloid face in vitreous detachment, 80
Hyaloideocapsular ligament of Wieger, 80
Hyaluronidase
   in experimental retinal detachment and reattachment, 240
   injection of intravitreal, 247, 258
Hypophysectomy, 347
Hypotony, 200

I

Illumination in examination of fundus periphery, 42
Impact, high-speed, deformation of pig and human globes by, 309-317
Implant material
   silicone, in surgical management of fixed folds and massive preretinal retraction, 203
   tissue tolerance and, 166
Implanted sclera in techniques of scleral buckling, 184
Implants
   in cryotherapy, relocation of, 138
   infection of, 231
   silicone; *see* Silicone implants
   over staphylomatous area, 213, 215
   twisted scleral, 192
Incarceration of retina during retinal detachment surgery, 228
Incision
   meridional scratch, in release of subretinal fluid, 207
   single scleral, in lamellar scleral undermining, 203
Inclusion bodies
   electron microscopy and, 274-276
   pigment epithelial, electron microscopy and, 276

Indenting effect in intrascleral buckling with inclusion of preserved sclera, 194

Indirect ophthalmoscopes, American Optical monocular, evaluation of, 352-353

Indirect ophthalmoscopy
in differential diagnosis of retinal detachment, 54
effect of light used in, 350-351
preceding biomicroscopy of vitreous cavity, 68

Indirect stereoscopic ophthalmoscopy
in contemporary period, 33
with scleral indentation, 39-49
improved scleral depressor in, 47-49
small-pupil ophthalmoscope in, 43-44
technique of, 39-43
use of scleral indentation in, 44-47

Infection
following retinal detachment surgery, 168
of implant, 231
postoperative, reduction of, in cryotherapy, 138
as postoperative complication of retinal detachment surgery, 230-231
and type of implant material, 215

Infectious endophthalmitis, 169

Inflammation
in complications of retinal detachment surgery, 224
postoperative, after scleral buckling procedure, 191

Inflammatory cells between vitreous body and retina in vitreous detachment, 80

Inflammatory detachment in differential diagnosis, 52

Inflammatory problems, cryotherapy and, 169-170

Ingram Ophthalmoscope, 128, 129

Injections
of air in treatment of giant breaks, 366-367
of silicone; *see* Silicone injection

Interpretation of photographic recordings in deformation of pig and human globes by high-speed impact, 311-314

Intraocular balloon in giant tears complicated by massive preretinal retraction, 182

Intraocular damage by contusion, experimental observations of, 305-317

Intraocular infection, postoperative, 231

Intraocular pressure
at end of surgery, 229
level of, 371-374

Intraocular pressure—cont'd
lowering of
after buckle, 374
in buckle for giant tear, 368

Intraocular surgery, previous, in complications of retinal detachment surgery, 224-225

Intraretinal separation, 52

Intrascleral buckling with inclusion of preserved sclera, 194

Intrascleral pockets, stuffing out of, with human sclera, 185, 187

Intrascleral segmental buckles of twisted scleral implants, 192

Intravitreal liquid silicone, follow-up of patients, 278-293

Intravitreal surgery
with liquid silicone, results of, 287-288
for reattachment of retina
indications for, 278, 283
technique for, 283-284, 287

Iris atrophy, small pupil in, 199

Irrigations for postoperative infection, 230

Iwanoff, 29

J

Jess, A., 34

Juvenile retinal schisis in differential diagnosis of retinal detachment, 64

K

Keeler Laser Ophthalmoscope, 128, 129

Keratocentesis and retinal detachment surgery, 229

Koeppe, L., 28, 29

Kolmer fixation, 253

Kolmer fixative, 247

L

Lamellar inclusion bodies of pigment epithelium, 274

Lamellar scleral undermining for fixed folds and massive preretinal retraction, 203

Lamellar undermining
diathermy, and tissue transplantation versus cryotherapy and full-thickness scleral buckling, 184-196
scleral, with diathermy and encirclage, indication for, 194

Laser in therapy of diabetic retinopathy, 344

Laser instruments, Campbell American Optical, 130

Laser ophthalmoscope, Keeler, 128, 129

Lattice degeneration
  advanced, 116, 118
  and age, relationship between, 334
  and anteroposterior position of lesions within eye, 334
  clinical importance of, 124-127
  continued observation in, 336
  cryotherapy versus lack of prophylaxis in retinal holes in, 337-340
  early stages of, 116, 117
  extent of area of involvement of, 119
  history of first eye in, 335
  location of degeneration in, 335
  location of lesion in, 119, 335
  prophylactic treatment of, 335-337
  of retina, 114-127
    clinical importance of, 124-127
    features of, 114
    histologic features of, 122-123
    stage of, and anteroposterior position of lesions, relationship between, 334
    tendency for tears in, 122
  tearing with, 334-335
  tendency for tears in, 122
  type of retinal lesion in, 335
  vitreous traction in, 336
Leber, T., 30
Lens
  contact; *see* Contact lens
  dislocated, small pupil in, 199
  insertion of, for vitreous cavity examination, 72-73
  opacities of
    in complications of retinal detachment surgery, 223
    or cornea in preoperative management, 198-199
Lenz, G., 32
Lesions
  location of, in lattice degeneration, 119
  trophic
    of inner retina, 91-95
    of middle retina, 95-99
    of outer retina, 99-101
  type of, in lattice degeneration, 335
  vascular, treated with cryotherapy, 370-371
  within eye, anteroposterior position of, and stage of lattice degeneration, relationship between, 334
Light sources with photocoagulation, 128-135
Linde cryosurgical unit, 141-142
  evaluation of, 351, 352
Lindner, K., 32, 33
Linnen, sclera marker of, 140
Liquefaction of vitreous gel, 80

M

Macrophages in retrolental space in retinal detachment, nature of, 354-357
Macula edema, recording of, 40
Macular puckering, 157
Maître-Jan, A., 27
Malignant melanoma
  and choroidal detachment, 165
  in differential diagnosis of retinal detachment, 56-58
Management
  of complex cases, 197-221
  of complications of intravitreal surgery with liquid silicone, 290-293
  of giant retinal breaks, 171-183
  of preoperative problems, 197-201
  surgical
    of choroidal coloboma, 220
    of fixed folds and massive preretinal retraction, 203
Marfan's syndrome
  relationship of, to Ehlers-Danlos syndrome, 217
  small pupil in, 199
Massive preretinal fibroplasia in complications of therapy of retinal detachment, 278-293
Massive preretinal retraction, 87-88
  in complications of giant tears, 181-182
  early stages in, 202
  established, 202-203
  and fixed folds
    problems during surgery and, 201-211
    special techniques for, 208-211
Massive vitreous retraction, 158, 233
Media, opacities of, in complications of retinal detachment surgery, 223-224
Melanoma, malignant
  and choroidal detachment, 165
  in differential diagnosis of retinal detachment, 56-58
Membrane of retina, internal limiting, composition of, 354
Membrane formation, preretinal, 157-160
Meridional fold, 7, 108-110
Meridional scratch incision in release of subretinal fluid, 207
Méry, 28
Metastatic tumors in differential diagnosis of retinal detachment, 61-63
Methylcellulose in contact lens for vitreous cavity examination, 72
Methylene blue in cryotherapy, 140
Meyer-Schwickerath, G., 34

Microscopic findings of ora serrata, correlation of gross features of topography with, 13-15
Microscopy
  electron, in experimental retinal detachment and reattachment, 258-277
  of fundus, slit lamp, 50-51
3-Mirror Goldmann prism; *see* Goldmann 3-mirror contact lens
Mittendorf's dot, 80
Monofilament nylon suture, reaction to, 166
Morgagni, J. B., 27
Morphologic features of ora serrata
  classification of, 5-10
  incidence of, 10-12
  table of, 8
Muller, H., 29
Müller, L., 31
Muscles, detachment of, during retinal detachment surgery, 227
M.V.R. in postoperative complications of retinal surgery, 233
Mydriatic mixture, 39-40
Mydriatics in preoperative management, 201

N

Nylon suture, monofilament, reaction to, 166

O

Occlusions of small peripheral arterials in retina or choroid detachment, 357-358
Ocular pressure in surgical procedures for fixed folds and massive preretinal retraction, 208
Opacifications in complications or retinal detachment surgery, 223
Opacities
  lens or corneal, in preoperative management, 198-199
  of media
    in complications of retinal detachment surgery, 223-224
    recording of, 40
Operative procedure in diabetic retinal detachment, 324-325
Operative risk in primary scleral undermining and primary full-thickness scleral buckling, 195
Ophthalmoscopes
  advantages of, in differential diagnosis of retinal detachment, 53
  American Optical monocular indirect, evaluation of, 352-353

Ophthalmoscopes—cont'd
  development of, 28-29
  Ingram and Keeler Laser, 128, 129
  small-pupil, 43-44, 197
Ophthalmoscopic appearance, pathogenesis and, of diabetic retinal detachment, 319-322
Ophthalmoscopy
  in contemporary period, 33
  development of methods of examination by, 28-29
  in differential diagnosis of retinal detachment, 53
  indirect
    effect of light used in, 350-351
    preceding biomicroscopy of vitreous cavity, 68
    stereoscopic; *see* Indirect stereoscopic ophthalmoscopy
  principles of, Helmholtz's monography of, 28
Optic disc
  average diameters of, 3
  topography of, and conventional fundus diagram, 22
Ora bay, 7, 10
Ora serrata
  average dimensions of, 4
  classification of morphologic features of, 5-10
  configuration of, 5
  morphologic features
    incidence of, 10-12
    table of, 8
  relationship of, to structures in anterior segment of eye, 4
  representation of, in fundus diagram, 22
  tags of retinal tissue at, 108
  topographic features of, localization and incidence of, 25
  topography of
    correlation of gross features of, with microscopic findings, 13-15
    overall, 13
  viewing of, with scleral indentation, 47
Oral zone of fundus periphery, 39
Orbital granuloma, chronic, 359
Oscillations, photographic recordings of, 313-314
Overshooting, photographic recordings of, 313

P

P[32] uptake studies in differential diagnosis of retinal detachment, 55-56

Pars plana ciliaris, viewing of, in vitreous cavity examination, 76
PAS, 247
Pathogenesis
development of concepts of, 29-31
contemporary period in, 34
early period in, 29-30
modern period in, 30-31
and ophthalmoscopic appearance of diabetic retinal detachment, 319-322
Pathologic changes following retinal detachment surgery, 147-170
Pathology, developmental, in choroidal coloboma, 217-218
Patient, preparation of, for vitreous cavity examination, 69
Paufique, L., 32, 33
Paving-stone degeneration, 99-101
Penicillin in experimental retinal detachment and reattachment, 242
Peripheral fundus; *see* Fundus, peripheral
Peripheral retina; *see also* Retina
tractional degenerations in, 103-127; *see also* Tractional degenerations of peripheral retina
trophic degenerations of, 90-102; *see also* Trophic degenerations of peripheral retina
trophic excavations of, 92-93
Peripheral retinal degeneration, 25
Peripheral tapetochoroidal degeneration, senile, 100, 101
Periphery of fundus, techniques of examination of, 39-51; *see also* Fundus, periphery of
Phakic eyes in vitreous cavity examination, 80
Phenylephrine hydrochloride, 201
in mydriatic mixture, 39, 40
Phosphate-buffered osmium tetroxide, 258
Phosphorus-32 uptake studies in differential diagnosis of retinal detachment, 55-56
Photocoagulation
and choroidal coloboma, 220
in comparison to cryotherapy for retinal detachment, 137-138
and cryoapplications, indications for prophylactic treatment with, 359
development of, 34
and diabetic retinopathy, 347, 348, 349, 350
with different light sources, 128-135
in posterior pole and changes elsewhere in eye, 344
in progressive diabetic retinopathy, 345

Photocoagulation—cont'd
as prophylaxis of diabetic retinal detachment, 326
in thin sclera, 215
in treatment of retinopathy, 294
Photocoagulator, xenon lamp, 134-135
Photographic recordings
in deformation of pig and human globes by high-speed impact, 309-311
of high-speed impact, graphic reconstruction of, 314-316
interpretation of, 311-314
Pig eyes, experimental damage to, 305-317
Pigment
in base of mass in malignant melanoma, 57
in choroid in metastatic tumors, 61
cryotherapy and dispersion of, 140-141
defect of, 218
at pigment layer of retina and choroidoretinal adhesion, 358
Pigment epithelial detachments, 55, 56
Pigment epithelial inclusion body, electron microscopy and, 276
Pigment epithelium
in experimental retinal detachment and reattachment, 252-255
lamellar inclusion bodies of, electron microscopy and, 274
and retina, 87
Pigmentation, retinal and choroidal, recording of, 40
Pilocarpine hydrochloride, 201
Pituitary
ablation, 348
ablative therapy as prophylaxis of diabetic retinal detachment, 326
destruction of, 349-350
Plantaris tendon
autogenous, in scleral buckling, 189
in scleral buckling procedures, success of, 192
in techniques of scleral buckling, 184
Polar hemorrhage, posterior, 55, 56
Polyak, S., 1
Polyethylene implant material, tissue tolerance and, 166
Polymyxin B sulfate, 208
Pomerantzeff, O., 33
Pomerantzeff's findings, small-pupil ophthalmoscope and, 197
Posterior pole
hemorrhage in, 55, 56
photocoagulation in, and changes elsewhere in eye, 344
recording landmarks of, 40, 41

Postoperative
  care for retinal detachment surgery, 361
  complications of retinal detachment surgery, 229-230
  exposure of silicone implants, prevention of, 208
  glaucoma, 231
  infections, reduction of, in cryotherapy, 138
  inflammation after scleral buckling procedure, 191
Posttreatment, cryotherapy and difficulty in recognizing treated sclera in, 139-140
Prednisolone, 201
Prednisone, 201
Preoperative complications of retinal detachment surgery, 222-223
Preoperative management of giant retinal breaks, 171-176
Preoperative problems, management of, 197-201
Preretinal fibrovascular proliferations in diabetic retinal detachment, 319
Preretinal membrane formation, 157-160
Preretinal retraction, massive; *see* Massive preretinal retraction
Pressure, intraocular
  at end of surgery, 229
  level of, 371-374
  lowering of
    after buckle, 374
    in buckle for giant tear, 368
Prevention of detachment and proliferation in diabetic retinopathy, 294-301
Principles
  of detachment surgery, 136
  of retinal surgery, fundamental, 223
Probe, danger of moving cold, 140
Procaine hydrochloride in mydriatic mixture, 40
Procedure
  operative, in diabetic retinal detachment, 324-325
  for vitreous cavity examination, 72-78
Projectiles in deformation of pig and human globes by high-speed impact, 309
Proliferations
  preretinal fibrovascular, in diabetic retinal detachment, 319
  prevention of, in diabetic retinopathy, 294-301
Proparacaine hydrochloride in insertion of lens for vitreous cavity examination, 72

Prophylactic treatment
  with cryoapplications and photocoagulation, indications for, 359
  of lattice degeneration, 335-337
Prophylaxis of diabetic retinal detachment, 326
Pseudohyaloid face, 80, 87
Pupil, small, surgical technique in, 199-200
Pupillary-block glaucoma, 288

R

Reattachment
  criteria for abandoning attempts at, 377-379
  day blindness after successful, 354
  after experimental retinal detachment, methods, clinical picture, and histology of, 239-257
  in experimental retinal detachment and reattachment, 255-256
  rates with lamellar undermining, diathermy, and preserved sclera, 192
Redetachment
  prevention of, 340-344
  after retinal detachment surgery, 231-234
Reoperation
  cryotherapy and, 138-139
  after scleral buckling procedure with human sclera, 190
Retina
  adhesions between vitreous and, 87
  attached, recording of, 40
  average dimensions of, 2-3
  average shape of, 3
  clinical correlations of, 21-25
  composition of internal limiting membrane of, 354
  cystoid spaces in, after retinal detachment, 276
  detachment of; *see* Retinal detachment
  difficulty in recognizing area of treated, cryotherapy and, 139-140
  in experimental retinal detachment and reattachment, 249-252
  high detachment of, 57
  hole in, 93-95
  incarceration of, during retinal detachment surgery, 228
  inner, trophic lesions of, 91-95
  internal limiting membrane of, composition of, 354
  ischemia of, 276
  in massive preretinal retraction, 87-88

Retina—cont'd
 middle, trophic lesions of, 95-99
 outer, trophic lesions of, 99-101
 peripheral
  degeneration of, 25
  tractional degenerations of, 103-127; *see also* Tractional degenerations of peripheral retina
  trophic degenerations of, 90-102; *see also* Trophic degenerations of peripheral retina
  trophic excavations of, 92-93
 pigment at pigment layer of, and chorioretinal adhesion, 358
 and pigment epithelium, 87
 regional anatomy of, 15-18
 in retinal breaks, 88; *see also* Breaks, retinal
 and retinal surgery, general summary on symposium of, 328-333; *see also* Retinal detachment surgery; Retinal surgery
 sensory, thickness of, 15
 surfaces of, technique for detecting extent and configuration of, in vitreous cavity examination, 74-75
 thickness of, variation of, 25
 topography and clinical correlations in, 1-26
  clinical correlations in, 21-25
  regional retinal anatomy in, 15-18
  retinal topography in, 1-15
  vitreous base in, 18-21
 transparency of, changes in, in cryotherapy, 137-138
 trophic lesions of, 91-101
 true giant rolled-over, results of surgery on, 367
 veins of, recording of, 40
 viewing of, in vitreous cavity examination, 74-75
 zones of, 2
Retinal anatomy, regional, 15-18
Retinal arteries, recording of, 40
Retinal atrophy, 150
Retinal breaks; *see* Breaks, retinal
Retinal degeneration, peripheral, 25; *see also* Lattice degeneration
Retinal detachment
 allergy or autoimmunological factors in pathology of, 357
 with choroidal coloboma, 219
 chronic open-angle glaucoma with, 200
 by contusion, clinical observations on, 302-305

Retinal detachment—cont'd
 definition of, 52
 diabetic; *see* Diabetic retinal detachment
 differential diagnosis in, 52-65
  specific problems in, 56-65
  techniques of examination in, 53-56
 evolution of concepts, 27-38
  assessment of contemporary period in, 33-35
  methods of examination in, 27-29, 33-34
  pathogenesis in, 29-31, 34
  treatment in, 31-33, 34-35
 examination with 3-mirror Goldmann prism, 353-354
 experimental, and reattachment, 239-277; *see also* Experimental retinal detachment and reattachment
 first description of clinical symptoms of, 27
 glaucoma associated with, 200-201
 high, 57
 horseshoe break in, 363
 inferior, after intravitreal surgery with liquid silicone, 291
 localized, preoperative management and, 198
 macrophages in retrolental space in, nature of, 354-357
 occlusions in small peripheral arterials in, 357-358
 and reattachment, clinical picture of experimental, 240-246; *see also* Experimental retinal attachment and reattachment
 recording of, 40
 recurrent, after intravitreal surgery with liquid silicone, 288
 surgery; *see also* Detachment Surgery; Surgery
  complications during, 225-226
  complications of, 222-234
  cryotherapy in, 136-146
  incarceration of retina in, 228
  pathologic changes following, 147-170
  postoperative care for, 361
  postoperative complications of, 229-230
  principles in, 136
  terminating operation in, 229
 techniques of examination in differential diagnosis of, 53-56
 therapy of, complicated by massive preretinal fibroplasia, 278-293
 total, and preoperative management, 198
 traumatic, clinical and experimental study of, 302-318

Retinal detachment—cont'd
types of, 242-243, 246
and vitamin A deficiency, 276
Retinal flap, posterior
inverted
and fixed to underlying retina, 180
with patient supine, 176-180
partial or complete inversion of, preoperative management in, 171-173
remaining unfolded, with patient supine, 176
Retinal folds, 108-110
Retinal hemorrhages during intravitreal surgery with liquid silicone, management of, 291
Retinal hole, 93-95
Retinal incarcerations, 228
planned, in giant break surgery, 366
Retinal ischemia, electron microscopy and, 276
Retinal lesions; *see* Lesions
Retinal pigmentation, recording of, 40
Retinal schisis in differential diagnosis of retinal detachment, 64
Retinal surgery; *see also* Retinal detachment surgery; Surgery
cataract extraction prior to, 198
fundamental principles of, 223
general summary on symposium of, 328-333
maintenance of corneal transparency during, 364-366
Retinal tag in ora bay, 10
Retinal tears, 110-114; *see also* Tears
full-thickness, 111-114
giant, complicated by massive preretinal retraction, 181-182; *see also* Giant retinal tear
partial-thickness, 110-111, 112
Retinal tissue, tags of, at ora serrata, 108
Retinal topography; *see* Retina, topography and clinical correlations in
Retinal tufts, 105-108
noncystic, 105
Retinopathy, diabetic; *see* Diabetic retinopathy
Retinoschisis, 52, 96-99
Retraction, massive preretinal, 87-88; *see also* Massive preretinal retraction
Retroillumination in differential diagnosis of retinal detachment, 54
Retrolental space, macrophages in, in retinal detachment, nature of, 354-357
"Ring callus," 87
Ringschwiele, 87
Rotter, H., 33
Rubenstein unit, evaluation of, 352
Ruete, C. G. T., 28

S

Saline in experimental retinal detachment and reattachment, 242
Salzmann, M., 1
Scarifier, Desmarres, in lamellar scleral undermining, 203
Scarring, scleral, 147, 150
Schepens, C. L., 28, 33, 34
depressor of, 44
ophthalmoscope of, advantages of, 53
Schisis, retinal, in differential diagnosis of retinal detachment, 64
Scissors for cutting vitreous membranes, 210, 211
Sclera
dehiscences of, 211, 212
difficulty in recognizing area of treated, cryotherapy and, 139-140
donor, in implants for thin sclera, 215
human
in stuffing out intrascleral pockets, 185, 187
in techniques of scleral buckling, 184
thin, 211-216
versus silicone implants, 194
Sclera marker of Gass or Linnen, cryotherapy and, 140
Scleral buckling; *see also* Buckle
full-thickness, and cryotherapy versus lamellar undermining, diathermy, and tissue transplantation, 184-196
intrascleral, with inclusion of preserved sclera, 194
procedures for
combined with scleral undermining, 137
development of, 34-35
with diabetic retinopathy, 346-350
in Ehlers-Danlos syndrome, 217
introduction of, 136
as prophylaxis of diabetic retinal detachment, 326
techniques of, with human sclera and plantaris tendon, 184
success of, 192
Scleral damage, minimal, in cryotherapy, 137
Scleral depression
in contemporary methods of examination, 33
information obtained by, 47
preceding biomicroscopy of vitreous cavity, 68
Scleral depressor
of Goldmann, 76

Scleral depressor—cont'd
 improved, 47-49
 of Schepens, 44
Scleral implants, twisted, intrascleral segmental buckles of, 192; *see also*
   Implants
Scleral incision, single, in lamellar scleral
   undermining, 203
Scleral indentation
 with indirect stereoscopic ophthalmoscopy,
   39-49
 use of, 44-47
Scleral lamellar undermining with diathermy
   and encirclage, indication for, 194
Scleral scarring, 147, 150
Scleral undermining
 cryotherapy in elimination of need for, 137
 lamellar, for fixed folds and massive preretinal retraction, 203
 and primary full-thickness scleral buckling,
   operative risk in, 195
Segmental buckle, Custodis-type, versus primary 360-degree band, 340-344
Segmental cryosurgery without drainage of
   subretinal fluid, 360-361
Senile peripheral tapetochoroidal degeneration, 100, 101
Senile retinoschisis, 64, 97, 98
Sensory retina, thickness of, 15
Shapland, C. D., 32, 33
Silastic sleeve in operative procedure for diabetic retinal detachment, 325
Silastic sponge in experimental retinal detachment and reattachment, 242
Silicone
 band in operative procedure for diabetic
   retinal detachment, 325
 characteristics, 235
 implants; *see also* Silicone
   choice of, 206
   in giant retinal breaks, 177
   prevention of postoperative exposure of,
     208
   reaction to, 168
   in scleral buckling procedures, 204
   in surgical management of fixed folds
     and massive preretinal retraction,
     203
   in techniques of scleral buckling with
     implanted sclera, 184
   tissue tolerance and, 166
 injection
   as absorbable vitreous substitute, 375-376
   into vitreous cavity, 235-238
     complications of, 237

Silicone—cont'd
 injection—cont'd
   into vitreous cavity—cont'd
     indications for, 235
     results of, 236-237
     technique for, 236
   intravitreal liquid, follow-up of patients
     treated with, 278-293
   liquid, 283
     overfilling, 288
   oil
     disadvantages of, 374
     injection of, in giant tear complicated by
       preretinal retraction, 181
     viscosity of, 236
   reaction to solid or sponge, 369-370
   rubber
     as implant in giant retinal breaks, 176
     molded, in comparison to silicone sponge,
       215
   sponge
     in comparison to molded silicone rubber,
       215
     reaction to, 369-370
   versus sclera implants, 194
Slit lamp, Haag-Streit model-900; *see* Haag-
   Streit model-900 slit lamp
Slit lamp biomicroscopy in vitreous cavity
   examination, description of, 69-71
Slit lamp microscopy
 in contemporary period, 33-34
 development of methods of examination by,
   28-29
 of fundus, 50-51
Small-pupil ophthalmoscope, 43-44, 197
Smith, R., 32
Sodium methicillin, 208
Staphylococcus albus, 168
Staphylococcus aureus, 168
Staphyloma
 equatorial, 211, 212
 retinal detachment surgery and, 227
Staphylomatous area, implant over, 213, 215
Stereopsis in fundus picture, 43-44
Stereoscopic ophthalmoscopy, indirect
 in contemporary period, 33
 with scleral indentation, 39-49
   technique of, 39-43
Sterilization
 of contact lens for vitreous cavity examina-
   tion, 72
 of transilluminator tip, 49
Steroid therapy, systemic, 201
Strampelli, B., 32

Sturge-Weber syndrome, 59
Subretinal fluid
    drainage of, 346
        cryotherapy in avoiding, 195
        indications for, 228
        segmental cryosurgery without, 360-361
    release of, in surgical technique for fixed folds and massive preretinal retraction, 207
Suprachoroidal space, expansion of, 160
Supramyd sutures in scleral buckling
    with autogenous plantaris tendon, 189
    with human sclera, 184
Surgery; *see also* Retinal detachment surgery, Retinal surgery
    biomicroscopy as aid in planning of, 88
    complications during, 225-226
    detachment; *see* Detachment surgery
    in giant retinal breaks, 176-182
        results of, 182
    intraocular pressure at end of, 229
    intravitreal; *see* Intravitreal surgery
    in management
        of choroidal coloboma, 220
        of Ehlers-Danlos syndrome, 217
        of fixed folds and massive preretinal retraction, 203
    previous intraocular, in complications of retinal detachment surgery, 224-225
    problems during, 201-216
    reattachment, criteria for abandoning attempts at, 377-379
    retinal; *see* Retinal surgery
    retinal detachment; *see* Retinal detachment surgery
    technique for
        in giant retinal breaks, 176-182
        for marked fixed folds and massive preretinal retraction, 203-208
        special, 208-211
Sutures
    mattress, in lamellar scleral undermining, 203
    reaction to, 166-168
    Supramyd; *see* Supramyd sutures in scleral buckling
Symposium on retina and retinal surgery, general summary of, 328-333
Syndechiae
    formation of peripheral anterior, in glaucoma associated with retinal detachment, 201
    posterior, small pupil and, 199

Syneresis, 80
Systemic disease with detachment in differential diagnosis, 53
Systemic steroid therapy, 201

T

Tapetochoroidal degeneration, senile peripheral, 100, 101
Tearing with lattice degeneration, 122, 334-335
Tears; *see also* Retinal tears
    with bullous detachment, localization of large, 362
    giant, lowering of intraocular pressure in buckle for, 368
    new, after silicone injection into vitreous cavity, 237
    tendency for, in lattice degeneration, 122, 334-335
    in tractional degenerations of peripheral retina, 110-114
Tendons
    autogenous plantaris, in scleral buckling, 189
    plantaris
        in scleral buckling procedures, success of, 192
        in techniques of scleral buckling, 184
Tetracaine
    in scleral depression, 47
    in transillumination, 49
360-Degree band, 340-344
Tissue tolerance to implant material and suture, 166
Tissue transplantation, diathermy, and lamellar undermining versus cryotherapy and full-thickness scleral buckling, 184-196
Tolentino chart, 79
Topography of retina; *see* Retina, topography and clinical correlations in
Traction tuft, zonular, 106-108
Tractional, definition of, 90
Tractional degenerations of peripheral retina, 103-127
    classification of, 103
    folds in, 108-110
    tears in, 110-114
    and trophic degenerations, 114-127
    tufts in, 105-108
Transconjunctival use of cryotherapy, 137
Transillumination, 49-50
    in differential diagnosis of retinal detachment, 54
    technique of, of Berrocal, 54

Transparency
  of cornea during surgery, maintenance of, 364-366
  retinal, changes in, in cryotherapy, 137-138
Transplant, vitreous, in detachment surgery, 376
Transplantation, tissue, diathermy, and lamellar undermining versus cryotherapy and full-thickness scleral buckling, 184-196
Trantas, A., 28, 29
  technique of, in scleral indentation, 44
Traumatic retinal detachment, clinical and experimental study of, 302-318
  discussion of, 316-317
Treatment
  of giant breaks with air injection, 366-367
  prophylactic, with cryoapplications and photocoagulation, indications for, 359
  of retinal detachment, evolution of concepts in, 31-33; *see also* Retinal detachment
    contemporary period in, 34-35
    early period in, 31-32
    modern period in, 32-33
  sites of, in diabetic retinopathy, 344-345
Trophic, definition of, 90
Trophic degenerations of peripheral retina, 90-102
  categories of, 91
  inner, 91-95
  middle, 95-99
  outer, 99-101
  and tractional degenerations, 114-127
Trophic excavations of peripheral retina other than vitreous base excavations, 93
Trophic lesions
  of inner retina, 91-95
  of middle retina, 95-99
  of outer retina, 99-101
Tufts in tractional degenerations of peripheral retina, 105-108
Tumors
  collar-button, 57, 58
  and conjunctiva vessels, coagulation of, 369
  metastatic, in differential diagnosis of retinal detachment, 61-63
  primary, in differential diagnosis, 52
Tyndall effect
  absence of, 80
  in normal vitreous, 79
  in vitreous detachment, 80

U

Ultrasound in differential diagnosis of retinal detachment, 56
Undermining, lamellar; *see* Lamellar undermining
Uptake studies, phosphorus-32, in differential diagnosis of retinal detachment, 55-56
Uveitis, secondary and acute, 201

V

Vascular disease, retinal or choroidal, in differential diagnosis, 53
Vascular lesions treated with cryotherapy, 370-371
Vessels
  conjunctiva, and tumors, coagulation of, 369
  fluorescein in, 344
Viscosity of silicone oil, 236
Vitamin A deficiency and retinal detachment, 276
Vitrectomy, total, microscopically controlled, 377
Vitreoretinal attachments, exaggerated, 111
Vitreous
  adhesions between retina and, 87
  normal, in vitreous cavity examination, 79-80; *see also* Vitreous cavity examination
  shrinkage of, after detachment operation, 376-377
Vitreous base, 18-21
  anterior portion of, 19
  description of, 2
  excavation, 92-93
  position of, 25
  posterior portion of, 19-21
Vitreous body, nature of, 34
Vitreous cavity
  anterior, viewing of, in vitreous cavity examination, 73
  examination
    preparation of observer in, 68
    preparation of patient for, 69
    technique of, 66-89
      changes observed in, 79-88
      description of slit-lamp biomicroscope and contact lens in, 69-72
      for detecting and tracing extent and configurations of surfaces of retina in, 74-75
      examination procedure in, 72-78
      general considerations in, 66-68

Vitreous cavity—cont'd
  examination—cont'd
    technique of—cont'd
      recording of findings in, 79
      viewing of retina in, 74-75
    recording of findings of, 79
  silicone injections into, 235-238
  surgery inside, 211
Vitreous detachment, 80, 87
  with collapse of gel, 80
  simple, 80, 83
Vitreous gel, liquefaction of, 80
Vitreous hemorrhage
  in differential diagnosis, 52
  in Ehlers-Danlos syndrome, 217
  after intravitreal surgery with liquid sili-
    cone, 288
  preoperative management of, 197-198
Vitreous injections, development of, 35
Vitreous opacities in complications of retinal
    detachment surgery, 223
Vitreous pull, continuous, in redetachment,
    prevention of, 340-344
Vitreous retraction, massive, 158, 159
  in postoperative complications of retinal
    surgery, 233
Vitreous substitute
  absorbable, 375
  nonabsorbable, 374-375
Vitreous traction in lattice degeneration, 336

Vitreous transplant in detachment surgery,
    376
Vogt, A., 32
Vogt's arc line, 80
von Blaskowicz, L., 31, 32
von Graefe, A., 29
von Helmholz, 1

W

Ware, J., 31
Weber, A., 31
Weve, H. J. M., 32, 33
"White with pressure," 368-369
"White without pressure," 368-369
White, mottled, flat mass in differential diag-
    nosis of metastatic tumors, 61-62
Wolff, H., 28, 29

X

Xenon-flash coagulation, 133-135
Xenon lamp photocoagulator, 134-135

Z

Zeiss slit-lamp in differential diagnosis of
    retinal detachment, 54
Zones
  of fundus periphery, 39
  of retina, 2
Zonular traction tuft, 106-108